# Perverse Romanticism

Aesthetics and Sexuality in Britain, 1750–1832

Richard C. Sha

The Johns Hopkins University Press
*Baltimore*

© 2009 The Johns Hopkins University Press
All rights reserved. Published 2009
Printed in the United States of America on acid-free paper
9  8  7  6  5  4  3  2  1

The Johns Hopkins University Press
2715 North Charles Street
Baltimore, Maryland 21218-4363
www.press.jhu.edu

Library of Congress Cataloging-in-Publication Data

Sha, Richard C.
   Perverse romanticism : aesthetics and sexuality in Britain,
1750–1832 / Richard C. Sha.
      p. cm.
   Includes bibliographical references and index.
   ISBN-13: 978-0-8018-9041-3 (hardcover : alk. paper)
   ISBN-10: 0-8018-9041-1 (hardcover : alk. paper)
      1. English literature—18th century—History and criticism.
2. English literature—19th century—History and criticism.
3. Romanticism—Great Britain.  4. Aesthetics in literature.  5. Sex in
literature.  I. Title.
   PR468.R65S53 2009
   820.9'145—dc22      2008013123

A catalog record for this book is available from the British Library.

*Special discounts are available for bulk purchases of this book. For more
information, please contact Special Sales at 410-516-6936 or
specialsales@press.jhu.edu.*

The Johns Hopkins University Press uses environmentally friendly
book materials, including recycled text paper that is composed of at
least 30 percent post-consumer waste, whenever possible. All of our
book papers are acid-free, and our jackets and covers are printed on
paper with recycled content.

*For*
*my parents,*
*Richard T. and Marjorie Y. Sha,*
*who wished for their son to go to medical school—this is as close as it gets!*
*and*
*Stuart Curran,*
*who taught me about honorable toil*

# Contents

# Acknowledgments

Fellowships from the National Endowment for the Humanities and the Huntington Library, in particular the Giles and Elise Mead and Andrew Mellon Foundation, were crucial to the research herein. At American University, Dean Kay Mussell generously supported research trips to the Wellcome Library for the History and Understanding of Medicine, British Museum, and the University of Glasgow Library and Hunterian Anatomical Museum. American University matched my NEH summer stipend and provided a sabbatical, making it possible for me to complete this book. Dean Kay Mussell provided a generous subvention for the costs of reproducing photographs in the book.

Almost every page of this book is beholden to librarians and staffs at major libraries. At the Wellcome, Lesley Hall bestowed every kindness upon a researcher. At the National Library of Medicine, Stephen Greenberg unstintingly answered the research questions of someone untrained in the history of science and medicine. Michael North, curator of rare books, translated many Latin and Greek passages. Michael Sappol not only read many of the articles that became this book but also encouraged their author. He and Stephen invited me to present my work at the National Library of Medicine's History of Medicine Seminar not once, but twice. I want to thank as well Anne Rothfeld and Elizabeth Fee. The music librarian got to supervise my reading of the British Library's Private Case materials. Dan Lewis, curator in the history of science at the Huntington Library, alerted me to recent acquisitions. Ginger Renner was a gracious hostess in Pasadena. At the Library of Congress, Daniel de Simone opened up to me and my classes Lessing Rosenwald's Library and Blake books. Greg Jecmen did the same for the Blake prints and drawings at the National Gallery of Art, Washington. In one word: heaven. At the British Museum, Judy Rudoe arranged for me to hold Richard Payne Knight's collection in my hands. Virginia Murray kindly combed the Murray Archives for materials relating to Byron's doctor, Pearson. Jill Hollingsworth, extraordinary librarian, is even a better friend.

For permissions to reprint manuscript material, I thank the Pierpont Morgan Library, the Wellcome Library for the History and Understanding of Medicine, the National Library of Medicine, the Huntington Library, and the Rare Book Library at the University of Glasgow. For permissions to use images from materials in their collections, I thank Alan Jutzi and the Huntington Library, the National Library of Medicine, Margaret Kieckhefer, Daniel de Simone and the Library of Congress, and John Windle. At the Johns Hopkins University Press, Michael Lonegro smoothly piloted the manuscript into print, despite a lengthy and complex vetting process. My copyeditor, Joe Parsons, saved me from many errors and infelicities. I am especially grateful to my readers (now, thankfully, no longer anonymous)—Frederick Burwick and Andrew Elfenbein—for helping to make this a stronger book. The book is markedly better for Andrew Elfenbein's detailed and generous yet critical reading of it.

My colleagues at American University have been a supportive bunch. Special thanks to David Culver, Deborah Payne Fisk, Madhavi Menon and her laughter, Chuck Larson, and Marianne Noble.

It is with pleasure that I record particular debts to Jonathan Loesberg, Alan Richardson, Alan Bewell, Ray Stephanson, Mandy Berry, Bradford K. Mudge, Anne Wallace, Bob Essick, G. E. Bentley, Frederick Burwick, the late Betty T. Bennett, Helen Deutsch, Jim Mays, George Haggerty, George Rousseau, Brian Mains, Myra Sklarew, Mark Lussier, and Michael Philips.

Jonathan Loesberg's magisterial *A Return to Aesthetics* made this book easier to write; his careful readings of every chapter made this a stronger book. I have tried to leave the clunk and haze on the cutting-room floor.

Alan Richardson has listened to many of this book's ideas at the MLA; he guided me to essential sources and wrote letters of recommendation. Mandy Berry's careful reading of my Byron chapter made it better. Unbidden, George Rousseau sent me an e-mail letting me know he liked one of my articles. I framed it and kept it on my desk to keep me going.

Alan Bewell taught me what to read and how to read it; in the final stage, he pointed me to the fascinating work of Joan Roughgarden. Bob Essick and G. E. Bentley told me what to look for as I began to think about medicine and Blake. Fred Burwick let me know of his enthusiasm for the project: here's to another breathless march around Grasmere Lake.

Brad Mudge shared his working notes on the Private Case in the British Library and improved the Blake chapter. Helen Deutsch invited me to share my work on Spallanzani at the Clark Library: I owe her some strawberry pie. Brian

Mains is an indispensable lunch companion. My late colleague, Betty Bennett, rewrote practically every sentence of my NEH fellowship application and made it successful. How I miss her wise counsel.

Marilyn Gaull gave me permission to reprint parts of chapter 2 from an article that appeared in *The Wordsworth Circle*. But her generosity and encouragement most sustained me during the rough patches. Thanks, too, for making it possible for me to speak at the Wordsworth Conference (where the "F word" is "Foucault"). Michael Philips showed me how to fake Blake; in a pinch it might pay some bills. David Krell answered my queries on Kant, and Andrew Cunningham and Joan Roughgarden also responded helpfully to my e-mails. Myra Sklarew shared her knowledge of neurology. Mark Lussier read the Blake chapter and strengthened it conceptually and stylistically. Whatever faults remain are mine alone.

For eighteen months, Arlene Sha cheerfully came home to an unshaven and sometimes cranky writer in his undershirt. Percy Shelley put it best: what would this all mean, if thou kiss not me? I'll stop strewing the books all over the house soon, I promise. And to my sons, Blake (aptly named) and Griffin (at this minute an aspiring writer), yes this book is finally done! Marie Berry, Arlene's mom, flew in to pick up the slack when I went away for research. I thank her for allowing me to have a home to come home to.

Hardest of all to specify are my debts to my parents and to Stuart Curran. My parents not only stepped in to pick up and take care of grandchildren but also cooked dinner on Tuesday nights. They so instilled in me the importance of education that I have become a lifelong student. Stuart Curran guided an undergraduate besotted in Blake, minted countless letters of recommendation in the more than two decades since then, and generously encouraged me throughout. I only hope that he will find this book's contents to be somewhat honorable.

Perverse Romanticism

# Introduction

*Perverse Romanticism* examines how sexuality and aesthetics—customarily treated as opposed concepts—were actually united in Romanticism by a common distrust of function. Aesthetics has long held the notion that works of art should avoid function (purpose, interest). In this book, I ask why functionlessness or perversity has been so valued in aesthetics and so lambasted in sexuality.[1] I also ask why Romantic writers such as Blake, Percy Shelley, Mary Wollstonecraft, and Byron thought that sexual liberation was possible, and I turn to the then contemporary scientific separation of sexual pleasure from function to think about how sexuality could then become a kind of Kantian purposiveness without purpose.[2] That is, rather than assuming that sex was necessarily a selfish pleasure, writers linked eroticism with a mutuality that had the form of purposiveness instead of with reproductive function.[3] To the extent that sexuality then separated pleasure from reproductive function, it became perverse, like aesthetics. The Romantics thus often insisted upon an eroticized aesthetics precisely to engage readers otherwise put off by an overly rational aesthetics, one that tried to give it an explicit purpose. Like the "prodigious pippin" Byron dangles in front of his reader—the one which "perversely clung/To its own bough" (*DJ eroticism counters industrialism*

6:76)—Romantic writers use eroticism to engage readers otherwise stupefied by the "savage torpor" of industrialism or encrusted by the weight of custom.[4] By distancing sexual and aesthetic pleasure from purpose, moreover, the Romantics could make eroticism a site for thinking about mutuality rather than hierarchy. Perversity thus demands nothing less than the reimagination of human relationships generally.[5]

Kant bracketed purpose outside aesthetics because purpose spoke merely to personal satisfaction and to interest. Such pleasures were "not brought about by the concept of freedom (i.e., by the prior determination of the higher power of desire by pure reason)" (Pluhar 30). Despite their inescapable subjectivity, aesthetic judgments could thereby claim "to be valid for everyone" (Pluhar 31) as long as one did not consider the causes of the beautiful form "in a will, and yet can grasp the explanation of its possibility only by deriving it from a will" (Pluhar 65). Aesthetics claims that pleasure without function (perversion) yields disinterested judgments or judgments brought about by the concept of freedom.

*aesthetic judgments / who / purpose / are aesthetic / judgments / unbounded?*

When applied to sexuality, this positive stance toward perversion allows us to revalue sexual perversion as a form of purposiveness: to see how sexual perversion obviates reproduction and the interests that reproduction serves, and to see the ways in which sexual acts never quite speak for themselves and resist being reduced to brute instinct. Insofar as Kant models a way of recognizing the essential and inescapable subjective origin of aesthetics—it is about the apprehension of beauty—and yet moving beyond that subjectivity toward something that can be understood as universal through an understanding of the purposiveness of form, he enables the imagination of sexuality as something more than personal satisfaction. Indeed, he makes it possible to see how sexuality must be apprehended without regard to crude reproductive purpose if it is to become idealized as a form of consent or of liberation. To the extent that reproductive function confers upon sexual acts heteronormativity, it also impoverishes sex by limiting it to function and animal instinct. Kant's concept of purposiveness furthermore unhooks aesthetics from the argument by design thereby helping to pave the way to understanding life itself in terms of purposiveness rather than in terms of Godly design: since purposiveness occurs in the mind of the perceiver who resists purpose for cognitive and ethical gains, aesthetics becomes a means to apprehension instead of an act of transcendence.[6] Hence, I am interested in how purposiveness is form of perversity and vice versa.

Where aesthetics gains from sexuality the possibility of a concrete mode of engagement in the world, sexuality can profit from the aesthetic distrust of purpose, as well as by the legitimating pedigree of this aesthetic distrust of purpose. Because the body was increasingly subsumed by a nervous physiology during the Romantic period, it was difficult to separate sexual from aesthetic sensation. Furthermore, this inability to separate clearly aesthetic from sexual sensation lent the ineffable potentiality of aesthetics some much needed empirical grounding. Where scientists found purposiveness to be such a useful concept because it did away with the need to deal with final causes, and confined science to the domain of the empirical by replacing divine purpose with the concept of the objective purposiveness of nature, aestheticians resisted purpose so that art could lead to universal apprehension instead of mere subjectivity and freedom instead of determinism. Biologists could thereby equate life with purposiveness and, as a result, could imagine a plan for an organism without having to specify one (R. Richards 71). Likewise, aestheticians could judge an artwork without having to specify the plan by which beauty is produced (R. Richards 71). Biology literally informs aesthetics: when they equated poems with organic beings, Romantic poets suffused their work with the purposiveness of life, suspending purpose. In the process, they made tradition and convention the organic building blocks of poetic form, transforming tradition into creative expressiveness.

Our sense of a binary opposition between sexuality and aesthetics has blinded us to a shared wariness of purpose between aesthetics and sexuality in Romanticism generally. Under the aegis of purpose, the body is denied free will, sexuality becomes subsumed under brute instinct, and aesthetics becomes selfish and determined. In a word, ideology. Thinking about sexuality without regard to purpose enables reflection about the forms that sexuality takes, along with skepticism about any claims that link forms to purpose. Thus, if heteronormativity is form, rather than a naturalizing of function or purpose, one can see it as ideology. Moreover, one can see it as a form of impoverishment: the reduction of sexuality to reproduction and animal instinct. However, despite this wariness of purpose, both scientists and aestheticians wanted this resistance to purpose to achieve apprehension: all stated hostility to purpose aside, purposiveness had a purpose. Even for Kant, aesthetic apprehension has a purpose, regardless of how it apprehends objects: it shows us how to look at the world as ethically meaningful without making the philosophically untenable claim that any transcendent force created that meaning.

Aesthetics cannot reject purpose completely because, as Marc Redfield reminds us, aesthetics is about *Bildung*, or cultivation.[7] The fact that Coleridge's teacher, Blumenbach, defined the "first cause of all generation, nutrition, and reproduction" (R. Richards 218–19) as *Bildungstrieb* further aligned organic purposiveness with aesthetics, making it easier to imagine an aesthetics that bracketed purpose. Whereas Blumenbach thought that *Bildungstrieb* actually existed, Kant considered it to be a useful idea, one that enabled the comprehension of how "organisms achieved species-specific goals" (R. Richards 19, 232). Aesthetics thus keeps purpose at bay at the risk of its own fecklessness, its own need to encourage *Bildung*. Of course, such declared hostility to purpose might in fact enhance its educative role in that readers were not generally receptive to works that had what Keats called "palpable designs" upon them (Rollins 1:224). Sexuality, too, as Foucault reminds us in *The Care of the Self*, is an exceptionally powerful form of stylistics: it is about the subjection of the body to an aesthetic regime, one assisted by medical notions of good health. The Romantics could thus profit from the ancient Greek argument that the self-mastery of the body and its pleasures paradoxically leads to liberation. Desire, of course, cannot be liberating when one is enslaved to desire: this is the problem with libertinism. Nor can inclination lead to freedom. Romantic sexuality and aesthetics are, then, best seen as forms of purposiveness with purpose because form enables the apprehension of liberation and mutuality even when self-mastery is the form of that liberation. The fact that Romantic writers linked sexual perversity with liberation meant that this purposiveness had a purpose: to imagine what mutuality and equality might look like.

Another key reason why aesthetics and sexuality seem to have so little to say to one another is an identity politics that narrowly construes perversion in terms of identity and simultaneously rejects the pervert as a legitimate identity since presumably no one would willingly subscribe to it. Clearly, in reclaiming the term "perversion," I do not wish to validate the "damning diagnostic power" (de Lauretis 61) of this term. Instead, I mean to remind us of how a resistance to function can be the basis of a meaningful critique of society, and that aesthetics has long been helpful for thinking about the limits of interest, purpose, and function. In giving up perversion, then, critics have given up not only pathology, but also a sense of how perversion works both for and against political change. Wishing away perversion, moreover, does not let us understand how we got to where we are today. The Romantic period is the one when function became central to the nascent science of biology, and this meant that perversion had important scientific, political, and aesthetic implications. I will show in my first chapter how the condom could not serve unambiguously as a contraceptive device as long as conception was thought to occur through an immaterial seminal aura. Barriers, after all, were no obstacle to auras. The Catholic scientist Spallanzani disproved the notion of seminal aura in the 1780s. And if, for example, reproduction could no longer justify sexual pleasure because such pleasure was merely ancillary to conception, then sexual acts that led to reproduction could no longer logically be elevated over others simply on the basis of function.

That the history of perversion—"turning aside from what is true or right" (*OED*)—is entangled within the history of subversion—"turning upside down" (*OED*)—further makes it rife for critical recovery.[8] Jonathan Dollimore suggests that the "perverse not only departs from, but actively contradicts the dominant in the act of deviating from it, and it does so from within" (*Dissidence* 125). Lord Byron's "perversely cling[ing]" apple, for instance, suggests that God is the great seducer, and that He is not unlike Don Juan. Dollimore thus reminds us of the lost histories of subversion that are buried under perversion.

As a form of "internal deviation" (*Dissidence* 124), the perverse thus has a unique destabilizing potential, one rendered ever more vexing given the role of the abnormal in eighteenth-century science. Medical and scientific knowledge were beholden to perversion insofar as anomalies were critical to the discovery of any knowledge. Without diseased or nonfunctioning organs, one could not know an organ's function in the first place. Indeed, the *OED* defines the medical application of perversion to be "an alteration of physiological function such that it becomes abnormal in kind rather than in degree; (also) distortion of a body part," and it dates this application of the term to as early as 1834.[9] Although literary critics have embraced the term subversion, "perversion" has proven less popular and key studies of the idea have avoided using the term in their titles.[10] What has enabled the elevation of one kind of turning over the other? The answer stems from the fact that perversion names as its enemy certain notions of the truth, notions that often condense around nature. Because contemporary critics have tarred Romanticism with the brush of ideological escapism, making it a purveyor of untruths, it is crucial to understand that writers of the period so often made war against notions of nature that attempted to justify hierarchy. Coleridge wondered how the "Crime against Nature" could be in other countries "a bagatelle, a fashionable levity."[11] One of these notions was that sexual pleasure was connected to function. Hence William Blake insists "Love seeketh not Itself to please,/Nor for itself hath any care" (E 19): for Blake's clod, at least, love as disinterest resists re-production of the self. Another was that aesthetics had to support the argument by design (Loesberg, chapter 1). Hardly quietist or escapist, Romanticism's interest in perversion suggests a far more radical politics, one that simultaneously had the capacity to challenge religious orthodoxies and societal hierarchies. Blake's "pebble," by contrast, reminds us that love is not automatically a form of selflessness, and thus we must work to equate love and disinterest. Read in this light, perversion in the Romantic period gains the possibility of fomenting meaningful social change especially when it recognizes that pleasure does not in itself necessarily amount to meaningful change.

Even marriage and the family were open to debate. Building upon Volney's claim that fathers were liable to become absolute despots in their own homes (1:75), Mary Wollstonecraft not only considered friendship a more durable ethic of care than marriage, but also considered parental affection as "the blindest modification of perverse self-love" (*VRW* 264).[12] Parental affection became perverse when it was a "pretext to tyrannise where it can be done with impunity" (*VRW* 264). She did not, however, give up on sexual intimacy. Julie Carlson has shown how Wollstonecraft weaved together textual and sexual intimacy, infusing both with mutuality rather than hierarchy (Carlson 2007 27). Byron lamented the power of "wealthier lust" to buy women in marriage (*DJ* 2:200), and he rued even more the day when criminal conversation allowed husbands to sue their wives' lovers for damage to their sexual property. Coleridge not only urged women friends to stay single so as to retain control over their property, but he also took umbrage at the fact that women bore the brunt of punishment for adultery.[13] In the end which was more perverse: the alternate forms of affection imagined by the likes of the Romantics? Or the norms celebrated by society? Indeed, Percy Shelley in *The Cenci* shows how patriarchal power and its demand for absolute obedience logically lends itself to father/daughter incest. Because the Count twice figures his incestuous rape of his daughter in terms of consent—"'tis her stubborn will/Which by its own consent shall stoop" (iv, i. 9) and "her coming is consent" (iv. i.101)—all forms of consent, especially sexual consent, are rendered meaningless. Leigh Hunt responded in his review of *The Cenci* that "we have thousands of Cenci's among us in a lesser way—petty home tyrants" (*Romantics Reviewed* C:II: 472). Because patriarchy threatened to make women's consent meaningless, and because Shelley believed women were sold into marriage, intergenerational incest was for him merely a logical outcome of marriage. As Wollstonecraft pointed out, the fact that women were being raised to be like children did not help matters.

The Romantic period understood what sexuality might gain from aesthetics and vice versa. The suspension or disregard of reproductive purpose allowed sexuality to rise above brute instinct and become idealized in terms of love, monogamy, equality, and mutuality. Heteronormativity thus has its price: the reduction of sex to reproduction and the consequent reduction of human beings to beasts. Hence, Coleridge thought that Malthus had reduced sexuality to an appetite, thereby eliminating free will along with the spiritual dimensions of sexuality. Although sexual desire is usually understood as a personal satisfaction or for the purposes of reproduction, and therefore the very antithesis to aesthetics, Byron considered his sexual generosity more virtuous than a selfish regard for one's one sexual virtue (Gross 107). Shelley figures sibling incest as an ideal form of love, equating sibling incest with aesthetic disinterest or selflessness, thereby uniting aesthetic and sexual perversity. Distinguishing between what he calls the "love of pleasure," a love he denominates as "self-centered self devoted self-interested; it desires it's [*sic*] *own* interest," and the "desiring of happiness of others *not* from the obligation of fearing Hell or desiring Heaven," which he equates with "Virtue Heaven disinterestedness" (Jones 1:173), Shelley collapses love and aesthetic disinterest to the end of warding off selfishness. Again in an 1812 letter to Godwin, the poet argued that "wholly to abstract our views from self undoubtedly requires unparalleled disinterestedness" (Jones 1:277). He can do so because he understands human sexuality ideally to be inextricable from selfless love. In our efforts to historicize sexuality we have encouraged a separation of sexual acts from affect, and thus made it more difficult to think of love, especially sexual love, in terms of aesthetic disinterest.[14] Shelley's problem is then how to make the immediacy of sexual passion disinterested without emptying it of passion.

Finally, since the term "perversion" in the Romantic period was not yet cemented into a distinct kind of medical personage, it had wide applicability and even wider potential leverage.[15] Because perversion was not subsumed by identity, the challenge was in making the charge of perversion stick. How to mobilize the destabilizing force of perversion? Hence, William Blake suggests that the Ten Commandments were themselves a perversion of the art of writing; for Blake, no God of forgiveness would have issued so many prohibitions. And Blake therefore considered a morality that subjected sex to the constraints of a law as being most detrimental to imaginative liberty. Precisely because even the idea of the normal was under construction during this period, perversion could not rely upon an unquestioned norm against which to measure itself. As biology attempted to stake out why living matter was different from dead matter into a specialized domain of knowledge, it struggled to name the normal constituents of life. And as I will show, the transition from a one-sex model to a two-sex model meant that sexual difference was itself open to debate.[16]

This book will demonstrate how a distrust of function or perversion could form the basis of a meaningful politics, erotics, and aesthetics. Skepticism about declared function enables Shelley, Hazlitt, Blake, Byron, and Coleridge to resist Malthus and the general effort of population to reduce human sexuality to reproduction and mathematics. Byron warned that Malthus "conducts to lives ascetic,/Or turning marriage into arithmetic" (*DJ* 15:38). Coleridge explicitly stated that Malthus's authority came "not from Human Nature, but Human Folly & inhuman prejudice" (*SW* 2:1374). At the same time, they had to resist Malthus's reduction of working-class sexuality to mere reproductivity, and consequent aestheticization of middle-class sexuality, or else sexuality would become an engine of class hierarchy instead of a means to liberation.[17] By depriving the poor of the "soothing, elevating, and harmonious gentleness of the sexual intercourse" (D. Clark 247), Shelley feared that Malthus would in fact degrade the poor to below the beasts.[18] And if Linnaeus and Erasmus Darwin made the erotic diversity of plants clear, their descriptions of plant wives turning to multiple husbands underscored that sexuality exceeds function. Blake and Shelley knew that when perverse desire became too comfortably ensconced within identity, the disruptive force of desire was necessarily contained. Hence, they were wary of any cementing of perversity and identity because that would limit change. Thus, for Blake, ultimately "Sexes must vanish & cease/To be" (*Jerusalem* 92:14 E 252). Moreover, their mutual distrust of selfhood, especially in the form of self-righteousness, further made them loath to think of identity as a container for the disruptiveness of desire. Yet this distrust of function could also prove therapeutic. In making function the enemy, one could contain anxieties about the value and importance of one's own poetry.

*Perverse Romanticism* further revisits the politics of Romanticism by asking how science has made sexuality—here encompassing desire and sexed bodies—a site for thinking about liberation. Science has always influenced the way in which we think about sexuality; moreover, to the extent that scientists then had to cope with the perversity of sexual pleasure itself since pleasure had no function, science then made it possible to think about sex in terms of mutuality instead of hierarchy. The anatomist John Hunter's first successful human artificial insemination, completed in 1776, demonstrated that pleasure was ancillary to function because syringes "could not meet with or communicate joy" (R. Couper

41). More recently, in *Evolution's Rainbow*, Joan Roughgarden has argued that same-sex sexuality is quite common in the animal kingdom, putting pressure on heterosexuality as the unquestioned norm, and that mating is less about sperm transfer than it is about the creation and maintenance of relationships, a point long anticipated by Percy Shelley when he insisted that "the act itself is nothing" (D. Clark 221). His resistance to the ontology of sexual intercourse empties it of Mathusian purpose. He elaborates, "The act . . . ought always to be the link and type of the highest emotions of our nature" (D. Clark 222). I suggest that the act only becomes meaningful for Shelley when it takes on the form of purposive mutuality: both "link" and "type" insist upon an aesthetic dimension to sexuality.

Science helped to make the Romantics far more reflective about sexual liberation than they are usually given credit for. It helped them to see the human body less in terms of a given materiality and more in terms of processes of materialization, processes subject to change.[19] They recognized to varying degrees that although liberation helped to define one's enemies, the mere elimination of one's enemies is not the same thing as liberty. In Romanticism, liberation does not simply amount to power extending its grasp. Only when Prometheus takes back his curse upon Jupiter will he become unbound; liberation goes hand in hand with forgiveness. More to the point, resistance need not be total to be effective. Prometheus cannot take back his curse until he recognizes that he himself is not unlike the tyrant Jupiter. That act of imaginative sympathy paradoxically enables a rejection of the cycle of power and destruction that Jupiter represents.

Above all, the Romantic poet's ability to stand inside and outside of desire enables a vantage point from where to gauge the extent to which mutuality or the dissolution of hierarchy has been achieved. To achieve such a stance, these writers must see sexuality without reference to reproduction. In Romantic studies of sexuality, too often the very possibility of such a vantage point has been lost to the immediacy of desire. Hence, for Blake, getting rid of sex under moral law does not entail liberty if sex is still selfish. One of the goals of this study is to show how self-conscious Romantic writers were when they turned to sexuality informed by science as a site for liberation. So attuned to negation is Prometheus at the outset of *Prometheus Unbound* that he cannot see love as a physical force in the world, whether manifested in terms of ether, or chemical attraction between particles, or magnetism, or infrared light.[20]

Two brief examples may begin to suggest the surprising degree of reflexiveness within Romantic accounts of perversity and sexual liberation. Shelley explicitly turned away from marriage because it furthered selfishness and the idea of women as property, and perversely turned toward the idea of sibling incest as a way of linking lasting eroticism with disinterest. If the unbreakable sibling bond meant that such eroticism could be lasting, the problem was that disinterest was not only antithetical to sexual passion but also that incest threatened to eradicate difference in the name of disinterestedness. Shelley claims, on the one hand, that "the conviction that wedlock is indissoluble holds out the strongest of all temptations to the perverse" (Reiman and Fraistat 2:253). Here Shelley aligns heterosexual marriage with the perverse and he can do so because marriage cannot achieve disinterest. Thus, although Annette Wheeler Cafarelli rightly takes Shelley to task for refusing to imagine that female prostitutes might be motivated by economics rather than desire, she is mistaken when she refuses to think about why Shelley gave up on marriage.[21] Shelley's rejection of marriage is not simply an inability to comprehend the condition of women; it is a principled refusal based on the fact that the form of marriage cannot lead to disinterest. On the other hand, he embraces erotic love, especially the love between siblings, as a paradigmatic and lasting relationship of equality. The poet therefore has Laon and Cythna remain passionate despite having grown up together but he is careful to direct their disinterest outwardly. Laon and Cythna fight for the social revolution of others. "Never will peace and human nature meet/Till free and equal man and woman greet/Domestic peace" (*LC* 2:37), Shelley trumpets.[22] Furthermore, the poet deliberately turns to sexual sensation to "break the crust of convention" of his readers. When we recall that Shelley thinks marriage fosters patriarchal incest in *The Cenci*, sibling incest becomes a temporary but necessary corrective to the patriarchal incest that is marriage.[23]

If Shelley suggests one way in which sexuality could become the ground for liberation while aesthetics could be the means of fomenting revolution, Anna Seward suggests another possible configuration of desire as the basis for social change. Seward argues in *Llangollen Vale* that the fecundity of female friendship outstrips the fecundity of romantic heterosexual love. Juxtaposing the gardening achievements of Miss Ponsonby and Lady Eleanor Butler with the sterile, if heteronormative, love of the Welsh bard Hoel and Petrarch, Seward uses landscape and spatial metaphors to detract attention away from teleology. However, by insisting upon the fecklessness of Hoel's love—Seward refers to Hoel's love for Lady Mifwany as "ill-starr'd" (3:74)—Seward suggests that reproduction can hardly grant heterosexual sex blanket normativity. To underscore this sterility, Seward writes, "Tho' Genius, Love, and Truth inspire the strains,/Thro Hoel's veins the blood illustrious flows,/Hard as th'Eglwyseg rocks her heart remains,/Her smile a sun-beam playing on their snows" (3:74). Notwithstanding the aid of genius, love, and truth, not to mention poetry, Hoel's passion has no impact on Lady Mifwany's heart. By contrast, the female friendship between Ponsonby and Butler results in the "bloom" of "Arcadian bowers" (3:76) and "all the graceful arts their powers combin'd" (3:76). Female friendship, then, is ultimately more fruitful than feckless heterosexual love, and Seward thereby suggests that reproduction is too narrow a criterion for fecundity. Because Seward herself wrote the beginning lines of Erasmus Darwin's *Loves of the Plants*, but could not take credit because of the sexual knowledge it would imply, Seward hints through an emphasis on the sexualized "bloom" of the "Arcadian bowers" (3:76), bowers being sites of lush vegetation and wayward sexuality, that female friendship is a closet for lesbian love.[24] What looks like an absence of function from the very limited criterion of reproduction, then, is really an opening up of function to include artistic and landscape cultivation for its own sake, purposiveness. Such lesbian purposiveness, then, undermines the very possibility of penis envy insofar as the phallus and heterosexuality have been exposed as lacks.[25]

My use of Percy Shelley and Anna Seward already suggests that the Romantics were far more perverse than we tend to remember them. As Daniel O'Quinn has perceptively noted, none of the six major male poets was a poster boy for heteronormativity.[26] And if, as Andrew Elfenbein has argued, Romantic genius itself came to be defined in terms of gender and sexual experimentation, perversity and genius were intertwined.[27] Furthermore, this study not only acknowledges the egregious affectivity of Romanticism, but it also acknowledges the purposive dimension to that excess. Such emotion was a much-needed counter to the otherwise disabling skepticism of the Romantics; without emotion nothing would get done.

In sum, perversion enables us to reimagine Romanticism from the ground up. It lets us appreciate the excessiveness of its aesthetics as a means to affective engagement. It allows us to contest vigorously the charge that the Romantics evaded or denied history even as their quietism gives way to radicalism. If the rewards of perversion were the active contradiction of the dominant from within, the risks were that the Victorians would pathologize Byron and Shelley in particular (Felluga). Nonetheless, the fact that they were pathologized meant that they provoked debate. More important, it enables us to consider how going after versions of nature that underwrote hierarchy was a political strategy. It enables us to see their investments in contemporary scientific debates about the function, if any, of sexual pleasure, and it permits us to rethink our criteria for liberation, especially since liberation is a negation rather than a manifestation of liberty. Although many have lamented the fact that Foucault insists that resistance is always co-opted by power, what would resistance without power achieve?[28]

Precisely because perversion seems to occur in a vacuum, this study insists upon the primacy of context. In particular, building upon a growing body of work that reminds us just how invested the Romantics were in science, it considers how science shaped the ways in which authors could consider human sexuality as a venue for thinking about social equality. The fact that previous studies of Romanticism and sexual liberation either universalize human sexuality or consider the body devoid of medical and scientific context, makes context all the more important.[29] Indeed, the Romantic disregard for reproduction acquires greater weight in light of the growing importance of function to biology. My point is that science's growing interest in the vitality and dynamism of the human body allowed that body to become a vehicle for liberation and apprehension instead of obstacles to them. Because function ultimately reduces bodies to separate functioning organs, body parts instead of wholes, scientists began to think of life in terms of a purposiveness that enabled holistic understandings of the body. Hence, three chapters focus on the ways in which science shaped human sexuality, showing that science could be used to deny femininity as real otherness and instead subvert the very opposition of masculinity and femininity. Another chapter considers perversion from the vantage point of aesthetics. Because this study is meant to be suggestive rather than exhaustive, it concludes with two chapters on canonical poets, showing how paying attention to perversion has its payoffs.

Chapter 1 considers how science shaped thinking about Romantic sexuality. In particular, I examine how scientists came to terms with an undeniable rift between sexual pleasure and reproduction. Such a gap enabled writers such as Shelley to imagine sex as a kind of purposiveness without purpose. Because he understands sex as a form of purposiveness, Shelley can thus question the uses to which others want to put it. I then historicize the Romantic interest in nonreproductive and antireproductive sex within the rise of function in the biological sciences of this period. Once pleasure is detached from reproduction, reproduction can be shown to be a heterosexual alibi of normativity.[30] Although historians of sexuality have argued that sexuality could not develop until the rise of psychiatry in the Victorian period and that until Victorianism, sexuality was inextricably linked to anatomy as destiny; I show in chapter 2 how this argument underestimates the incoherence of localization, the need to connect functions to organs or to structures like the instinct. The gap between the location of function into organs or instincts allows Romantic writers to resist anatomy as destiny.

Chapter 3 then develops the implications of Thomas Laqueur's argument that the Romantic period was the one in which a two-sex model of complementarity begins to replace a one-sex model of hierarchy whereby women were inferior men. Throughout, my primary interest is in the conditions of possibility that enabled Romantic writers to imagine the sexed body not as an albatross, but rather as the site of radical potential. Once again competing standards of the norm thus deny perversion a single standard against which to measure departures from the norm. I then turn to Mary Wollstonecraft and Mary Robinson's interest in neurology, because the nervous body had the potential to efface difference instead of underscore it. As a vast system of neural networks connecting mind and body demonstrated, Cartesian dualism obscured a basic similarity between the sexes. Finally, I consider how anxieties about the very facts of sexual difference are rehearsed in then-contemporary treatments of puberty and hermaphroditism.

If the first three chapters emphasize sexual perversity yet argue that sexual perversity was understood in terms of Kantian purposiveness without purpose, chapter 4 examines key treatments of aesthetics in the period by Burke, Coleridge, Longinus, Winckelmann, and Payne-Knight. By calling Romantic aesthetics "perverse," I aim to capture the reasons why the Romantics turned away from an overly rational aesthetics and turned perversely toward an insistent sexuality within their aesthetics, creating an eroticized aesthetics that sought to blur the lines separating poet and audience through a common nervous physiology. Such blurring demanded readerly engagement rather than disinterest. Once again, Romantic purposiveness therefore has a clear liberating purpose.

My final chapters show how perversion revises our sense of how Blake and Byron imagined sexual desire and difference. For Blake, perversion was a central concept. I trace how he uses the term in his writings, arguing that he uses the term to enhance epistemological uncertainty: how do we know perversion when we see it? Instead of framing perversion as being automatically disruptive, Blake demands that we think about the consequences of perversion since sex must lead to self-annihilation if it is to be truly redemptive. Blake thus understands even perverse sexuality as a form of purposiveness. The purpose of this aesthetic framing of sexuality is to make sexuality a form of liberation without insisting that mere perversity alone indicated liberation had been achieved. Chapter 6 situates Byron in the context of puberty and Brunonian medicine, arguing that the radical instability of the body makes it an insecure foundation for sexual identity and even gendered hierarchy. Byron thus makes the Epic epicene, lacking fixed gendered characteristics or violating accepted gender roles.

If this study argues that Romantic writers were more thoughtful about sexual liberation than the critical record shows, it does not attempt to sanitize the record. By recognizing the aesthetic dimensions of sexuality, dimensions occluded by identity, Romantic writers and scientists enabled sexuality to become a means to apprehending if liberation has occurred and for whom, even when their own practices fell short. Becoming a liberator thus did not mean simply the question of being a liberator. The question was not who am I, but what forms of sexual liberation should I encourage and how?[31] My point is that these writers know that they need to, on the one hand, suspend the automatic linking of sexuality and reproduction so that sexuality can be a form of liberation. By contrast, that suspension of reproduction is for the express purpose of linking intimacy with freedom. This double movement captures their idealism and skepticism about sexuality's role in liberation; moreover, this aesthetic vantage point gives them the possibility of seeing the ways in which "the value of sexuality stems from its ability to demean . . . the seriousness of efforts to redeem it" (Bersani "Rectum" 222). When Blake connects Orc, liberation, and rape, for instance, he insists that there is nothing inherently liberating about sexuality. This vantage further allows them to anticipate Elizabeth Povinelli's powerful charge that "intimate love . . . state[s its] opposition to all other forms of social determination even as it claims to produce a new form of social glue" (190).

As my reference to Orc already suggests, if the history of Romantic sexual liberation is about hope and achievement, it also encompasses loss and failure. As long as such loss and failure act as spurs to further thinking and refinement, they need not remain historical waste products. Indeed, Heather Love has recently urged queer theorists to come to terms with such negative "backward" feelings as loss and failure simply because those feelings can be a much needed reminder of the history of repression that is bound up with and indeed generative of hopes for future liberation.[32] Thinking about perversion and its histories is a key part of such a project. Such backwardness, she hopes, will enable us to rethink forms of political agency.

Each Romantic writer had his or her own blindnesses. As Jonathan Gross has pointed out, Lord Byron's liberalism had its distinct limits: he worried that although libertinism would put an end to patriarchy, it might also lead inevitably to radicalism.[33] While Percy's Shelley's equation of sibling incest with a durable form of passion attempted to think through sexual equality, it also threatened to deny difference. That Cythna changes her name to Laone—merely adding an "e" to Laon's name—highlights this problem. And Helen Bruder reminds us that Blake was aware of the cost of his gender attitudes.[34] Nonetheless, because the notion of sexual liberation is now so often rejected out of hand, I have tried to make the case that the positions of these writers were often more nuanced than we have credited them to be.[35] In much the same way that equality must be approached negatively—that is, in terms of "not taking irrelevant distinctions into account" (Appiah 193)—liberation allows one to see one's enemies, and needs not be total to be effective. To the extent that perversion and liberation gave the Romantics the possibility of reimagining even the most basic of human relationships, it gave them hope for a better, if not always reproductive, future, one that was neither necessarily escapist nor necessarily "colonizing of the feminine."[36]

# CHAPTER ONE

# Romantic Science and the Perversification of Sexual Pleasure

During the Romantic period, the sciences of sexuality and of sexual pleasure (neurology, botany, natural history, biology, and anatomy) acknowledged the perverseness of human sexuality, its resistance to reproductive telos and discipline. This conception of perversity helps explain why the Romantics constructed what Blake called "the lineaments of gratified desire" as a potential, if problematic, site of social liberation. This scientific uncoupling of sexual pleasure from reproduction opens up the possibility for sexuality to become a site of liberation. Such reminders, moreover, may help Romanticism move out from under the shadow of a Romantic ideology that impoverishes it by reading Romantic politics in terms of a transcendence that offers false imaginative consolations for social problems. By contrast, I ask why the Romantics linked sexuality with liberation and why, after Michel Foucault, it is so difficult to take seriously the notion of sexual liberation, to see sexual liberation as more than mere hedonism. Attention to Romanticism's sexual liberation instead of transcendence will result in a less escapist Romanticism, one that sought nothing less than the transformation of basic human relationships.[1] Such reorientation may remind us of how science in the Romantic era was about so much more than a monolithic discourse of Foucauldian "biopower."[2] It is against Foucault that science could enable resistance as well as domination.

Foregrounding the perverseness of pleasure suspends the automatic linking of pleasure with either the conservation of or undermining of power.[3] By turning to science, I am able to explain why Romantics as diverse as Byron, Blake, Anna Seward, the Shelleys, and Wollstonecraft begin to organize their emancipatory politics around the axis of sexuality and indicate how much has to be in place—contra Barthesian readings of *jouissance*/desire—for sexuality to become linked with liberation. Percy Shelley, for example, was skeptical of "the purposes for which the sexual instinct are supposed to have existed" (D. Clark 223). And although critics have chided Wollstonecraft for her sexual prudery, she argues for a "true voluptuousness," one that "proceeds from the mind" and takes the form of "mutual affection, supported by mutual respect" (*VRW* 316). Even though that desire masks itself as presocial, it is actually antisocial, which means desire is constructed but also functions against construction. Rather than assuming, like Barthes and Marcuse, that *jouissance* is a ground that always already disrupts the repressive work of civilization, I ask what enables the Romantics to enlist various constructions of the body and desire in service of social liberation. In brief, I suggest that they turn to science to construct a notion of sexual pleasure that is separable from reproduction and marriage and, in so doing, construct desire and pleasure so that they can enable personal autonomy, meaningful consent based on shared erotic pleasure, the choice of whether or not to reproduce, and conscious opposition to both organized religion and the enemies of democracy. It was to this end that the radical Richard Carlisle hoped that "the sexual commerce . . . may be made a pleasure, independent of the dread of conception that blasts the prospects and happiness of the female" (41). That fertility rates "rose with increasing speed throughout the eighteenth century until they peaked in 1816" meant that there was much to dread (Cook 11). In any case, apprehending sex without regard to purpose enabled it to become a form of equality.

To the extent the sciences of sexuality then understood pleasure to be perverse—turning away from the supposed naturalness of function—the scientific enterprise helped connect sex with liberation. Science has always had an important influence on the ways in which we think about our bodies and its pleasures.[4] The influence of vitalism in the Romantic period meant that at very least sexual desire could be transgressive and unpredictable since even if human bodies were subject to natural laws, the operation of natural laws upon the vitalist body now meant that the body actively modified those laws (Temkin 1977 361). Vitalism was the belief in fundamental differences between the living and nonliving, differences that could not be reduced to chemical or mechanical laws but could be located in a living principle or in structural and organizational differences. For Coleridge, "to explain organization itself we must assume a principle of Life independent of organization."[5]

Vitalism made it imperative to study reproduction.[6] Because clocks could not reproduce themselves and organisms could, life became increasingly divorced from death and sexuality became a means to understand that living principle. Vitalism frustrated all forms of mechanism because organisms reproduced themselves. Because vitalism stressed interconnections between individuals and the species, as well as sympathies between species, vitalist thinkers began to turn away from thinking of organisms in terms of absolutism and hierarchy and instead began to think in terms of images of consent and sympathy linking all forces of nature (Reill 154). Vitalism thus had a democratizing edge to it,[7] one enhanced by the breakdown of the body into vital organs that did not need centralizing control.

The shift in vocabulary from generation to reproduction, moreover, meant that the biblical associations and hierarchical kin relations associated with generation began to give way to a more democratic language of reproduction, a language that leveled distinctions between humans and beasts but insisted upon interconnections between animals and man.[8] In his *Natural History* (1749), the Compte du Buffon substituted reproduction for generation; the word entered into English in the 1780s. This unfortunately paved the way for women to be linked more with other animals than they were with humankind. Nonetheless, whereas generation imbued sexuality with hierarchy, reproduction simultaneously loosened the strictures of hierarchy and condensed that hierarchy in terms of gender. This condensation of hierarchy into gender would make gender a place to think about hierarchy and the extent to which hierarchies were necessary or natural.

The reach of vitalism was deep, and it began to make serious inroads to such disciplines as natural history and even chemistry: the index of this was that chemistry was clothed in the language of reproduction and affinity. Before 1750, like particles were thought to attract like. After the middle of the century, opposites were taken to attract. As chemicals and elements began to be understood in terms of reproduction, affinity was heterosexualized and the erotic affinities of difference became paramount.[9] Vitalism also suffused botany. It is no accident that the word "sexuality" originates in reference to plants, for they helped make sexuality visible.[10] Unlike humans, who hid their genitals, plant genitals were open to inspection without any sophisticated technology. Whereas Linneaus used the morphological differences between male and female plants as the basis for his taxonomy, Buffon took him to task for categorizing on the basis of superficial similarities. Despite their fundamental disagreements, both made sexuality central: Linneaus by using sexual organs of plants as the basis for taxonomy, Buffon for making reproduction the criterion for a species. Animals that could not reproduce with one another could not by definition be of the same species.

Vitalism helped effect a shift away from preformation and toward epigenesis, and this shift too helped to make sexuality rife for liberation. Preformation was allied with theological absolutism since God had preformed all human beings within the ovary of Eve or the sperm of Adam, but epigenesis in the late eighteenth century became widely accepted over preformation because it defined each new birth as a new formation, a theory that accounted for variability but implied the existence of an invisible vital force that could organize living matter into complex forms. As Peter Reill puts it, "Epigenesis threatened established authority, questioning foundations established to worship God and venerate social hierarchies" (159–60). The reasons for this growing acceptance of epigenesis were that nature was increasingly understood to be self-generating, that preformation had a hard time accounting for variation and monstrosity, and that preformation could not explain resemblance between parents and offspring. But if epigenesis helped divorce God from matter by necessitating that parts of the body be produced successively, it gave the Romantics a way of thinking about the purposiveness of life without a predetermined form or purpose.[11] In short, life itself was perverse.

Because vitalism put such a primacy upon connectedness and sympathy, it is but a small step away from Romanticism and its reliance upon feeling. Vitalism, therefore, relied upon metaphors of human interaction and was a key means by which society turned to the nature of living things to rethink its social contracts. In the same way that electricity could galvanize dead bodies into a semblance of life, the French and American revolutions could have an electrifying effect on the body. Vitalism promised an always shifting dynamic body and so made bodies susceptible to change even as it endowed life with a purposiveness instead of purpose. Thus, if sexuality objectified the subject for himself in Foucault's formulation,[12] vitalism mandated that living beings resist the status of object and opened the door to sexual subjectivity.

Although vitalism would seem to play a crucial role in the development of what Foucault calls biopower insofar as life thereby "enters into the order of knowledge and power," I want to underscore key differences (Foucault *HS* 1: 142). In order for vitalism to be connected with liberation, it cannot be reduced to Foucauldian biopower, which he defines as a two-fold strategy of suffusing life with power. On the one hand, the body as machine was reduced to instrumentality. On the other hand, the body as species mandated control over population, fertility, mortality, and health.[13] Foucault continues, "Broadly speaking, at the juncture of the 'body' and 'population,' sex became a crucial target of a power organized around the management of life rather than the menace of death" (*HS* 1:147). For one, not only did vitalists reject the notion of the body as predictable machine, insisting upon its ability to self-generate, but they also had an epistemological skepticism that resisted the transformation of life into knowledge and power.[14] Caspar Wolff, the discoverer of the female ovary in humans, admitted that there were complexities to generation beyond his deductive procedure.[15] Perhaps the most famous anatomist and man-midwife of his day, William Hunter began his 1784 anatomical lectures by "avowing great ignorance, in many of the most considerable questions relating to animal operations; such as, sensation, motion, respiration, digestion, generation, & c. In my opinion all these subjects are much less understood, than most people think them."[16] Two, in making life a principle that could not be delivered by empirical science, vitalists endowed life with purposiveness but not purpose, a conceptual maneuver that enabled life at very least to be in excess of function if not at odds with it. When coupled with the vitalist distancing of the living principle or life force from God, vitalists opened the door to bodies and organs not reducible to function. The gap between organ and vital force is the place where instrumentality is challenged. To the extent that vitalism and attention to the nature of the life force made sexuality central to living things, vitalism also offset physical determinism.

It is no accident that in the Romantic period, physiology, the study of living bodies, would come to define itself against dead anatomy and supercede it. The important surgeon and anatomist John Hunter would even locate life in the coagulating powers of the blood: the dynamic and fluid nature of the blood as life meant that the body could not be a static entity. It was Hunter's assertion that the testicles and ovaries produced fluids—what we now know to be hormones—that led to the manifestation of physical sex. Even then, sex was not a fixed thing. Indeed, when John Abernethy, president of the Royal College of Surgeons and teacher of William Lawrence, Percy Shelley's friend and doctor, credits Hunter with the vitalist claim that "life does not depend on organization" (1815 14), he makes it clear that anatomy is far from destiny, that physical determinism does little to explain human life. That by the end of the eighteenth century sex was thought to take place in the head, not the genitals, meant that sexuality could now become central to psychology.

In a larger view, we can profit from the complex, flexible, and often ironic ways in which Romantic scientists and poets understood the body and sex. Girded by Foucault and his keen awareness of how science passes itself as knowledge/power, social constructionism has long made the body and science enemies insofar as it claims that by making something socially constructed we have thereby made it open to change.[17] Nature and the body, by contrast, are considered impervious to change. The fantasy of biological fixity has had an even more unfortunate influence on the history of sexuality, where the standard Foucauldian wisdom is that the move from sex to sexuality—from sex as acts, or merely as one dimension of human life that may include sexual subjectivity, to sex as a totalizing feature of identity—did not take place until the advent of sexology in the 1860s, when the homosexual became a personage.[18] To take an important recent example of this kind of history, Arnold Davidson's *Emergence of Sexuality* insists that sexuality could only emerge as a coherent style of reasoning with the advent of psychology in the nineteenth century.[19] Before sexuality emerged, there was sex, a regime under which anatomy was destiny. This not only makes Romantic sex mere foreplay to the real thing but also the conflation of sex with anatomy rigidifies sex so that it seems antithetical to liberation. This chapter will show why the Romantics could not think in terms of biological or sexual fixity and why "one's sexual identity" was not "exhausted by anatomical sex" in the Romantic period (Davidson 36).

Eve Kosofsky Sedgwick has challenged this easy binary opposition between the fixity of biology and the elasticity of culture by asking what makes us think that culture is any easier to change than biology (1990 41). Recent developments in science suggest that it is high time to rethink biological fixity from the ground up and look at the nuanced ways in which science recognizes the role of culture. To wit, Matt Ridley has pointedly refuted the fantasy that biological genes determine behavior. He argues in *Genome* that "our biology is at the mercy of our behavior" (1999 157) and points to how behavior changes the levels of cortisol in our bodies. Because cortisol works as an on/off switch for genes, behavior in effect changes biology. Neural Darwinism suggests that neural networks are shaped by behavioral choices. Hence, Steven Pinker highlights the fact that "innate structure evolve[s] in an animal that also learns" (1997 177).

Anticipating Ridley and Pinker, the Romantics knew that neither the body nor science were given enemies because they understood that ontological narratives can be used for liberating ends, that living bodies were in the state of dynamic flux, that biology hardly excluded culture, and that desire was elastic. Sensationalist psychology sought to understand how custom and habit were inscribed upon the body, whether through vibration or through association. The schoolboy Coleridge worried about habit's ability to become "securely grafted . . . on . . . nature" (*Shorter Works* 1:4). Because scientists had to be so careful to avoid the charge of materialism, they thought carefully around physical determinism, arguing that living bodies were essentially different from dead ones and that the existence of organs only indicated propensities or perceived effects, not realities. Coleridge, for instance, warned that "visible surface and power of any kind, much more the power of life, are ideas which the very forms of the human understanding make it impossible to identify" (*Hints towards the Formation* 35). By essentializing an epistemological gap between visible surface and powers, Coleridge made it more difficult to think of biology in terms of Ozymandian fixity. Our tin ear to the nuances of science says more about our need to make science about logocentrism and the tyranny that results from it than it does about the limitations of science itself. That natural history was really an allegory of human history meant that sexuality could be understood as an allegory of power. We see this most clearly in William Blake, who equates that "false/ and generating love" with the "pretense to destroy love" (*Jerusalem* 17:25–26 E 161). Finally, Karl Figlio has shown how the biomedical sciences in the eighteenth century "focuss[ed] increasingly upon the limits and methodology of knowledge, rather than upon the existence and essence of substances" (1975 183), and this methodological shift enhanced Romantic skepticism about the fixity of the body, especially ideas that sought to naturalize hierarchies.

## Romantic Science and the Perversification of Pleasure

By "perversification," I mean the ways in which the seemingly natural and normative connection between pleasure and function was undermined, an undermining that allowed sex to be thought of as a form of purposiveness.[20] The sciences, by contrast, helped separate reproduction and pleasure. Romantic poets and scientists thus claimed that pleasure was either an unnecessary or insufficient cause of reproduction and suggested that there was no necessary causal connection between pleasure and reproduction. This uncoupling of sexual pleasure from reproduction makes it possible to link pleasure with liberation. Linnaean botany, conversely, helped undermine the prevailing wisdom that perverse or unnatural forms of sexuality were by nature unproductive; Linnaean botany gave the lie to the uselessness of perverse forms of sexuality by showing how productive plant polygamy, hermaphroditism, and gender bending could be. From the Abbe Spallanzani's work on artificial insemination and on the minute amount of spermatic fluid needed to achieve "efficacy," through the famous anatomist John Hunter's removal of a sow's ovary to see what, if anything, happens to fertility as a result, to the localization of sexuality to the brain and the imagination, this double breach between normative pleasure and reproduction, and between perverse pleasure and sterility, became increasingly difficult to ignore. If this scientific perverseness made sexual pleasure, contra Foucault and Thomas Laqueur, a potential and meaningful site of antagonism against church and aristocracy, then perhaps the symptom of this cultural anxiety was the obsessive condensation of unproductive sexuality onto masturbation.[21]

To explore this perversification within Romantic science is to see how cultural norms are both maintained and challenged.[22] Perversity's location at the center of heterosexual pleasure means that the unnatural/natural binary refuses to stabilize. Although we now perceive the perverse to be completely alien to dominant culture in part because we take for granted the pathology of perversity, science in the Romantic period struggles to come to grips with the fact that perversion is within heterosexual pleasure, that it refuses to remain external to mainstream sex. Perversity in this period thus resists pathology in part because, as Georges Canguilhem has brilliantly shown, the science of pathology is instrumental to the consolidation of the norm. Scientists therefore had to construe the norm from pathological specimens. Perversity's very inherence to culture, thus gives it the potential to challenge dominant values: in particular, the role and value placed on function itself. The fact that it does so from within threatens the very idea of the norm in ways that Foucault's notion of "'reverse' discourse"—whereby "homosexuality began to speak on its own behalf" (*HS* 1:101)—simply cannot account for. I want to emphasize here as well Sedgwick's caution that consequences of positions cannot be anticipated in advance because they cannot be known in advance (1990 27–39).

The sciences, of course, were then far from cordoned off from the learned middle class in the way they are now, in part because aesthetic apprehension and scientific apprehension were not considered to be opposites (Richards 12). Coleridge, for example, read, owned, or had access to books by most of the scientists discussed here. He not only often attended medical lectures (Coffman and Harris), but also wrote an essay on physiology called *Hints towards the Formation of a More Comprehensive Theory of Life*.[23] Romantic culture's emphasis on feeling and on a mind-body reciprocity led scientists and poets to explore human sexuality in unprecedented ways. They asked what sexuality could tell us about the interaction between the body and mind, especially because many believed as did Coleridge that the "plastic life or the power of the Germ [seed] . . . is the manifestation of distinct essence in the all-common Matter" (*Shorter Works* 2:873). Was pleasure necessary for reproduction, and, if not, what might sexual intimacy have to teach us about human equality, genuine intersubjectivity, and freedom? And was sexual desire a biological imperative? The stakes were indeed high in the answer to this question: the rationalist Godwin's insistence that it was not did not stop Malthus from making "passion between the sexes" one of the incontrovertible laws of human nature. Blake, Coleridge, and the Shelleys consorted with scientists and doctors like George Fordyce, Mary Wollstonecraft's midwife; James Gillman; and the radical surgeon William Lawrence; and doctors such as Erasmus Darwin turned to poetry to make sexuality the most important feature of organic life (A. Richardson 7). Galvani's popular lectures on medical electricity became fodder for *Frankenstein*, whereas Gall's and Spurzheim's phrenological lectures were forms of public entertainment.[24] Even though more popular medical writings on sexuality such as *Aristotle's Masterpiece* ostensibly instructed readers on how to achieve fertility, Godwin and Wollstonecraft studied it to avoid pregnancy (St. Clair 500–501). Although they thought they were separating sexual pleasure from function, the ensuing birth of the future Mary Shelley reminds us that everyone then had some stake in sexual knowledge.

Science helped bring together the Romantics' interest in democracy and sexuality. Scientists often came from backgrounds of religious dissent: by 1750, the finest physicians were dissenters by religion (Porter 1997 and Bynum 4). That so many physicians rejected careers in the clergy meant that science was informed by an "ecclesiastes interruptus." These backgrounds made many scientists of the period keenly aware of the unjust benefits derived from hierarchies within the profession and without. Dissent also made many interested in a fundamentally democratic body, a shared body and nervous system, rather than a body differentiated by class. At the same time the French Revolution showed that the king's body was just a body and could be beheaded, poverty was no longer considered to be a natural state (Arendt 14–15). Hence, sensibility in this period shifts from being an elite marker of distinction to a generally human quality. And the Romantics thereby began to insist that the poet's feelings differ from those of others not in kind but in degree. Where Jan Golinski has shown how Priestley "turned to the public manifestation of phenomena produced by instruments . . . as a potent means to undermine the illegitimate authority of corrupt religious and political institutions" (96), Alan Richardson has argued that materialist theories of the brain underpinned much of revolutionary Romantic culture (2). Dorothy and Roy Porter foreground the breakdown of hierarchies in the medical profession of the eighteenth century and the pluralist dimensions of medicine (18–19, 26–28), and Roy Porter elsewhere shows the links between social and medical radicalism (1992). John Keats's teacher, Astley Cooper, expressed Jacobin ideas in his medical lectures (de Almeida 104). Thomas Beddoes in particular was so ardently devoted to the French Revolution that he quit his post as reader in chemistry at Oxford to open his Pneumatic Institute outside Bristol (Porter 1992 216). If Romanticism can be understood in terms of revolution, then, the sciences of sexuality played a major role in the ideological ferment of the age. I rehearse these examples to remind us that science could have a more vexed relationship to what Foucault calls "biopower" than Foucault's collapse of sexuality and power allows for.[25]

I begin with Albrecht von Haller, the most influential physiologist of his age, because he was the first to argue that the genitals and breast nipple had a "proportionate degree of sensibility" (1755 30), meaning by this that they "transmitted impressions to the soul" (1755 23).[26] Refuting the Scottish physician Robert Whytt's 1751 claim that the mind had no influence on the genitals—that erection and ejaculation could be explained by "spontaneous" muscular irritable contractions—Haller suggested in his *Dissertation on the Sensible and Irritable Parts of Animals* (1752–53 in Latin; 1755 English translation by S. A. Tissot) that the brain and mind and especially the imagination triggered tumescence. Whereas Whytt linked the genitals to "spontaneity," a term that Whytt used to signify "not with any conscious exertion of the mind's power," Haller insisted upon a connection between sensibility and the soul, and noted that "the soul is a being which is conscious of itself" (1755 38). "Spontaneity" thus threatened to debase human will into mere animal instinct. For Haller, "irritability is independent of the soul and the will" (ibid.). Whytt, by contrast, claimed that "men do not eat, drink, or propagate their kind, from deliberate views of preserving their species, but merely in consequence of the uneasy sensation of hunger, thirst, etc." (288). Later, in his *Observations on Nature*, Whytt ascribed erection to the "stimulus communicated to the nerves of the genital parts by the semen" (27). By making sexual desire a kind of unconscious reflex response to an "uneasy sensation," Whytt could rely upon a predictable sentient principle—a ubiquitous immaterial soul that could feel stimuli and respond purposefully—that would in the end both prove the existence of God and do God's reproductive bidding (Rocca 98).

Haller's contention that the genitals were connected with sensibility and consciousness, by contrast, opened the door to human interference with God's fiat to be fruitful and multiply. Whytt's spontaneity, his making of sexuality as a science of immediacy, had its price insofar as the body had little choice but to reproduce. Haller further links man's soul with rebellion when he writes, "The brutes, properly so called are restrained by wise laws, which in them are invariably executed; whereas, on the contrary, the soul frequently rebels against these laws, in man" (1755 xxx). Haller understands "voluptuous ideas [as] the most proper stimulus to put them [the constriction of veins] in motion" (1755 45); these ideas come from the conscious mind, over which we have control. Only when sexuality became tethered to the brain could sexual liberation become reflective and therefore meaningful because it could now be part of a deliberate strategy. And once a kind of muscular irritation no longer explains sexual desire, that desire becomes less predictable and less "spontaneously" reproductive.

John Hunter, the famous anatomist and surgeon, would later explicitly detail potentially perverse consequences of this nascently conscious sexuality: performance anxiety, the possibility of deceiving others that one is a man of gallantry when one has "no passion for the female sex" (1861 269) and an aestheticized but potentially sterile sexuality.[27] Hunter, we might recall, was called in to examine Byron's clubfoot; Hunter recommended a special shoe that would help him to walk (Marchand 1957 1:25–26), and Coleridge singled him out for praise as a scientist whom "mankind would love and revere" (cited in Knight 1998 101). In 1786, Hunter argued that impotence depended upon the state of the mind: complete action in those parts [of generation] cannot take place without perfect harmony of body and mind" (1786 201). In his posthumously published *Essays and Observations on Natural History* (1861), Hunter elaborates on the connections between conscious desire and deceit: "no man is so fond of being thought a man of gallantry as he who has no passion for the female sex, yet would feel proud if it were conceived he had always some intrigue on his hands, even at the expense of the reputation of the innocent; while the man who is really passionately fond of the sex, and perhaps their dupe, would rather choose to hide that turn of mind, as if it were a defect" (269). Could Hunter have had Byron in mind with his first example? Sex is here understood as a conscious ploy: the one who has no erotic feelings for women is the one most eager to parade signs of his heterosexuality. Insofar as Hunter figures heterosexuality/gallantry as a performative compensation for its lack, perversion inheres at the very center of culture, even masquerading as the norm.

Hunter also allows us to see that the very aestheticization of sexuality is also its perversion: "A man has an appetite to enjoy a woman; but if the mind has formed itself to any particular woman, the appetite or enjoyment can be suspended till the object is presented; and the more the mind interferes, the greater stress will be laid upon this relation: the mere sexual enjoyment will be almost forgot, and the whole pursuit will be after the particular quality of the appetite" (1861 273). Here the mind is in danger of blocking conception—it "interferes," "suspends," and almost allows the forgetting of appetite—even as it aestheticizes sexual enjoyment into taste. The problem with this aestheticization—a Kantian rendering of sexuality into a kind of purposiveness without purpose—is of course that lusting after quality is perilously close to being perverse: Hunter clarifies that the "natural man" will thereby be refined away. Zizek frames it this way: "Our libido get[s] 'stuck' onto a particular object, condemned to circulate around it forever" (62). Perversity became aligned more closely with nature when Kant insisted that the assumption that there is nothing gratuitous in the world and that all is for good had no place in the natural sciences other than as an enabling fiction (Larson 179). Because science had no insight into transcendental principles and acts but could not do without the principle of purpose in relation to the products of nature, nature was purposive. This perspective gave scientists a heuristic device that could guide them when mechanical principles were inadequate (Larson 181); nonetheless, Kant made it clear that purposiveness could not be constitutive of nature (Pluhar 379). Hunter continues, "The temporary appetites, as venery, become in time blunted . . . and he begins to lose the substance in pursuit of the qualities, refining away the natural man becoming rather ideal, whence arise 'taste,' 'graces,' etc." (1861 270). As taste transmogrifies the materiality of the body into the ideal, the danger is that the body and its pleasures will melt away into the thin air of Godwinian perfectibility.

Hunter had a longstanding distrust of the mind's taste and its role in redefining the sexual enjoyment. In 1786, in the first edition to his *Treatise on the Vene-*

*real Disease*, he ignited a firestorm of controversy when he claimed that masturbation was actually less harmful to the body than natural intercourse for the
sake of intercourse. His critics were so shrill in their criticism that Hunter ex-
purgated these remarks in the second edition of the work, published in 1788.
Here is what Hunter initially wrote:

> I think I may affirm that this act [masturbation] in itself does less harm to the con-
> stitution in general than the natural. That the natural with common women, or as
> such as we are indifferent about, does less harm to the constitution than when it is
> not so selfish, and where the affections for the woman are also concerned. Where
> it is only a constitutional act it is simple, and only one action takes place; but where
> the mind becomes interested, it is worked up to a degree of enthusiasm, increas-
> ing the sensibility of the body and disposition for action; and when the complete
> action takes place it is with proportional violence; and in proportion to the vio-
> lence is the degree of debility produced or injury done to the constitution. (200)

Hunter makes the astounding claim that sex with a woman you love or find
beautiful is actually more harmful to the constitution than masturbation or sex
with a common woman (prostitute). Once the mind becomes involved in the
sexual act, sensibility is intensified and the violence that ejaculation does to
the body is also intensified. By a medical standard, then, a standard that judges
the relative healthiness of the activity, heterosexual intercourse with someone
you love or find beautiful is actually more perverse than masturbation, because
the pathological consequences of sex with affection are much more dire. More
shocking was the fact that Hunter was thus flouting the accepted medical belief
that sex with love actually helped to restore the losses to the spermatic economy. Even though Hunter links bourgeois sex with pathology, he nonetheless
facilitates the creation of what Gayle Rubin calls the "charmed circle" of sexuality whereby heterosexual reproduction is accorded more validity and humanity than nonreproductive sex. The very need to distinguish between "simple"
sex as merely constitutional (sex) and "complex" sex as affectionate (sexuality)
helps to make affectionate heterosexual intercourse fully human, if diseased.
The upshot of all this is which is more perverse, masturbation/prostitution or
middle-class married reproductive sex?

   If Haller's linking of sensibility to erections of the breast nipple and penis insinuated a gap between sexual pleasure and reproduction, one intensified by
John Hunter, Lazzaro Spallanzani's work on artificial fecundation—what we
would today call artificial insemination—and on the semen widened that gap

considerably. This is despite the fact that Spallanzani mistakenly thought that the semen was responsible for conception, not the sperm, which he thought were merely parasitic worms. In his *Tracts on the Nature of Animals and Vegetables* (1799), Spallanzani speculated that although the vermiculi were "not immediate authors of generation," some of them might "cause . . . venereal pleasures" (193). Once pleasure is no longer enslaved to reproduction, sexual liberation becomes possible because desire can now be its own end. Percy Shelley orders Spallanzani's work in "either English or Italian" in December 1812 (Jones 1:344). Shelley was not only skeptical of "the purposes for which the sexual instinct are supposed to have existed"—namely, reproduction—(D. Clark 223), but also wrote in a still-unpublished manuscript that "any student of anatomy must be aware of an innocent, small and almost imperceptible precaution by which all consequences [of sexual intercourse] are prevented" (Pierpont Morgan Library, New York MS MA 408).

The Catholic scientist Spallanzani's unwitting divorce of sexual pleasure from reproduction was fivefold. By clothing frogs in taffeta shorts and by placing open vessels of semen within another vessel to the sides of which the eggs had adhered, permitting any aura to escape near eggs, Spallanzani proved definitively that there must be physical contact between semen and egg in order for reproduction to occur. He thus showed in 1780 that there was no such thing as seminal aura, an immaterial means of fecundation. Charles Bonnet had already conveyed to his friend his doubts that an immaterial aura could have such material effects. Because William Harvey could not see any trace of male semen in the female genital ducts of the mammals and birds he dissected, Harvey insisted that male semen had no material contribution at all to make to the egg, but rather was the provider of an energizing essence—the legacy of Aristotle's *pneuma*—by which the egg became fertile, an essence that was free to dissolve away the moment matter had been vitalized. Until Spallanzani disproved the notion of seminal aura, condoms could not be considered an effective form of birth control because an aura could presumably transcend any physical barrier. Condoms were considered primarily "armor" against venereal contamination. In Edmund Curll's *The Potent Ally*, for instance, a poet praises the *cundum*: with it, "he fears no dangers from the doxies, / . . . and scorns their poxes" (27). The demonstrated materiality of the semen meant that it could be stopped using various barrier methods.[28]

Spallanzani also queries why the "tenacious and amorous embraces, which sometimes last 40 days" of frogs continue so long after fecundation (1769

46–47); his research into how little semen was actually needed for reproductive "efficacy" meant that sexual pleasure was enormously wasteful; his experiments to determine the strength of the spark of life in which he added liquids like oil, wine, and lemon juice to the semen or exposed semen to tobacco fumes could be used, contra Spallanzani's intent, to prevent that very efficacy, and his substitution of a warmed syringe filled with semen implied that pleasure might merely be ancillary to reproduction. By putting an end to the Aristotlean theory that the active sperm infuses the otherwise inert menstrual blood of the female with life, a theory made popular in the eighteenth century by the best-selling book of sexual knowledge, *Aristotle's Masterpiece*, Spallanzani strengthened the cause of ovism—the idea that all life was preformed in the ovary—and thereby undermined one key biological basis for male superiority.[29] Haller had insisted that the female belongs entirely to the female, that, entire, it exists before fecundation.

Much of Spallanzani's 1780 *Dissertations Relative to the Natural History of Animals and Vegetables*, translated into English in 1784 by the father of the poet/physician and friend of Coleridge, the elder Thomas Beddoes, sought to clarify and quantify the nature of "the prolific virtue of semen." Part of what he was trying to understand was why frogs continue to mount and remount the female even after seminal discharge, why their "ardour" so exceeds function. Spallanzani marvels, "Such is the ardour of the males, that after the discharge is finished, and they have quitted the female, they will return to her again, and embrace her for several hours" (2:34). To his consternation, that ardor could outweigh the need for safety, hunger, and severe pain. Even after Spallanzani amputated both thighs of his male frogs and pricked them repeatedly with needles "till blood issued out at every puncture" and beheaded them, they would not give up their embraces (2:72–74). Neither pleasure nor function could explain such intense sexual desire, making normative desire perverse. When normal heterosexual pleasure cannot claim ontological priority over perverse or functionless pleasure, desire cannot be reduced to an engine of repression or biopower. Moreover, when reduced to reproduction, sex becomes animal instinct. Heteronormativity thus simultaneously normalizes and bankrupts human sexuality.

Spallanzani also wanted to figure out just how much semen was necessary for conception. He writes, "Three grains of semen mixed with twelve or eighteen ozs [*sic*] of water will communicate to the mixture its prolific virtue" (cited in Gasking 135). This led him to determine that the weight of the particles of semen spread throughout the water drop was merely one three billionth of a grain. He concludes not only that "the quantity of seed which effects impregnation is small beyond conception" (1784 2:216), but also that "the surplus does not contribute at all to fecundation" (2:170). "I cannot therefore imagine," Spallanzani admits, "what purpose the surplus of seed can serve, and am obliged to consider it useless" (2:170). Spallanzani then asks if this "discovery may be extended to man" (2:217). He posits that this extrapolation is "in some measure probable" (2:171).

What then to make of this perverse expense of spirit, this waste of semen? Erasmus Darwin would suggest that "waste" was really a form of providential "wise superfluity," the way that nature "ensured the continuance of her species of animals" (*Zoonomia* 1801 2:209), although he later argues that excess nutrition is the cause of monstrosity (2:228). One might ask how a wise superfluity was also the cause of monstrosity. Spallanzani briefly suggests that the excess seed might act as a stimulant to the fetus's heart and as a kind of nutrition for the fetus (1784 2:173, 174), although he had eleven years earlier raised considerable skepticism about this theory because the "juices of the mother" often provide both "stimulation and nutrition" and because "the eggs of tadpoles [had] unfold[ed] themselves considerably before fecundation," meaning that circulation and therefore life had to already be in effect for nutrition to have occurred (1769 45). Spallanzani argues, "We are obliged to infer that these maternal juices are themselves that kind of stimul[i] of which the seminal liquor is supposed to be in birds. Consequently the heart in the germ of the tadpole, must beat sufficiently to produce a circulation of fluids, without an insuperable impediment from the solid" (1769 45). The "uselessness" of the majority of male semen coupled with his paradoxical sense of the seed's active fecundating power engenders a panicked justification of waste. Why else would Spallanzani return to an already rejected hypothesis, one that was contraindicated by much of his own empirical evidence and his own commitment to ovism? Given his insistence that "truth can only be attained by the constant success of repeated experiments (1784 2:62), what would lead him to violate his own standards of truth? Certainly returning to the theory that sperm stimulated the fetus compromised the activating powers of the female.

Spallanzani's conundrum is this: on the one hand, as an ovist, he wants to insist that "the young belong originally to the female" (1784 2:161). For this reason, he made no distinction between unfertilized eggs and tadpoles, calling them by the same name (Gasking 135). Also for this reason, Spallanzani dismissed spermatic worms as mere parasites, preferring instead to credit the seminal fluid with the fecundating virtue. Even though Spallanzani went to great lengths to prove the animality of sperm thereby refuting Buffon's argument that sperm operated blindly and mechanically, and despite the fact that this animality could look like the living principle, his faith in ovism leads him to render spermatic animality in the form of a negation of life—a parasitical life—rather than life itself. The analogy of sperm to parasite helps Spallanzani to make sense of animality that is not to be mistaken for the origin of life. Although he had tried to ascertain the function of these worms, even momentarily entertaining the possibility that the worms "cause the venereal pleasures," Spallanzani conceded that this is "beyond the sphere of human knowledge," forgetting that he had already designated any references to "the mysteries of generation" as an excuse for "idleness" (1799 193–94; 1784 2:iii). On the other hand, he cannot ignore the fact that the female cannot create life without contact with the semen, a fact that might justify male activeness over female passivity. Therefore, Spallanzani trumpets the fact that "previously to the influence of the seed, there was a beginning of motion and life" (1784 2:161).

Spallanzani must, however, immediately qualify such feminine powers of activation because females cannot create life on their own. The experimenting priest thus solves his conundrum by insisting that "the young belong originally to the female, while the male only furnishes a fluid, which determines them to assume motion and life" (1784 2:161). Here semen determines life. He elaborates, "I would not indeed assert that these little organized bodies are without motion before they experience the action of the masculine liquor. . . . Growth implies nutrition, nutrition the circulation of fluids, and circulation depends upon the pulsation of the heart. I therefore conceive, that, previously to the influence of the seed, there was a beginning of motion and life, but in a degree exceedingly dull and languid, from the extreme slowness of the movement of the fluids" (2:161). He concludes, "Hence tadpoles would never be so rapidly evolved, or attain that sensible animation, which we denominate life, if they were not subjected to the influence of the seminal fluid" (2:161).

By creating a distinction between weak feminine powers of activation and strong masculine powers of activation, Spallanzani can have his ovist cake and eat it, too. Although he must concede that female activation is weaker than male activation, and although he initially asserts that semen "determine them to assume life," Spallanzani does not quite credit males with bestowing life; rather, he makes a nominalist distinction between the activating powers we can see and therefore associate with life and the activating powers we cannot. He underscores that the distinction is one of name only when he writes, "The influence

of the seminal fluid . . . raises them [tadpoles] from a state of apparent shapeless-
ness and immobility, and produces a due unfolding of the limbs, and evident
motion, and active life" (2:161).[30] The difference between "apparent immobility" and "evident motion" reminds us that just because weaker activation does
not look like activation, this does not mean that females are not responsible for
life. After all, both growth and nutrition precede masculine activation. Although Spallanzani's backhanded crediting of females with activating life begins
to unravel a gendered hierarchy that insisted that males are active and females
are passive, his emphasis on the stronger and more visible masculine powers and
his sense that female activation was more passive than male activation could be
used to support the very gender hierarchy he sought to undermine. These gendered distinctions are very much with us to this day: in *Im/Partial Science* (1995),
microbiologist Bonnie Spanier shows how biology textbooks still inscribe feminine passivity onto the egg and masculine activeness onto the sperm when in
fact the egg has active cilia that draw in the sperm.

Such justification of waste was all the more necessary given Spallanzani's successful artificial insemination of a female spaniel. Spallanzani claimed that he obtained the seed of a male dog by "spontaneous emission" (1784 2:250).[31] Using
a syringe warmed to body temperature, Spallanzani injected nineteen grains of
semen into a bitch in heat, who had remained in isolation. Three whelps were
delivered. Spallanzani proclaimed, "I have no difficulty in believing, that we
shall be able to give birth to some large animals, without the concurrence of the
two sexes, provided we have recourse to the simple mechanical device employed
by me" (2:198), and he blustered, "I have succeeded as well, as if the male himself had performed his function" (2: ii). Such a "simple mechanical device," then,
had the power to supplement procreative pleasure and helped demonstrate that
female sexual pleasure was unnecessary for conception to occur, and that so long
as semen could be obtained by "spontaneous emission," male pleasure too might
be ancillary to reproduction. As the Scottish doctor, R. Couper, put it, "Syringes could not communicate or meet with joy" (41).

In John Hunter's *Observations on Certain Parts of the Animal Economy* (1792),
one experiment helps to underscore further the perversification of normative
sexual pleasure. This essay had already appeared in the Royal Society's famous
*Philosophical Transactions* (1787). To determine whether women's limited fertility
can be explained by a natural period of fecundity, or whether "repeated acts of
propagation" wear out the ovaries, Hunter removes one ovary from a sow to see
if the number of pigs produced differs from the output of a perfect sow. Blake

identifies Jack Tearguts as John Hunter in his manuscript of the *Island in the Moon;* Blake may have met him through Joseph Johnson's radical circle or through his apprenticeship with James Basire, the official engraver to the Royal Society. Blake's choice of "Tearguts" indicates his knowledge of Hunter's medical experiments even as it renders Hunter into an object of satire. What those medical experiments made clear was that bodies and culture were far from mutually exclusive categories. Hunter showed that the perfect sow produces eighty-six more piglets than the spayed sow: only eleven more in the first eight farrows, but seventy-five more in farrows nine through thirteen. "It appears," Hunter concludes, "that the desire for the male continues after the power of breeding is exhausted in the female; and therefore does not altogether depend on the powers of the ovaria to propagate" (88). By unhooking sexual desire and pleasure from the ability to propagate, Hunter suggested that sexual pleasure in fact might be perverse. Hunter's medical casebooks reveal that he saw male patients "troubled by Erections and Emissions in [their] sleep" (66) because of strictures in the urethra; these nocturnal emissions indicated that pleasure might have no necessary connection to function. Moreover, by showing that repeated acts of propagation do not wear out the ovaries, Hunter weakened the connection between perverse sex and sterility. Having more sex than nature intended was believed to defy reproduction: this was the cultural logic that explained why prostitutes were thought to be barren.

Hunter did not stop with experiments on ovaries. He dealt the seeming natural connection between sexual pleasure and reproduction a more serious blow in 1776, though the results of the first successful human artificial insemination were not published until twenty-three years later in the Royal Society's *Philosophical Transactions* in Everard Home's "An Account of the Dissection of an Hermaphrodite Dog." Home, John Hunter's brother-in-law, was entrusted with Hunter's manuscripts after his death. A man suffering from hypospadias— a deficiency of the urethra behind the scrotum—could ejaculate, but only behind the scrotum. He married and, of course, could not sire children. Hunter advised the husband to prepare a warm syringe to collect the semen and inject it into his wife's vagina. A successful syringe-induced pregnancy ensued. Although this result would seem to make married heterosexual pleasure definitively perverse, in Home's published account of the experiment Home makes it clear that "the female organs were still under the influence of coitus" (1799 162). The sundering of sexual pleasure from reproduction was far more subtle. Home only discusses this insemination at all to refute the notion that "imperfection[s] in the structure of the penis" necessitate defects in "the more essential organs of generation" (161–62). Hunter's patient had a defective penis/urethra but not a defective testicle. Hunter's success is used to separate the penis, the defective organ that gives the wife pleasure, from the more essential testicles, which make the emission. A failure in one does not indicate a failure in the other; hence, is pleasure truly tied to function? In any case, Hunter's experiment showed conclusively that perversions—defects of nature—are not necessarily sterile.

Perhaps John Hunter's demonstration of the perversity of sexual pleasure was not lost on the anatomist William Cruikshank, who sometimes lectured in the place of William Hunter and later carried on in Hunter's Windmill Street School with Matthew Baillie after Hunter's death. Refuting the notion that pain was divine punishment for sexual abstinence, Cruickshank claimed "to be of the opinion that abstinence from venery is not punished but Haller has different sentiments on the subject and says that it is punished in females by epilepsy and hysteria & c but to this Mr. C replies why should a woman have these disorders, when she's married, if these arise from abstinence?"[32] When pain can no longer be seen as divine punishment for not having sex, can pleasure be a form of divine reward?

At the same time as artificial insemination becomes possible, the nerves, the organs of sensation and pleasure, are being increasingly pathologized and feminized. If leisure, luxury, sensibility, urbanization, and passivity conspire to refine the leisure-class body, this refinement also makes that body effeminate and perversely sterile. Nerves begin the eighteenth century as masculine signs of strength or virtue and end the century pathologized and feminized into consumption, the uterine furor, menstrual irregularities, and that catch-all pathology, nervous diseases.[33] This enormous shift in thinking about nerves from strength to pathology, from masculinity to feminization, serves to make normative pleasure in Romanticism always on the verge of the perverse. Indeed, neurologists such as Charles Bell, James Vere, and Thomas Laycock suggest that the very aestheticization of the body of feeling is simultaneously a movement toward perversion and pathology. If the nervous system had the potential to heal the Cartesian split between mind and body (Figlio 179), that potential was compromised by the insistent threat of disease. Vere, governor of Bethlehem Hospital, argued that nervousness involved a conflict between lower-order instincts and moral instincts. Such a conflict made sexual desire central to health. Laycock listed ungratified desire, excited love, disappointed affection, and the fashion for women's cinched-up waists as the underlying causes of nervous diseases for fashionable women (142). He therefore recommended marriage as the cure for hysteria (142). Even a key cure for nervous diseases, opium, helped make sexual pleasure perverse. At the same time that it helped to excite venery, it dulled the semen (Youngquist 93). Moreover, Dr. John Jones claimed that an opium high was even better than a sexual high, the effects comparable to "a permanent gentle Degree of that Pleasure, which modesty forbids the naming of" (cited in Youngquist 93).

Although the phrenologists Gall and Spurzheim insisted that "the function of the cerebellum is to manifest the instinct of reproduction" (Gall 1838 xxxii), their relocation of sexual desire from the testicles to the cerebellum or little brain had perhaps the unintended consequence of making that desire perverse on at least two levels. One, by insisting on mankind's free will, they undermined this instinct. Two, they also separated sexual desire from parental love. Spurzheim declared that the cerebellum was part of consciousness itself, linking it with "phrenic life" as opposed to "vegetative life" (*Anatomy* 25). Gall's ideas were well known in Britain at least since 1800 (Cooter 7), and Spurzheim lived and lectured in London from 1815 to 1832.[34] They also made it clear that, although man has "no power over the existence of desires and inclinations which depend upon his organization and the circumstances stimulating it," the fact that he has multiple cerebral organs of higher order means that he can choose among motives and therefore determine himself (Temkin 1947 285). That the brain was far from an organic unity meant that choice was possible. Of course, such self-determination was compromised by the strength of feelings produced by even a moderately sized cerebellum (Gall 1838 xix). After connecting small cerebellums with effeminacy verging on sodomy, Gall notes that Kant had a small cerebellum (1838 24). To refute charges of materialism, Gall insisted that the existence and size of organs only spoke to the "possibility, not the reality of any passion" (Crabb Robinson 90), and in later works he insisted not only that it was the struggle against one's own propensities that amounting to moral merit (*Origin* 6:9) but also that "the genital functions are for the most part subject to the will" (1838 4). Wordsworth's and Coleridge's friend, Henry Crabb Robinson, published an English translation of Gall in 1807 (Richardson 2001 36).

Spurzheim shrewdly gentrified the organ of sexual desire—*Zeugungstrieb*—into the more polite "organ of amativeness" (Cooter 78), and he did so because "it is inaccurate to choose a name according to any abuse of an organ . . . there can be none of libertinism . . . the names should express only the propensity" (*Physiognomical System* 280). He later explained that "amativeness" was in fact more accurate than "propagation," because this instinct "often acts without there being any intention to continue the species, and is also satisfied in various ways incompatible with such a purpose" (*Doctrine* 134). Here the substitution of "amativeness" for "propagation" allows the organ to move from reproductive purpose to a Kantian "purposiveness without purpose" insofar as amativeness exceeds generation and reproduction can be irrelevant. Lest he be accused of advocating a kind of perverse amativeness, however, Spurzheim hastens to add that "the disorderly satisfaction of the amative propensity undermines the health of individuals, even of the species; and I think that as soon as young persons understand the difference and the distinction of the sexual functions, they should be taught the laws of propagation" (*Doctrine* 135). Where Foucault sees the Romantic period as one of "perverse implantation," an explosion of perversions so that sex can intensify its power, Spurzheim suggests that it was one of heterosexual implantation insofar as he insists that propagation is far from innate: it must be taught. If perverse amativeness is ontologically prior to propagation, and propagation has to be taught, then how can perversion remain unnatural?

By situating the part of the brain devoted to parental love next to the organ of amativeness, Gall and Spurzheim sought to finesse the relationship between the two organs: desire will lead to parenting. The fact that they made these functions separable, that Spurzheim renamed the organ of desire the organ of amativeness as if the name change alone would change the nature of the organ from selfish indulgence to feelings for others, however, meant that pleasure was biologically incommensurate with function. Moreover, when they acknowledged that men had larger organs for desire while women had larger organs for parental love, they implied that, at least in the separate sexes, pleasure was perverse. Crabb Robinson's translation of Gall went so far as to highlight the "inverse ratio" between the "organ of sexual passion" and the "organ of parenting," insisting that licentious mothers were generally bad mothers (89). In calling attention to this inverse ratio, Gall explicitly refuted the idea that these two organs were too closely connected "to be distinguished from it" (89). My point here is that Gall and Spurzheim deliberately separated desire from parenting and that this separation could be liberating to the extent that amativeness did not naturally or even necessarily lead to reproduction. Anticipating Freud's sense that we are all perverts, "amativeness" thus inserted a perversion of both sexual object and sexual aim within human desire.

If this gap between desire and parenting did not cause enough problems,

Gall conceded that "the function, or tendency of the activity of an organ, is graduated according to the degree of its development or excitement" (*Origin* 1:216). This meant that if the organ were too little developed, "impotence, indifference, or even aversion to the other sex" could result (ibid.). Gall further argued that a "really large" cerebellum would destroy "connubial bliss" (1838 xix), which implies that marriage would not always be able to domesticate the sexual passions. He also had the audacity to claim that "everyone knows there is no proportion between fecundity and the inclination to sexual embraces" (1838 17). Hence, Gall warned, "too ardent a flame may present obstacles to fecundation" and continued that "there are men and women who perform the act of cohabitation only as an act of duty" (1838 17, 23). He added, "I am acquainted with women . . . who, although they have borne several children, have never experienced the least sensation of pleasure" (17).

Of course, Gall enabled his phrenological system to compensate for such an absence of proportion between desire/pleasure and fecundity: he showed there was a proportion between the size of one's cerebellum and the sexual inclination even if that proportion could no longer predict reproductive success. Lecturing in Paris in 1810, he blamed "excessive development of the cerebellum" for sodomy, making it clear that he felt sodomy was akin to bestiality.[35] By 1835, Gall made "individuals who are tormented with a singular predilection for their own sex" exceptions to his system, remarking instead that they "have in general a small head, delicate features, dimpled hands, and developed breast; whilst females, on the contrary, are masculine in appearance and in manners" (*Manual* 157–58). The connections between sexual desire and fecundity were further sundered by Gall's recounting of the fact that some like to be hanged so that they can produce erections. These examples perhaps led him to conclude that "men have always been, and will always be, inclined to all sorts of perverse actions; they have always been, and will always be, tormented by carnal desires" (*Origin* 1:212). In sum, Gall and Spurzheim underscored numerous gaps between normative sexual pleasure and function, gaps encapsulated in the phrenological axiom that "structure does not reveal function" (Spurzheim *Anatomy* 204), and they did so in part to avoid charges of materialism and atheism as well as to preserve free will. In this, they were perhaps less than successful: Doctor J. P. Tupper's *Inquiry into Doctor Gall's System* (1819) concluded that his "system furnishes a most fertile source of excuses for the commission of crimes, and is subversive of all civil and social order" (165).

Because neurology emphasized the vast neural networks that connected parts of the body, it made it possible to see the anus itself as an erogenous zone. Although Erasmus Darwin insists that "pleasurable sensation" is "necessary to copulation" (2:261) in *Zoonomia* (1794), he undermines this connection between pleasure and copulation when he points out that although male nipples "erect on titillation like those of the female" they "seem to be of no further use" (1: 171) and when he discusses priapism (3:77, 3:411). Switching to the more scientific Latin, Darwin also notes that "from their first swaddling clothes, boys' penises may be reached for more frequently; though love has not yet awakened" (1:46), and this implies that pleasure has no necessary connection to reproduction.[36] Alan Richardson comments that "the suggestions of polymorphous or ambiguous sexuality . . . find resonance in Darwin, who postulates an 'original single sex' . . . that accounts . . . for the human male's possession of seemingly useless nipples" (2001 62).

But once pleasure has been located in the anus, it has become definitively perverse. Erasmus Darwin concludes his three-volume *Zoonomia* with an example of a fifty-year old gentleman who had applied to Darwin for help because of imperfect erections. Darwin writes,

> A gentleman about 50 years of age, who had lived too freely, as he informed me, both in respect to wine and women, complained that his desire for the sex remained, and that he occasionally parted with semen, but with the defect of a perfect tensio penis, and that he had tried 20 drops of laudanum, and 20 drops of tincture of cantharides on going to bed without effect; and that as the debility or irritability of the system in this case rather than any mental affection seemed to be part of the cause, he was advised to stimulate the sphincter ani by the introduction of a piece of root ginger, as is done by the horse dealers to sale horses. And however ridiculous the operation may appear, he assured me, that it succeeded; which I suppose might be owing to the sympathy between the sphincter and the penis; which is often the cause of the painful sensation in the former, when a stone at the neck of the bladder affects the latter; and conversely when painful piles affect the rectum, a strangury is sometimes produced by sympathy. (3:505–6)

Although it is true that Darwin recommends the stimulation of the anal sphincter in the service of heterosexual sex, the passage above is nonetheless interesting because it emphasizes the sympathy between the anus and the penis, thus explaining how sodomy can be a form of pleasurable sex, and brings beasts and men in proximity to one another (he learns about this technique from what horse dealers do to their horses to advertise their virility). Despite the fact that anal stimulation is in service of heterosexual sex, Darwin makes a point of noting the procedure's "ridiculousness" even as he erases his own presence when he dispenses the advice: Darwin noticeably turns to the passive voice at the moment of advice, claiming "he [the patient] was advised."[37] The neurological connection between the anus and penis thus perversely binds together sodomy and heterosexuality, excrement and sexuality, and sodomy and sexual pleasure.

Railing against sodomites, the poet Charles Churchill decries the fact that "Women are kept for nothing but the breed / For pleasure we must have a Ganymede" ("The Times" 20). Freud would later comment that the position of the genitals—*"inter urinas et faeces"*—was a decisive factor in human sexuality (cited in Dollimore *Sexual Dissidence* 257). Darwin's argument is part of the genealogy of how the anus and the genitals became sexual.

My emphasis thus far has been to show how Romantic science enabled scientists and poets to understand normative sexual pleasure as increasingly perverse and make it separable from reproduction. Medical interest in nocturnal emissions, the titillation of the male nipple, and the clitoris, an organ of pleasure with no known function in reproduction, made it clear that pleasure did not necessarily have a function. Now that pleasure had no natural role, it could be constructed as a liberating force rather than as a discovered ground of reality. Such perversification of pleasure was intensified by the multiple strategies of birth control available in the Romantic period: in *A History of Contraception*, Angus McClaren had detailed herbal contraceptives, the sponge and other barrier methods, the condom, coitus interruptus, abortion, and extended lactation (65–87).[38] Wordsworth's "The Thorn" alludes to infanticide as a possible means of eradicating the consequences of sexual intercourse. Francis Place began distributing his practical contraceptive handbills in 1823 to the working classes from Manchester to London, and it was Place who prompted Richard Carlisle to write *Every Woman's Book*, in which he advocated contraception so that the working classes could have pleasurable intercourse without fear of the consequences.

I now focus briefly on Linnaean botany and its introduction into England because Linnaean botany, popularized by Erasmus Darwin's *Botanic Garden* (1791), puts lie to perverse forms of sexuality being unproductive. Compounding the gap between normative sexual pleasure and function in this period was a second gap between perverse sex and sterility. Together, these gaps showed that perversity was more about social convention than it was about naturalness: although perversion masks itself as a violation of nature, it is in fact only a violation of outdated social conventions. If heterosexual pleasure was functionless, and if perverse sex could lead to reproduction, then was function a stable natural ground upon which to valorize certain sex acts over others? Linnaean botany thus made it clear that nature herself was teeming with perverts. Moreover, in *The Elements of Botany* (1775), an exposition of the Linnaean system, the author comments that "no luxuriant flowers are natural, but all monsters; full flowers are eunuchs, and therefore always miscarry; . . . proliferous flowers increase the deformity" (152). The irony is in the fact that the very flowers that we consider most beautiful are really the ones that are the most monstrous. Not only were many female flowers thought to be "seductive harlots" (Browne 159), but also parent plants incestuously mingled with their offspring (Teute 325).

The perversity of plants is, however, much more complicated than the foregoing suggests. James Jenkinson's *Generic and Specific Description of British Plants* highlighted the "promiscuous use" of even staid British plants (1775 xvii). And in the botanical society of Lichfield's sponsored translation of Carl Linneaus's *Families of Plants* (1787), plants were divided into a productive sexual system based almost entirely upon the arrangement and number of male parts, which included hermaphrodite flowers (flowers with stamens/husbands and pistils/wives in the same flower); flowers with as many as twenty males together; polygamous flowers (husbands and wives who live together with their concubines); clandestine flowers, flowers with hidden sexual parts; and flowers that reproduced with "feminine males" or stamens that were inserted on the pistils.[39] Polygamous flowers were further divided into: equal polygamy and spurious polygamy, with spurious polygamy—where the "beds of the married occupy the disk, and those of the concubines the circumference"—being yet still further divided into superfluous polygamy, frustraneous polygamy, necessary polygamy, and separate polygamy (lxxx). That polygamy could be necessary in cases where the married females are barren and the concubines fertile meant that bourgeois marriage might not be the best means of reproduction if either the husband or wife were barren or sterile.

It is the category of spurious but necessary polygamy that most renders absurd social conventions that legitimate one form of sexual activity over another. For one, since plants have no legitimating ceremony how does one distinguish between married plants and a male plant and his concubine? Second, what makes the relationship of a male plant and his concubine spurious if multiple sexual partners are deemed natural? And, yet, even within the defiance of social conventions lies the reinscription of those very conventions: the very need to make distinctions between polygamy among married couples, and polygamy between married couples and concubines hints that, although Botany flirted with the idea of a natural pornotopia,[40] a never-never land where sexuality is untainted by social reality, even polygamy could not do without what Gayle Rubin calls a "charmed circle" whereby certain acts are accorded more validity than others.

All of this "natural" erotic diversity put considerable pressure on the notion that reproductive sex between married couples was the only kind of procreative and therefore legitimate sex because flowers so successfully reproduced under so many differing "domestic" arrangements. Clandestine flowers in particular were perhaps a gibe against the 1753 Clandestine Marriage Act, which made all marriages illegal unless banns had been publicly proclaimed in the couple's parish previous to the ceremony. This was to discourage the wealthy from marrying without parental consent. If flowers "married" clandestinely, why should the clandestine marriage of human beings be illegal? Not even Erasmus Darwin's technically perfect rhyming couplets, insisting on the propriety of pairs, could monogamize the kinds of plant polygamy that the doctor, father of two illegitimate daughters himself, so eagerly cataloged in his *Botanic Garden*. Indeed, Darwin's couplets had much to discipline. Darwin was careful to praise the virtue of the monogamous Canna or Indian reed and to wag his finger at more licentious forms of "plant hymen" (*BG* 4:183). As Fredrika Teute points out, Darwin's "sexual-social fantasy was not just the provenance of men; women partook of liberation too" (333). Alan Bewell comments that "by the 1790s, botanical pastoralism took a decidedly revolutionary turn, as it began to question explicitly the universality of European sexual customs and attitudes, notably the institution of marriage and concepts of sexual difference" (1996 184–85).[41] And Janet Browne highlights the radical implications of Darwin's materialism: "there was a great deal of ambiguous materialism, possibly even atheism, in Darwin's outspoken rejection of traditional Anglican ethics in favor of the supposed sexual freedoms of classical antiquity" (161).

Linneaus's and Darwin's critics recognized how botany was naturalizing erotic diversity; they sought to counter this by insisting upon the perversity of Linneaus's terms or the sloppiness of his scientific methods. Critics thus called attention to the "harlotry" of plants and the promiscuousness of pollen, arguing that nature could hardly have intended such perverse forms of sexuality (Schiebinger 30). Spallanzani insisted that botany would have been better served had Linneaus first determined whether the husbands he cataloged had "performed their office," before he erected a system of classification that relied so heavily on counting husbands (1784 2:424). Colin Milne, author of *A Botan-*

*ical Dictionary* (1778), carped that, although many have extolled the ease of Linneaus's system, that ease "only exists in theory"; moreover, "none of the classes are [*sic*] completely natural, though some . . . might have been rendered such, without any material violence to the principles of the method" ("Chart Showing the Sexual System of Linneaus"). Not only is Linneaus guilty of perverting plants, but his very system of classification also is enshrining perversion—"material violence" to nature—within science itself.

In light of all these radical implications of the loves of the plants, it is no accident that Byron and his circle code their homosexuality in botanical terms. Charles Matthews writes to Byron, "I take it that the flowers you will be most desirous of culling will be of the class nogynia" (cited in Crompton 1985 129; Dyer 568). In one fell swoop, Byron and his friends could attack religion, return to a liberating classical sexuality, one that could conceive of pederasty as being a higher form of love than married heterosexual love, and undermine heteronormativity.

## Foucault, Science, and Sexual Liberation

Now that I have laid out some of the medical grounds for why sexuality could become coupled with liberation during Romanticism, we are equipped to reexamine Foucault's legacy for the history of sexuality in the Romantic period. Michel Foucault has almost single-handedly made sexual liberation seem like a quaint delusion. Foucault's skepticism about sexual liberation is grounded upon two premises. The first is that the repression/liberation binary opposition reduces power to working in a crude juridical form and thus cannot address how pleasure becomes power. Hence, Foucault argues that "saying yes to sex is not saying no to power" (*HS* 1:157). But this is not news to scientists working in the Romantic period: Franz Gall warned his readers not to mistake pleasure for liberty. Gall insisted, "It is this satisfaction which misleads the individual, and makes him imagine that in this case he acts with freedom" (*Origin* 1:212). Nor is it news to Percy Shelley, who equated unbridled lust with tyranny, or to Byron, who warned that "headlong passions form their proper woes" (*DJ* 5:6). Foucault has influenced the historian of sexuality Jeffrey Weeks to dismiss sexual liberation as a "delusion, a God that failed" (13).

Foucault's second ground for skepticism is based on his sense that liberation movements have accepted the basic principle that there is such a thing as "life," about which knowledge can be had, and that sexuality is one area of such knowledge. For Foucault, sex is not a ground reality beneath the historical formation of sexuality: getting beyond sexuality to sex does not in fact move beyond power. Hence, he writes, "the rallying point for the counterattack against the deployment of sexuality ought not to be sex-desire, but bodies and pleasures" (*HS* 1:157).[42] One might ask here how it is that "bodies and pleasures" stand outside of "biopower" while sexual desire doesn't. Foucault seems to suggest that while pleasure is a form of power, it is not a form of knowledge, and he therefore thinks it can be a rallying point for resistance. His archeology of the sciences accordingly shows again and again how science as a discipline organizes the "truth games" of sexuality without allowing them to be seen as truth games.[43]

The Romantics anticipated both of these skepticisms, yet they still held onto the possibility of meaningful sexual liberation. But why? If pleasure and sex as well as sexuality exist within a grid of power/knowledge, there is no need to give up liberation in favor of pleasure because both pleasure and liberation have the same possibilities and liabilities. The Romantics realized that pleasure and sexuality could be worked for both resistance and domination.

Like Foucault, the Romantics too could be skeptical that sexual liberation was meaningful liberation. If the gaps between normative sexual pleasure and function helped to make sexual liberation seem possible, this gap also enabled the Romantics to recognize the gaps between pleasure and liberation and between liberation and liberty. In Percy Shelley's concepts of "anarchy" and "wanton," referring to a spoiled and lascivious child (Reiman and Fraistat [R&F] 2002 266), an individual guided by the whims of desire, he consistently denounces a libertine sensualism that is merely hedonism. Where Blake's notion of Beulah points to the fecklessness of vegetative sex and sexual permissiveness, his depiction of Vala as "Sexual Death living on accusation of Sin & Judgment" (*Jerusalem* 64:22 E 215) indicates his acknowledgment of how sex becomes power. Moreover, Blake suggests that because women are falsely taught to value chastity as a virtue, it is difficult for them to know their own desires. And although feminist critics have argued that Blakean sexual liberation is for men only, Blake has female Earth acknowledge that "free Love [can be] with bondage bound" ("Earth's Answer" E 19).[44]

For Blake, sexuality can be liberating only if it leads to self-annihilation, the loss of all forms of self-righteousness including male egotism. Byron's emphasis on the youthful Don Juan's effeminacy undermines any neat equation of pleasure and subversion. Nor do the Romantics understand sexual desire and pleasure as intrinsically liberating; in fact, they insist that sexual permissiveness can mask oppression under pleasure and that sexual intimacy is short-lived and must be subsumed under a more durable form of caring. Percy Shelley deliberately contrasts the tyrant Othman's rape of Cyntha with the pastoral, mutual, and incestuous embraces of Cyntha and Laon precisely to underscore the potential abuses of desire. If the Romantics bought into the notion that despots, Oriental or otherwise, invariably manifested their political tyranny in sexual terms, one's sexual conduct could be a symptom of a larger despotism. Shelley's paradoxical definition of wisdom and love as "but slaves of equality" (Laon's Song of Liberty, RI, stanza 3), signals his skepticism that desire is necessarily tantamount to liberty. Shelley in fact argued that "the conviction that wedlock is indissoluble holds out the strongest of all temptations to the perverse" (R&F 2:253). Because marriage encouraged selfishness and the idea of women as property, Shelley turned instead to sibling incest as a paradigmatic sexual relationship of equality.

Consider too Thel's highly ambiguous entry into sexual knowledge—her final acts are to shriek and flee—not to mention Orc's rapes. By linking sex and rape, the poet entertained the notion that "the value of sexuality itself is to demean the seriousness of efforts to redeem it" (Bersani "Rectum" 222). Blake shows that, if desire is an impetus for revolution, the disruptiveness of desire cannot be controlled even by the liberator. Blake thus anticipates a charge that Jonathan Dollimore levels against queer activists: desire is only disruptive for everyone else since the queer activist is never undone by desire. Dollimore thus muses that the "rhetoric of liberation" in much queer theory "is a cover for the self-empowerment of a politically conservative kind," a kind of empowerment that contains desire under identity (*Literature* 25). Blake's Orc, by contrast, is constantly on the verge of becoming another (Jesus, Luvah, etc.). For Blake, desire will not be contained by identity and ego, and it potentially shatters them both.

The Romantics also understood the gaps between liberation from something and the general condition of freedom. Hannah Arendt incisively claims that "liberation may be the condition of freedom but by no means leads automatically to it; that the notion of liberty implied in liberation can only be negative; and hence, that even the intention of liberating is not identical with the desire for freedom" (*On Revolution* 22), and her point was hardly lost on Romantic artists. Percy Shelley in *Laon and Cythna* shows that recently liberated peoples often resort to vengeance and murder in the name of justice: once freed from the Tyrant Othman, the people cry, "He who judged let him be brought/To judgement! blood for blood cries from the soil ... " (5:32). Laon intervenes, however, demanding, "What call ye justice? Is there one who ne'er/In secret thought has wished another's ill?—/Are ye all pure?" (5:34). Of course, Shelley's insistence that the failures of the French Revolution did not undermine the idea of revolution itself leads the poet to ask in his Preface, "Can he who the day before was a trampled slave suddenly become liberal minded, forbearing, and independent?" Shelley further recognized that the criteria of liberation can be set so high that they are unreachable: "such a degree of unmingled good was expected as it was impossible to realize" (Preface). The poet's central image of "An Eagle and a Serpent wreathed in fight" thus serves as a reminder that liberation and domination are inextricably intertwined. That both the serpent and the eagle symbolize liberation and repression furthers Shelley's anticipation of Foucault, that liberation is not freedom, but is, contra Foucault, a necessary step on the way to freedom. Although the serpent initially serves as an emblem of freedom, by Canto 9 it becomes an emblem of hate in the "snaky folds" of the heart (9:21) and "serpent Custom's tooth" (9:27). By giving custom serpentine teeth, Shelley overturns Burke's claim that custom was the foundation of British Liberty.

For the Romantics, it was difficult to imagine biological sex as a ground reality for the simple reason that biology itself was a nascent discipline, only just beginning to understand the implications of life and the differences between the physical sciences and biology. Not only did vitalism complicate the very possibility of a ground reality, since that ground was always in flux, but the skepticism explicitly within science itself also further ironizes that ground. That medical jurisprudence as in its formative stages—Samuel Farr published the first English book on medical jurisprudence in 1788—meant that such disciplines were just beginning to teach others what the bodily signs of consent, murder, especially infanticide, or false pregnancy and how to interpret them.[45] Whereas Foucault thought of the natural sciences as his enduring enemy because they constrain sex and sexuality and yet naturalize these constraints, I have tried here to suggest how the Romantics could perceive the sciences to be helpful to liberation because the sciences (1) repeatedly showed the resistance of sexual pleasure to reproductive function, a resistance that made it difficult to consolidate heterosexual sex into heteronormativity; (2) had more nuanced and flexible understandings of ontology and ontological narratives than we now do; and (3) demonstrated that historical constructions could facilitate both resistance as well as power/knowledge. To the extent that it was possible for the Romantics to see sex as a Foucauldian truth game, Blake, Hunt, Shelley, and Byron realized that they could use the insights of science for their own liberating ends. Yet this does not mean that embodiment could not be therapeutic because it might locate utopianism within the body and make subversion biological, thereby rendering it difficult to eradicate.

Fredric Jameson may help us to think about how sexual liberation then could be meaningful. He argues that, in order for pleasure to become "genuinely political, if it is to evade the complacencies of hedonism—[it] must always in one way or another also be able to stand as a figure for the transformation of social relations as a whole" (74). Building upon Jameson's work, I suggest that Romantic writers and scientists recognized how others used sex as a powerful form of allegory for political power, an allegory that is occluded by claims to naturalness and transparent representation. By turning to sexual intimacy to think about meaningful consent and genuine intersubjectivity, Blake, Hunt, and the Shelleys made pleasure an allegory for human relationships generally. Hence Blake, on the one hand, links Orcian revolution with sexual desire yet, on the other hand, insistently demarcates between fallen and unfallen love, thus rendering sex multiple and allegorical. I have argued that, because Percy Shelley could not imagine sodomy as pleasurable in his essay on the "Manners of the Ancient Greeks," he therefore could not imagine that anyone would consent to it.[46]

Why, despite these considerable skepticisms, did the Romantics cling to sexual liberation? Insofar as liberation mandated that repressors be identified, the Romantics found the targets of Malthus, the church and state, enabled them to channel fruitfully their liberating energies. Hannah Arendt reminds us that the "fruits of liberation" are the "removal of restraint" and the ability to move about freely: "these are the [very] condition of freedom" (25). And whereas Foucault insisted that liberation did not dismantle power, but merely extended its grasp (Dean 283), the Romantics found the always shifting ground of the sexed body made it possible to "perceive subordination, where differentials of power seem necessary, as oppression, a site of potential antagonism" (Laclau and Mouffe 153). Indeed shifting representations of the body made it possible to see how subordination masks oppression, how gender inequality is no longer justified. In the words of Ernesto Laclau and Chantal Mouffe, the Romantics could now "identify the conditions in which a relation of subordination becomes a relation of oppression and thereby constitutes itself into the site of an antagonism" (153). Laclau and Mouffe's example, we should recall, is Mary Wollstonecraft, who pointedly argued that women must have physical exercise; she reasoned that if women were allowed to arrive at "perfection of body, . . . we may know how far the natural superiority of man extends" (*VRW* 182–83). The sciences thus made it possible to "propose the different forms of inequality as illegitimate and anti-natural, and thus make them equivalent as forms of oppression" (Laclau and Mouffe 155). As Shelley's Cyntha puts it, "Never will peace and human nature meet/Till free and equal man and woman greet/Domestic peace" (*Laon and Cythna* 2:37). Because Cyntha must have power in order to dethrone the tyrant Othman, Shelley sees liberation not so much as a liberation from power, but as a reorganization of how power works.

Part of the reason why historians of sexuality such as Weeks are so skeptical of sexual liberation is that he was and we are so removed from an eighteenth-century philosophical tradition that understood pleasure itself as a moral category. Locke's moral hedonism stipulated that pleasure is good and pain is bad; Burke sought to solidify these distinctions in his *Enquiry into the Origins of the Sublime and Beautiful*. Our own skepticism that pleasure is feckless or merely self-indulgent thus renders a work like Jeremy Bentham's *A Table of the Springs of Action* as being impossibly strange. Bentham grounded virtue in pleasure and vice in pain.[47] And he concluded that "legislators, moralists, and divines, finding [sexual desire] operating, to so great an extent, and with so efficient a force, in opposition to their views and endeavors, make unceasing war upon it" (18). If Bentham helps us to see why sexual desire would logically become a primary site of antagonism in this period, he also reminds us that pleasure could achieve moral ends. Bentham also puts further pressure on Foucault's privileging of bodies and pleasures as opposed to liberation, since pleasure is so clearly tied to knowledge. Of course, when Bentham has to concede that the pederast finds "intense pleasure" in "odious and disgusting acts"—"it gives him pleasure" ("Essay on Paederasty" 94–95), pleasure would prove to be a problematic ground for morality. He thus justifies the decriminalization of sodomy on the grounds that the desire for severe punishment of sodomy is based upon an even more unnatural (more unnatural than sodomy) hatred of sexual pleasure and the fact that the punishment, hanging, inflicts more harm than the offense itself. "Moral antipathy is the more ready when the idea of pleasure, especially of intense pleasure, is connected with that of the act by which the antipathy is excited" (95), thunders Bentham.

In sum, Romantic skepticism about sexual liberation makes it possible to revisit and revalue this concept and necessary to rethink the extent to which pleasure can lead to positive social change. By replacing function with a kind of purposive, if perverse, mutuality, the Romantics made it possible to use sexuality as an index of mutuality and, in so doing, gauge the extent to which liberation had been achieved and for whom, especially since the gaps between liberation and liberty were a given.

I now turn to the work of the sociologist Anthony Giddens because it suggests both a counter-narrative to the Foucauldian history of sexuality and the possibility of thinking about sexual liberation as meaningful. Whereas Foucault's skepticism about sexual liberation is helpful for articulating the Romantic' own skepticism about it, Foucault has made the reasons for the Romantic valuing of sexual liberation opaque. Giddens allows us to understand why.

Giddens himself critiques Foucault on the grounds that "power moves in mysterious ways in Foucault's writings, and history as the actively made achievement of human subjects scarcely exists" (24). Moreover, because Foucault writes a history of sexuality without intimacy, Giddens argues that Foucault cannot acknowledge the democraticization of sexuality. In *The Transformation of Intimacy*, Giddens argues that plastic sexuality, sexuality freed from the needs of reproduction, began in the late eighteenth century as a means of limiting family size, and he insists that plastic sexuality is necessary for emancipatory intimacy, "a transactional negotiation of personal ties by equals" (2–3). Giddens is not blind to the "deep psychological, as well as economic differences between the sexes [that] stand in the way of the achievement of an ethical framework for a democratic personal order" (188), but he argues that this utopian ideal is offset by what he sees as a "trend of development of modern societies toward their realization" (188). Changes in sexual attitudes have been emancipatory even if they have not achieved emancipation (172). In constantly weighing the utopic elements of sexual liberation against measurable political change, both Giddens and the Romantics well before him, I suggest, make an important if unacknowledged contribution to the achievement of emancipatory intimacy as the basis for societal liberty, even if their own practices fall considerably short of this ideal.[48] Blake's depictions of fellatio in *Milton* thus eroticize what otherwise might remain an abstract concept, brotherhood. And when Coleridge wrote in his notebook, "I desire because I love, and [I do] not imagine I love because I desire" (no. 3284), he anticipates Giddens insofar as he rejects a necessary connection between sex and power and chooses instead the possibility of mutual love as the basis for social relations. As Shelley's *Laon and Cythna* and *Queen Mab*, Byron's *Manfred* and *Don Juan*, Anna Seward's "Llangollen Vale," and Blake's *Jerusalem* all attest, the Romantics were at least theoretically committed to what Giddens calls a "pure relationship," a "situation where a social relation is entered into for its own sake, for what can be derived by each person from a sustained association with one another; and which is continued only so far as it is thought by both parties to deliver enough satisfaction for each individual to stay within it" (58). As Romanticism continues to reevaluate the impact of gender on its canon, we would do well to remember this possibility. And as more nuanced understandings of the role of science and sex in the Romantic period are attained, we might gain a richer sense of its contexts, politics, aesthetics, and pleasures. Finally, the Romantics might help us to think about how liberation and sexuality became linked in the first place so that both together might enable some meaningful resistance.

I give the final word to Hannah Arendt, who writes of the age of the American and French revolutions that "the eagerness to liberate and to build a new house where freedom can dwell, is unprecedented and unequaled in all of human history" (28). Perhaps in the Romantic period that house could be the human body.

# CHAPTER TWO

# Historicizing Perversion

## Perversity, Perversion, and the Rise of Function in the Biological Sciences

That Percy Shelley's skepticism about the "the purposes for which the sexual instinct are supposed to have existed" (D. Clark 223) appears in his treatment of Greek pederasty shows the poet refusing to elevate one kind of sex act over another on the basis of purpose. Likewise, William Blake vehemently denied Emanuel Swedenborg's point that "Organs and Viscera" of man's body correspond to "Thing[s] in the created Universe . . . not with them as Substances, but with them as Uses" (*Complete Poetry and Prose of William Blake* [E] 607), noting instead that "Uses & substances are so different as not to correspond" (ibid.). This resistance to use and reproduction—whereby Romantic sexuality ideally becomes a kind of Kantian purposiveness without purpose—can be explained in part by the fact that physical intimacy could not symbolize equality within the then accepted understandings of gender and their relation to reproduction. For physical intimacy to symbolize equality, sex had to be a common search for shared pleasure, and could not be for reproductive purposes. As Percy Shelley put it, "Love makes all things equal" (Reiman and Fraistat 2002 296). The radical Richard Carlisle said it thusly: "Sexual commerce . . . may be a pleasure, independent of the dread of conception that blasts the prospects and happiness of the female" (41).

Historicizing this interest in nonreproductive and antireproductive sex within the rise of function in the biological sciences in this period reveals that the Romantic period is the one in which function not only becomes central to the life sciences but also attains primary causal explanatory power over structure.[1] Why did biologists then begin to insist upon the necessary relationship of structure to function, with function increasingly serving to explain structure? How did this expanded explanatory role of function shape the possibility of a scientific concept of a perverted identity? By wedding functionlessness to pathology, scientists and physicians medicalized sexuality, converting reproduction into the sine qua non of health while resisting connections between identity and the perverse. At the same time, however, because pathological knowledge was so vital to claims of normality, functionlessness would not remain confined to disease. Without understanding the historical rise of function in the biological sciences of the Romantic period, Romanticists are unable to account for how and why perverse sexuality could then become such a powerful metaphor for equality.

My larger aim here is to put pressure on the influential historiographical premise that the nineteenth century witnessed a shift from perversity to perversion: from thinking about perversity as a vice, and therefore a category whereby deviant sexual acts stemmed from an individual's morally depraved character, to explaining perversion in terms of psychology and identity, thereby enabling medicine simultaneously to invent, individualize, and explain the pervert. In the *Emergence of Sexuality*, Arnold Davidson has recently captured the difference between perversity and perversion by arguing that sexuality could only come about when perversion shifted in the nineteenth century from being localized in organs, subject to the anatomo-clinical gaze, to belonging to the instinct, and thus under the purview of psychiatry. Before sexuality, there was sex, and anatomy was destiny. After sexuality, the moment when psychiatry localized desire in the instincts, the sodomite became a person. The problem with Davidson's epistemic shift between sex and sexuality and with his historical epistemology of the pervert is that they both ignore the moment when function became central to biology as well as underestimate the complexity of localization. When sensory function is localized in the nervous system, the idea of psychological integrity and the indivisibility of the personality becomes the guiding principle of physiological analysis (Figlio 179).

Hence, on the one hand, Romanticism is when the neurological groundwork is laid for sexuality to become identity: the Romantic body becomes an especially dense network of the organs of pleasure. On the other hand, the rise of function in this period makes it more difficult to think in terms of the pervert. A historical understanding of how and why function came to have such a central role in biology undermines Davidson's thesis that sexuality could only become a valid style of reasoning when psychiatry localized sex in the instinct and—voilà!—the pervert was born. The rise of function in biology suggests a more nuanced historical emergence, one whereby the absences Davidson relies upon to prove sexuality did not occur before 1869 are calculated absences rather than ontological absences. I am therefore using the nexus of biology, localization, and function to consider the ways in which scientists made it more difficult to think in terms of a perverted identity and the implications of this resistance for understanding why Romantics such as Blake, Byron, and the Shelleys could believe in perverse forms of sexuality—sex without reproduction—as a means to liberation.

The fact that anatomy still has an important role in medical education, long after its supposed decline, undermines the convenient Foucauldian rupture between anatomy and psychiatry that Davidson relies upon. Physiology and neurology, moreover, provide important if neglected missing links between anatomy and psychiatry—sex and sexuality—for the history of sexuality. Growing recognition of the gaps between structure and function in medical science meant that even anatomical localization was far more complex than Davidson recognizes, insofar as anatomical localization is often, especially in Romanticism, more about the idea of localization than about any actual locus. Nor should we forget that localization itself was a tool of pathology, a way of understanding disease. To appropriate it as a way of making sense of sexuality—to localize sexuality—implies that sexuality can be subsumed under disease.

The Romantic period's understanding of sexuality as a kind of purposiveness without purpose has recently been corroborated by the biologist Joan Roughgarden. Roughgarden surveys how widespread homosexuality is in the animal kingdom and argues that mating is not about reproduction and sperm transfer (2004 171). Rather, she insists that mating enhances cooperation because it occurs a hundred to a thousand times more often than is needed for conception. Moreover, she argues that many secondary sexual characteristics are to facilitate homosexual matings (171) and that these matings also enhance cooperation. By separating sexual pleasure from reproduction and by linking it instead with purposive mutuality, Romantic writers such as Hunter, Blake, Byron, and Shelley made it possible to think about sexuality as a form of disinterestedness rather than selfishness. The upshot of Roughgarden's work is that we will have to rethink what counts as the norm and what counts as pathological.

## Playing Hocus Pocus with the Locus

That physiology to 1800 was largely a theoretical discipline rather than an experimental one meant that corporeal localization occurred in language as opposed to the body. Truth occurred in bodily language and thought, not in the body, insofar as physiological demonstration was in logic, not in bodies. In an important series of recent articles, Andrew Cunningham has argued that until the turn of the nineteenth century physiology was essentially a theoretical and therefore noble science, one ground not in the vulgar knife of the anatomist, but rather in the pen of the physiologist. As evidence, Cunningham proffers the fact that Haller understood physiology as a "narration of the motions by which the animated machine is moved" (cited in Cunningham 2002 654). "What Haller does not do when investigating function is start from experiment on the live animal" (656). Cunningham does not ignore the importance of investigative experiments in Haller. Rather, he insists that Haller is an old physiologist who relies upon old anatomy to ground his knowledge. Cunningham writes, "Anatomy suggests to physiology: . . . anatomical practical investigation" serves to buttress "physiological theoretical conclusion" (2002 658). Whereas old anatomists proceeded from structure to function, extrapolating through reason the relations of structure to function, the new experimental physiologists such as Flourens and Magendie "begin with function and then seek its explanation in the organism" by doing vivisections on animals (Cunningham 2002 661). This means that, whereas in the first half of the Romantic period localization threatens to evaporate into language since function must be extrapolated from structure, in the second half the need to begin with function and then work back to structures—reversing the previous way of doing things—meant that the body was still a precarious locus to the extent the traffic between structure and function has merely shifted direction, leaving the gap between the two intact. That is, although the new physiology post-1800 begins in the body with vivisection, the need to correlate function to structure still meant that language had a key role in localization.

Part of the problem with localization was the fact that eighteenth-century medicine was reliant upon symptoms, subjectively felt, rather than more scientific and objective forms of knowledge like lesions or organs (Bynum 30). This problem was exacerbated by medical examinations that relied upon the patient's words as opposed to bodies: decorum in this period mandated that the physician not examine the body too closely or too directly. The upshot of this was that medical localization was really in language rather than in bodies. W. F.

Bynum cites the example of Queen Caroline, whose death might have been prevented; had her abdomen been physically examined, her hernia would have been properly diagnosed (34).

Given the age's preference for understanding diseases holistically and in terms of common physiological principles, especially those of vitality, localization becomes even more vexed in the Romantic period. Bynum writes, "Although Cullen admitted that disease sometimes could be local (one of his four classes of disease was locales), he conceived the human body as an integrated whole, so that individuals, not organs or body parts, were the actual loci of disease" (16). Cullen's nosology shaped the beliefs and practices of thousands of doctors for the next fifty years (Porter 1997 262). Because Cullen had "no knowledge of the essence of nervous power, he equated it with an aetherial fluid which was also the basis of light, heat magnetism, and electricity" (Porter 1997 260). Cullen's localization of diseases in the nervous system thus diffuses disease throughout the body and winds up becoming an abstraction only to be recontained in the idea of nervous fluid. John Brown, his pupil, defined health in terms of neither too much nor too little excitability and this also meant that localization was throughout the body. Brown boasted that he was the very first physician to treat "the human body as a whole" (cited in Canguilhem 1988 47).[2] John Abernethy agreed with a holistic approach to disease, arguing that local problems must be treated by attention to the general health of the patient (Ruston 85). Such stress upon general health as the cure to disease brought an aesthetics of the self very much in line with medicine of the period, but it did not do much to actualize localization.[3]

This medical emphasis on holistic treatment, however, was countered by the surgical and pathological need to specify localization. Giovanni Battista Morgagni's *The Seats and Causes of Disease* (1761) refined an organ-based approach to disease. Morgagni's work was first translated into English in 1769. By correlating symptoms to anatomical lesions, Morgagni shifted the emphasis from subjective symptom to anatomical site (Porter 1997 264). Hence his three-volume work begins at the head and descends into the lower regions of the body. In spite of this topographical organization, however, because few diseases had isolated disorders, Morgagni had to admit that "as there are very few diseases . . . , to which some other disorder is not join'd, or to which many different symptoms are not added; for this reason every observation of such a disease, after having been given at large under the head whereto it particularly belongs, ought, without doubt, to be made mention of under other heads to which it likewise relates in some measure" (1:xvii). Like Hydra, one heading spawns others. Loci thus become infinite. To make matters worse, how does one distinguish between a primary seat and ancillary seats of disease? Morgagni himself could not quite re-solve this dilemma: his treatment of venereal infection, for example, cites more than twenty-four other letters that treat the subject, each letter nominally de-voted to a particular locus in the body. The upshot of this is that no part of the body seems immune from this disease (2:343–45). Even the structure to his work undermines the possibility of a stable seat for disease. After a chapter on universal disorders, a category that by definition vitiates localization, Morgagni launches into a supplement to his earlier letters, a supplement that suggests the inadequacy of his original localizations. To wit, in one of these supplements de-voted to the disorders of the genital parts, Morgagni performs an exhaustive au-topsy of a woman who died of apoplexy. After meticulously documenting her brain, heart, and thorax, he finally gets to the part in question, briefly mention-ing that she "labour'd under a uterine fluor" (3:563–65). Once again global at-tention to the body outweighs attention to the specific part.

James Hamilton, the younger, professor of midwifery in Edinburgh Univer-sity, republished Morgagni's influential plates in 1795: the result of which was that the ontology of locus was rendered even more perplexing by Hamilton's di-vision into predisponent, exciting, and proximate causes of disease. Hamilton's main claim to fame was that he eventually prevailed in his recommendation that training in midwifery be mandatory for all physicians. The first category of causes referred to the circumstances that make the body susceptible to disease (xxi) like a delicate habit and florid complexion, the second to the circumstance "on the application of which to the body disease follows" (xxi) as when violent passions of the mind are excited or too much food is eaten, and the third, cir-cumstances from which the symptoms of the disease arise as in laceration of the lungs (xxii). Whereas predisposition localized disease in the whole body and its habits, the exciting cause led to a circumstance with effects anywhere on the body, and even beyond the body in "external circumstance" (xxiii). More trou-bling is the fact that proximate causes could be at some distance from the cause of the disease. Proximate causes cannot be located without "intimate acquain-tance with the structure and functions of the human body.—But as such knowl-edge is yet in a very imperfect state, the proximate cause of diseases is still in-volved in so much obscurity, that it is discovered only in those disorders which are seated in a single organ, and in some particular part of the structure of that organ" (xxiii). Proximate causes, then, are finally located outside the domain of knowledge. Thus, when Hamilton localizes fever to the entire "sanguiferous system" (4), the course of treatment would logically be leeches or bloodletting; nonetheless, his locus once again subsumes the entire body. To the extent that these three kinds of causes might each point to different loci, Hamilton helped muck up localization in the name of refining it.

The great pathologist Matthew Baillie himself faults Morgagni for "taking notice of smaller collateral circumstances, which have no connection with them or the disease from which they arose" (vii) in his *Morbid Anatomy*. Baillie's awareness of gaps between circumstances and disease reinforced his distrust of symptoms as a means to localization. Baillie writes, "Person who previously had attended very accurately to symptoms, but was unacquainted with disease, when he comes to examine the body after death . . . will acquire a knowledge of the whole disease" (v). As if to prevent the subjectivity of symptoms from tainting scientific knowledge of disease, even Baillie's syntax insists upon distance be-tween symptoms and disease, symptoms and knowledge: each appears in a sep-arate clause set off by commas. Baillie continues, "When a person has become well acquainted with diseased appearances, he will be better able to make his re-marks, in examining dead bodies, so as to judge more accurately how far the symptoms and appearances agree with each other; he will also be able to give a more distinct account of what he has observed, so that his data shall become a more accurate ground of reasoning for others" (v–vi). Far from being irrelevant to the understanding of disease in living human beings, dead bodies offer the only reliable correlation between diseased appearance and symptoms. Baillie wants the dead body to replace the patient's unreliable articulation of symp-toms. Having closed the gap between bodies and symptoms with dissection, however, Baillie opens another gap between structure and action. He argues, "Knowledge of morbid structure does not certainly lead to knowledge of mor-bid actions, although one is the effect of the other. . . . Morbid actions going on in the minute parts of an animal body are excluded from observation" (ii). The problem is that structure may have little to do with action beyond cause and ef-fect. And while effects are visible, they may or may not tell us something about morbid action, which is invisible. Baillie thus makes it clear that localization is very much limited to what can be seen by the medical practitioner.

By now, one might despair of ever finding a real locus. More problems arise. Was disease to be localized within organs or tissues? Xavier Bichat located pathology in the body's twenty-one kinds of tissues: "The more one will ob-serve diseases and open cadavers, the more one will be convinced of the necessity of considering local diseases not from the aspect of the complex organs but from that of the individual tissues" (cited in Porter 1997 265). Rather than identifying tissues using a microscope, Bichat "used techniques of maceration and chemical reactivity" to identify tissues (Coleman 21). Under Bichat, visible localization was at odds with technique in that such maceration required the grinding up of tissues. Nor was chemical reactivity immediately visible to the eye. Since the word "organ" is etymologically related to "tool," Bichat thereby threatened to make organs themselves oxymorons because it was the tissues that were the real tools, not organs. Here, we should recall Blake's insistence upon separating organs from their uses. Coleman puts it this way: "the study of organs was consequently but a first approximation as well as a very imperfect one to the essential truth being sought, the irreducible structural and active elements of vital organization" (21). Localization to tissue type was just steps away from cell theory, which envisioned the cell as the basic unit of organic structure and function (Coleman 23). Bichat's sense of the continuity of the normal and pathological (Bynum 45), furthermore, meant that the disciplinary boundaries between physiology and pathology now threatened to collapse. As we have already seen with the nervous etiology of all diseases, localization could also work falsely to telescope disease into one organ: Broussais, for instance, thought all diseases stemmed from the gastrointestinal tract. The state of knowledge about a certain system within the body thus had considerable impact upon the kinds of localization that could be imagined. Localization had to have a kind of therapeutic and epistemological payoff, making treatments of disease easier or better or lending knowledge where none was to be had.[4] Often that payoff was more important than having an actual corporeal locus.

## Instinct

As sex moves from organ to instinct, the word "localization" has shifted even further from the literal to the metaphorical. Etymologically related to "tool," the very word "organ" mandates localization and offers the promise of material embodiment of function. Professor of anatomy and surgery to the Royal College of Surgeons, William Lawrence hinted that if thought were not understood as the brain's function, then the brain itself would become a perverse organ (*Lectures on Physiology* 97). Yet an "organ of generation" that does not generate is an ontological oxymoron, a paradoxical concept that invites blockage to notions of perverted identity. Inasmuch as instinct serves as a synecdoche for innateness, the localization of sexuality from the organs to the instinct further diffuses localization to a corporeal idea, not to any precise site. Because sexuality is so often reduced to genitality, the embodying work of synecdoche is usually taken for granted. Yet this very gap between literal and metaphorical locus, part for whole, allows sexuality and the pervert to emerge, a gap that is even further intensified once we examine how "instinct" was understood in the period.

Instinct has a complex history, one that has not been well served by the notion of an epistemological break between localization in organs to instinct.[5] If there is no clear shift from organ to instinct, the binary opposition between sex and sexuality collapses. Because "instinct" then straddled the bodies of brute animals and the mind's reasoning abilities of humanity and between conscious intent and acts without an end in view, the localization of sex to instinct brought with it many problems. For one, it initially meant a switch of scientific disciplines from physiology to comparative anatomy, natural history, and zoology. For another, it threatened to level distinctions between beasts and human beings. By contrast, the fact that instincts were often ascribed to the divine wisdom operating in the natural world implied that the study of instincts was a theological rather than scientific matter. Third, to the extent that instincts equated to a divine wisdom that eschewed function or purpose—instincts, most agreed, were done without any end in view—these natural impulses provided a vehicle for thinking about the role and value of function instead of presuming its value. Because localization presumed function, the notion of sexual instincts enabled skepticism about function, at least as it was understood by human beings. Instincts paradoxically brought sexuality closer to a Kantian purposiveness without purpose insofar as the instinct to perpetuate the kind was not knowingly pursued. Such a link made it possible to imagine a value for nonfunctioning or perverted organs if not beings.

To wit, the 1771 entry in the *Encyclopedia Britannica*, likely written by the influential man-midwife William Smellie, defined instinct as: "an appellation given to the sagacity and natural inclinations of brutes, which supplies the place of reason in mankind."[6] Smellie highlights the nominal status of instinct: it is emphatically an "appellation," giving the term roots in language, not the body. Moreover, the absence of clear differences between the instinct of brutes and the reason of mankind threatens to make human beings disturbingly animalistic. Perhaps for this reason Smellie insisted in his article on instinct in the *Transactions of the Royal Society of Edinburgh* (1788) that human instincts "receive improvement from experience and observation, and are capable of a thousand modifications. One instinct counteracts and modifies another, and often extinguishes the original motive to action" (43). He offers the example of "devotion [being] an extension of the instinct of love, to the first Cause or Author of the Universe" (43). Under Smellie's view, then, localizing sex to the instincts highlighted man's relationship to animals and not difference from them, a relationship that Smellie heightened when he ended this article with a concession that "the instinct of brutes are likewise improved by observation and experience" (43). Yet any actual locus of the sexual instincts soon evaporates into love which in turn evaporates into the first cause. Moreover, Smellie's acknowledgement of the fact that one instinct can be counteracted by another, canceling out the original motive, meant that the instincts in human beings were potentially perverse insofar as any originating function is lost.

James Perchard Tupper believed that even plants had instincts. In his *Essay on the Probability of Sensation in Vegetables* (1811), he submitted that "Instinct is a particular disposition or tendency, in a living being, to embrace without deliberation or reflection, the means of self-preservation, and to perform on particular occasions such other actions as are required by its economy, without having any perception for what end or purpose it acts, or any idea of the utility or advantage of its own operations" (16). Tupper argued that plants demonstrate their instincts when they turn toward the sun and climb or attach themselves to trees and other objects or vary the placement of their roots in accordance with quality of soil. If "instinct" had no perception of end or purpose, then it was uncannily like Kant's aesthetic insofar as aesthetic apprehension does not pay attention to actual ends.

Although Tupper begins his essay by defining instinct clearly against volition, when he describes the instincts of man, who has the "greatest number of instincts" (95), he admits that he may no longer be able to distinguish between instincts and volition (95). "Some instincts possess so much of the external character of reason and intelligence" that many animals "seem to indicate by several of their actions, the exercise of reflection" (96). Furthermore, there is a "close resemblance between results of intelligence and design in rational beings" (97). Animals are imbued with some degree of rational power (110). Instinct in animals will "appear to accommodate itself to particular circumstances, as from design; but it is no more the result of design on the part of the agent, than the first action of sucking of the new-born viviparous animal" (110–11). Because instinct in animals looks uncannily like design, all Tupper can do is acknowledge a resemblance, one that may or may not lead to knowledge. Here, the implicit contrast between surface and depth whereby all Tupper can comment on is "external character" of the appearance of it hints that his remarks might extend beyond epistemology.

Tupper's essay points to the lasting influence of the great chain of being. Plants, animals, and humans are suffused with instinct; here, however, the natural hierarchy promised by that chain is in the process of breaking down. The vegetarian Shelley thus could extend the notion of rights to animals (Ruston 95). Through instinct, Tupper collapses differences and insinuates an essential equality among all living beings. The price of this collapse, however, is that mankind loses any claims to specialness, and the value of deliberation and reflection, along with function, is undercut. Because the deity operates without a need for considerations of utility, why did function come to accrue such importance in the sciences of this period?

Coleridge would later suggest in his contributions to J. H. Green's "A Course of Lectures" that "may it not be said with truth, that all the Instincts of the Animal World are united in man, in a higher form?" (*Shorter Works* 2:1390–91). Differences between animals and humans and even insects thus were of degree, not kind. Man's instinctive need to "federate," by which Coleridge means to develop social compacts, "began as his sexual instincts" but is "not, however, determined thereby" (2:1394). Whereas in neutral or worker bees, "its sexual organs are sacrificed to the unity of the state" (2:1395), humans engage in much more complex forms of confederation through will, and this is what endows them with personality: "Man alone is a Person" (2:1396–97). Because Coleridge here defines personality on the basis of a resistance to sexual instincts, a resistance that is complicated by the fact that mankind embodies a unity of animal instincts in higher form, he unintentionally opens the door to the pervert. Personality is contingent upon a resistance to sexual instincts; a will that resists instincts allows for the possibility that man might seek forms of sexual confederation beyond reproduction. I use "unintentional" because Coleridge at times censured both male and female homosexuality.[7] Despite his censures, Coleridge here denigrates function, referring disparagingly to "tool-animals . . . creatures that act on external bodies by particular instruments." In man, by contrast, tools are merely "aids of his own formation & acquirement" (2:1397).

In Philip Bury Duncan's pamphlet "On Instinct" (1820) and in Thomas Hancock's *Essay on Instinct, and Its Physical and Moral Relations* (1824), we witness the continued supremacy of the idea of locus over actual locus. Duncan begins his pamphlet quoting the British Encyclopedia for a definition of instinct: instinct is defined as "that power of the mind by which, independent of all instruction or experience, without deliberation, and without having any end in view, animals are unceasingly directed to do spontaneously whatever is necessary for the preservation of the individual or the continuation of the kind" (1). By localizing instinct in the mind, Duncan distinguishes between the mind as idea and the material organ of the brain, a distinction whose purpose becomes fully clear when Duncan launches into metaphysical explanation of how specks of instinct become mingled with degrees of reason and then those with "divine infusion" (32). Because the mind is a structuring principle and not a material locus, instinct can evaporate into theology. Materialism, we should recall, was linked with atheism.

To the extent instinct comes to be defined in terms of acts "without deliberation, and without an end in view" (Duncan 4) and a "power operating above the conscious intelligence of the creature" (Hancock 52), sexual instincts become proximate to the Kantian idea of purposiveness without purpose. Because they are not done through volition, instincts embody purposiveness that only has a purpose from the vantage of the Creator. Because "actions performed with a view according to a certain end are called rational, the end in view being the motive for their performance" (Duncan 6), instincts are outside the domain of rational function. One unintended consequence of this exile is that the value of volition and debate, doing things to accomplish a function, is potentially open to question insofar as God does not need to resort to reason/volition or consciousness of function in the natural world. Hancock raises this issue implicitly when he claims that "every thing under the guidance of instinct in the natural world, is maintained and regulated with consummate wisdom:—there is no want of harmony,—no disorder" (185). Hancock therefore dismissed the possibility of the perfectibility of mankind because "reason cannot feel the evidence of the divine spirit" (195). Reason, function, and purpose, it would seem, cannot possibly supplement the harmony regulated by God through instinct.

Hancock nonetheless attempts to make reason acknowledge divine spirit in his culminating metaphor of the mind to the ovum. He writes, "The rudiments of life and lineaments of organized structure, observable in the embryo, are analogous to the underdeveloped characters of the mind" (280). Rejecting the Lockean notion of the mind as a tabula rasa, Hancock insists that "the assimilating powers of the mind . . . are analogous to the assimilating powers of the body, or of a seed" (283). The mind then is analogous to the seed, the component of generation. The instinct, then, can be given a material locus through the figure of analogy and the notion of the mind as an analogous embryo. So, too, is the instinct brought close to the products of generation, the embryo. Because both the embryo and seed underscore a materiality endowed with vitality, they are the best metaphors Hancock can find to give the mind and instincts a biological correlative. Thus, the actual locus of instinct resides in the figure of analogy.

In light of their declared preference for spontaneity over labored composition, the Romantics might be expected to have placed much stock in instinct insofar as the very word denotes "innate impulse" (*OED*) or spontaneity. Graham Richards suggests another reason why the Romantics might be expected to be invested in instinct: the Romantic cult of childhood, which stipulated children to be the best philosophers. Richards cites the example of John Gregory's popular *Comparative View of the State and Faculties of Man with Those of the Animal World* (1765), which at once claimed that children are beholden to instinct, and that this was hardly a bad thing since "the voice of Nature and Instinct . . . is the surest guide" (Richards 229). Although Charlotte Smith twice links the wheat-ear, a Sussex bird that builds its nests in stone quarries, with instinct (lines 9 and 17), she denigrates instinct by comparing the bird to those "with distorted view/ Thro' life some selfish end pursue,/With low inglorious aim" (Curran 196). No "mute inglorious" Miltons here.[8] It is also thus perhaps surprising that Blake refers to instinct only once in his entire written corpus, and he does so in "King Edward the Third" when he has Dagworth accuse William of being a "natural philosopher" who "knowest truth by instinct," an argument for the value of innate knowledge if there ever were one (*Poetical Sketches* E 48). Dagworth, by contrast, only sees limited value in instinct, preferring instead the light of reason.[9]

Byron, on the one hand, uses "instinct" to name a biological essence in human beings that is seemingly immune from culture. Hence in *Don Juan*, he invokes instinct to bring back the reader to the "another Eden" of Juan and Haidee. Byron writes, "Alas! There is no instinct like the heart—/The heart— which may be broken: happy they!" (4:10–11). On the other hand, Byron makes it clear that instinct can prevail here only because of the lack of cultural restrictions on love and marriage: pastoral brackets their love, suffusing it with literary artifice. By figuring "another Eden," Byron ironizes instinct because it cannot refer to a tabula rasa of the body before culture. That tabula rasa bears the literary hand of pastoral. Although the poet localizes instinct in the heart, which itself could be a euphemism for the genitals, the fact that he radically enjambs the heart, and by extension instinct, breaking it into two stanzas, implies that instinct can only bear the residue of nature, not the imprint of nature itself. Like the heart, natural instinct is irretrievably broken by culture. Moreover, because instinct here also refers to sexuality before the fall of man, it is necessarily bound up with postlapsarian consciousness even at the moment of second origin. Because the patriarch of this Eden is a pirate, and not God, Byron saturates instinct with irony, and this makes instinct a locus of essence against itself.

When Don Juan masquerades as a female, Byron ironizes instinct once again.

Upon being inspected by Dudu, Juan "knelt down by instinct" as if to pray (5:95). Because Dudu recalls the Hindi word for milk, Juan is reduced to infantile sucking. Juan straddles sexual difference, a straddling that threatens to erase instinct, at the very moment when he is motivated by instinct, a figural juxtaposition that suggests nature must rub up against culture. In much the same way as Byron ironizes instinct, we find Shelley skeptical of the "supposed purposes" behind the sexual instinct (D. Clark 223). In sum, because Romantic artists and scientists understood instinct as operating between nature and culture, it provides the idea of locus rather than a means to local embodiment.

## Cuvier and the Rise of Function

Now that I have rehearsed some of the many complexities of localization, we are well equipped to understand why function became so important to the biological sciences in this period. While function had an important role in physiology before him, it was Georges Cuvier who made functional integrity of the organism the very basis for biological science. Cuvier was the first to raise harmony of structure and function to a general principle of biology (Russell 34). His lectures on *Comparative Anatomy*, translated into English in 1802, was organized by functional systems, and his system of classifying was built upon a hierarchy that was itself based upon the "subordination of functions" (Appel 41). Because Cuvier's functionalism lent an implicit support to the traditional argument for the existence of God, the argument from design, his works were enthusiastically received in Britain (Appel 41). This connection of function to the argument from design suggests that underlying the Romantic resistance to reproduction was a secular refutation of God's design, a refutation that brought Romantic sexuality even closer to Kantian purposiveness without purpose insofar as Kant's aesthetics made it possible to apprehend design even without a designer, intelligent or otherwise (Loesberg). Cuvier's systematic insertion of function into taxonomy helped to make nonfunctioning organs and beings oxymorons, or nonsense. Basing the "nature of each animal . . . on the relative energy of each of its functions" (*CA* 2:3), Cuvier furthermore helped make function coextensive with identity. When he insisted that deviations in one organ manifest themselves over multiple organs, Cuvier at once limited the range of deviations from the normal that were possible and made it difficult to link nonfunctional sexuality with identity since it had to have implications across organ systems. "For it is evident that a proper harmony among organs that act upon each other is a necessary condition of existence for the creature to which they belong," writes Cuvier (cited in Gould

294). By making harmony between properly functioning organs a "condition of existence," Cuvier thrust the pervert outside ontology. And when he argued that animals share basic plans because they carried out a similar combination of interrelated functions (Appel 45), he undermined the foundation of structuralist morphology, insisting that structural relations had less explanatory value over correlations between parts of an organism than function did (Gould 268). In Cuvier's hands, function acquired a kind of global explanatory power over structure, making it difficult to conceive of a perverted being.

When Toby Appel, a historian of science, argues that "there was no place in Cuvier's thinking for useless organs" (Appel 41), Appel has only begun to describe how Cuvier helped to make a biological concept of a perverted identity difficult to imagine. Having exiled the pervert from the realm of ontology, Cuvier goes so far as to bracket nonfunctionality outside of epistemology: "all other considerations to which an organ, whatever be its rank, may give rise, are of no importance, so long as they do not directly influence the function it exercises" (*CA* 1:64). From Cuvier's point of view, anything which did not speak to the function of an organ was not knowledge. Hence, he bracketed nonfunctionality or perversion outside of epistemology itself.

Cuvier already helps to make clear that, as function acquires increased explanatory power in the biological sciences of the nineteenth century, it becomes more difficult to understand functionlessness at all, and almost impossible to understand functionlessness outside of pathology. William Lawrence recounted how Blumenbach had labeled the tadpoles of the Surinam toad monsters because he could not comprehend the function of such a tail (*Lectures on Physiology* 46). Indeed, to the extent that life itself became understood as the sum total of functional processes in the body, the perverse became connected with death. Yet, as George Canguilhem reminds us, it was only when organs ceased to function or functioned badly that the relations of structure to function could be fully understood. Canguilhem sums this up by stating, "The scientific study of pathological cases becomes an indispensable phase in the overall search for the laws of the normal state" (51). In light of the fact that biological knowledge in the Romantic period was in fact beholden to the perverse, Cuvier's bracketing of perversion outside of epistemology threatened to undermine completely the foundations of that knowledge.

Cuvier further claimed that "all animal functions appear to reduce themselves [in the body] to the transformation of fluids" (*CA* 1:33). In so doing, he not only provided the means by which function could circulate influence over the entire body, but also once again undermined the claims of structuralist morphology by suggesting that structure was at odds with the liquefied essence of function. By manifesting function in the body as a liquid, Cuvier allowed for a kind of dynamic or vitalist materialism, one that might have no correspondence with physical organs. This absence of a clear physical embodiment of a correspondence between function and bodily organ meant that function might not be easily localizable in the body. This absence also meant that biological function was coming closer to the idea of purposiveness to the extent it was not directed to any specific aim but rather to a general behavior that does not appear aimless.[10] Cuvier's liquefied and vitalist function meant that localization was holistic and did not necessarily rely upon a one-to-one correspondence between structure and function. In fact, Cuvier's liquid function implies that there might be an insurmountable gap between organ and function, a gap that undermines the possibility of localization. The very notion of a liquefied function indicates the problems endemic to basing the emergence of sexuality upon a shift in localization of sex from anatomical parts to the instinct.

That Cuvier insisted upon an analogy between the functional role of each organ in the body to the role of each organism in the universe also meant that nonfunctioning organs had cosmic implications. "There are some [functions] which, in constituting animals what they are, fit them for fulfilling the part nature has assigned to them in the general management of the universe" (*CA* 1:18–19). Cuvier continues, "each animal may be considered a partial machine, co-operating with all the other machines, the whole of which form the universe" (*CA* 1:19). Perversion thus now had the potential to upset the order of the universe.

As we might expect, Coleridge soundly rejected Cuvier's emphasis on function, largely for its materialism. In Coleridge's view, Cuvier had been infected by his French upbringing and was so "modified by his habitat as to fall into the old sophisms of materialism respecting the Brain and c[.] as organs of Thought, in the sense that Thought is a function of the Brain" (*CN* 3:4357). Coleridge further mocks the reductiveness of functional accounts when he writes, "The heart is an organ of circulation, for what more natural than that a bilocular Hollow squeezed together should propel the fluid contained therein?—but is it therefore the Organ of the battle of Waterloo?" (ibid.). The virulence of Coleridge's attack can be explained in part by the fact that Cuvier's materialism and functionalism threatened the very notion of a stable identity or of human agency insofar as functioning organs seemed at the expense of free will (Richardson 2001 12).

Yet, even those biologists who opposed the rise of function lent little help to possibility of a perverse identity. This is in part because structuralist morphologists, those who insisted on the priority of form over function, did "not deny the evident utility of most organic structures" (Gould 268). They just believed that function did not have ontological priority over form. Edward Russell, a historian of science, frames the debate between Cuvier and the morphologists as the difference between asking is "form merely the manifestation of function" or is "function the mechanical result of form"? (2). The key point here is that neither side of the debate completely rejects function: notwithstanding the fact that the morphologists think that function can give rise to misleading analogies, they concede that form has something to do with function even as they deny function's principle explanatory power.

## Geoffroy: Let There Be Monsters

One of the main opponents to the priority of function over form was Cuvier's rival, Geoffroy St. Hilaire.[11] Geoffroy thought that functionalism not only debased the creator by ignoring the unity of design and the beauty of homologies, but also led to error. Working intensely with the bones of the shoulder girdle in fishes and finding a homolog to the wishbone in birds, Geoffroy showed that the functionalist belief in the existence of such bones for the purpose of flight was false (Gould 299). Geoffroy also argued that unity of plan precedes particular modifications to suit individual functional requirements (Appel 4). Nonetheless, even Geoffroy could not banish function from his morphologies because he could not explain structures abstractly without some recourse to function (Appel 203). Geoffroy was a trenchant defender of what he called transcendental anatomy (*anatomie transcendante*). Transcendental anatomy further shows the complexities of localization: by yoking together transcendence and the body, Geoffroy enabled the body to serve as metaphysical figure and corporeal ground. Geoffroy's concept of "principle of connections" pushed the body further in the direction of metaphysics, because it insisted that anatomical homologies had to be "identified by the relative position and spatial interrelationships of elements, rather than primarily by form" (Gould 300).

Cuvier responds to Geoffroy that morphology provides misleading information, since resemblances often only provide "external" information (CA 151). Yet even Cuvier acknowledges the explanatory power of morphology when he must explain why males have nipples. Nonfunctioning organs were generally lumped under the category of rudiments, "to exemplify the prevalence, in animal organization, of a mechanical principle, of the adherence to a certain original type or model" (Lawrence *Lectures on Physiology* 44). Cuvier writes, we "perceive a part, or vestige of a part, in animals where it is of no use, and where it seems left by nature, only that she might not transgress her general law of continuity" (*AE* 66). Whereas in theory Geoffroy's sense that the unity of plan and homologies were incommensurate with function opens the door to a perverted identity, in practice Geoffroy is careful to limit the kinds of deviations from that unity of plan that are possible. He demonstrates this most clearly in his theorizing of monstrosity. Indeed, Geoffroy was the very Frankenstein of monstrosity, going so far as to invent the science of it: teratology, but even Geoffroy's monsters can't be perverts, because they are still beholden to function even by its absence.

Until Blumenbach, monsters had been regarded as aberrations of nature (Appel 126). Blumenbach envisioned a formative force that regulated both the development and form of each class of animals, a force inseparable from matter but irreducible to it. By refusing to materialize this force, Blumenbach thus raised another barrier to localization insofar as there was now a gap between structure and the structuring force. Monstrosity was especially important to Blumenbach because it helped to show the variations of this formative force (Appel 270, note 85). Building upon Blumenbach's argument that monsters "were the results of modification of the normal forces of nature" (Appel 126), Geoffroy argued that monsters conform to laws of unity, morphology. Monsters, he insisted, were merely "preturbations in normal development" that occurred "when an accidental lesion modified the action of the nisus formatives (formative force)" (cited in Appel 127). Dismissing the popular notion that the female imagination was responsible for monstrosity because something had violently impressed itself upon the mother's imagination (*PA* 500–505), Geoffroy developed instead a theory that "amniotic adhesions" were the cause of monstrosity (Persaud 9) and argued that anomalies were merely "exceptions to the laws of naturalists, not to the laws of nature" (Canguilhem 1989 133). Because monsters were his most extreme category of anomalies—very complex ones "that make the performance of one or more of the functions impossible" (Canguilhem 1989 134)—Geoffroy's ability to align them within the laws of nature was no mean feat. His theory that monsters were due to "arrests of development" in otherwise normal organs enabled those retarded organs to "resemble to a greater or lesser degree, the form of the organ in an animal lower in the scale of being" (Appel 127). To the extent that those arrests corresponded to a place in the scale of beings, then, monstrosity did not upset God's unity of plan. Describing an ancephaletic child, Geoffroy insists, "however, this confusion has its limits: a certain order reigns even in this disorder" (*PA* 21; translation mine). The bases for his confidence in the triumph of order are the fact that "irregularities do not change the form" and that these irregularities "never change the relations between the parties" (*PA* 21). While Geoffroy took enormous pains to link anomalies with the laws of nature and not with the perverse, the problem he faced was that lapses of function were necessary to make anomalies register to consciousness. Despite his protests to the contrary, Geoffroy's taxonomy of anomalies and his science of monsters thus relies upon the perversion of function because the complexity of anomaly was gauged by the degree of functional disruption. Geoffroy's normalizing of monsters thus threatens to unravel the moment when his taxonomy of irregularities imposes its own order upon them.

For all of his interest in making even monsters testify to God's unity of plan, Geoffroy does allow for a perverted sexual identity when he invents a new psychological term, "heterotaxy," a term that describes modifications in the inner organization, that is, in the relations of the viscera without modification of the functions and external appearance (Canguilhem 1989 135). Geoffroy introduces the notion that something can have "harmful or disturbing influence on the exercise of functions," even when there is no material manifestation of that disturbing influence (Canguilhem 1989 134). Geoffroy's invention of a psychological anomaly, one that has no material trace, is part of a complex genealogy whereby sex circulates between sexual organs and sexual instinct. That functions are neither modified nor localizable, except to the ambiguous place called "inner organization," enables "heterotaxy" to anticipate the pervert.

## Neurology, Sexuality, and Localizing Sexual Function

Cuvier and Geoffroy have highlighted the complexities involved in localizing function in the body. If the great physiologist Albrecht von Haller's 1751 insistence that the penis and breast nipple were "sensible"—and therefore are processed by the brain/soul—made it possible to localize sexual desire in the brain, ever more detailed and lavish maps of the human brain in this period seemed to defy any necessary relationship of structure to function. Although the eminent neurologist Charles Bell believed fervently in the power of structure to declare function, when it came to the brain he had to deal with its relative amorphousness and lack of clear outlines, and he did so by preferring to illustrate the brain's clear vessels and cavities (Compston 45) and by dividing the brain into four brains (*New Idea* 17). The tenacious Cartesian legacy whereby the mind was not to be reduced to the brain raised even more problems for the idea of localization, as did the growing recognition of the multiple functions and interconnectedness of the brain. One way out of these difficulties was to conceive of the brain in terms of structuring principles like a sensorium commune (Figlio 180–83) or the imagination, with eighteenth-century roots in a localizable image-producing capacity of mind, rather than an actual structure. Of course, earlier mechanistic explanations of the imagination as a picture-producing structure had the distinct advantage of deferring location into the physical laws of the universe.

By endowing the imagination with the ability to create rather than re-arrange, the Romantics furthered localization as an idea rather than a place because they endeavored to accord imagination metaphysical powers. Localizing the sexual instinct in the brain thus situates sexuality at the crossroads between physical organ and metaphor, and localization itself threatens to degenerate into mere metaphor. This metaphoricity of the imagination was especially suggestive to the Romantics because late eighteenth-century medical accounts of the imagination generally sought to pathologize it, equating it with delusion, irrationality, and masturbation.[12] Again it is this shuttling back and forth between organ and something like instinct that allows sexuality to emerge. Part of the genealogy of the instinct was the structuring principles like the imagination that preceded it, principles that were physiological ideas that could remain unencumbered by local details.

Since a meticulous dissection of her body could reveal no anatomical irregularities, it was precisely the imagination that had to be taken to task in the infamous 1755 case of Catherine Vizzani, a woman who lusted after other women, going so far as to masquerade as a footman and to wear a leather dildo. Her case was translated by none other than John Cleland. Indeed, the imagination from a medical standpoint was a lightning rod for medical illnesses that could not otherwise be explained. Parr's *London Medical Dictionary*, for example, went so far as to localize "all the evils flesh is heir to" in the imagination (s.v. nervous fever 2:252). And, whereas in women, the mother's imagination was blamed for all sorts of peculiarities in infants (Parr s.v. imagination 2:7), in men the imagination was the primary culprit in impotence. "The imagination broods over fancied ills, till the whole system is disordered" (Parr s.v. impotence 2:8).

Vizzani took the name of Giovanni Bordoi, fell in love with a woman, and sought to marry her. The sister of Vizzani's lover, however, discovered the plans and threatened to tell the uncle if she was not taken to Rome with the couple. The uncle nonetheless discovers the plan to elope and has servants detain Vizzani at gunpoint. Not to be daunted because of her "masculine spirit and masculine desires" (34), Catherine brandishes a gun and is fatally wounded in the leg. Upon perceiving her recovery to be doubtful at the hospital, Vizzani then unfastened "a leather contrivance, of a cylindrical Figure, which was fastened below the abdomen, and had been the chief instrument of her detestable imposture" (36) but not before she secured promises that her sex would not be revealed until after her death. Upon her death, her body was taken to a surgeon, Giovanni Bianchi (1693–1775), professor of anatomy at Siena, who dissected her. Because her clitoris was found to be of a normal size, even slightly smaller than normal, and because her hymen was not yet imperforated, Bianchi could not localize her perverse desires in her anatomy. Bianchi went so far as to remove her parts of generation from her body and bring them to his house, where he noted that "the clitoris of this young woman was not pendulous, nor of any extraordinary size, as the Account from Rome made it, and as it is said to be that of all those females, who, among the Greeks, were called *tribades*, or who followed the practices of Sappho; on the contrary, hers was so far from any unusual magnitude, that it was not to be ranked among the middle-sized but the smaller" (43–44). Of particular note is the fact that, although Bianchi's title announces "anatomical remarks on the hymen," he is really more interested in her clitoris. His substitution of the hymen for the clitoris might be explained by the fact that gender mandates women's bodies to be the objects of male penetration: her intact hymen, however, testifies to the possibility that sexuality is not limited to penile penetration.

That Vizzani's body has no story to tell about her perverse desires, on the one hand, affords Bianchi considerable relief since he can now "acquit nature of any Fault in this strange creature" (54). On the other hand, the illegibility of this desire upon her body leads the surgeon to localize that desire in her perverse imagination: "It should seem, that this irregular and violent inclination by which this woman render'd herself infamous, must either proceed from some error in nature, or from some disorder or perversion in the imagination" (53). The imagination thus allows Bianchi to promise yet defer ocular proof of the legibility of perverse desire upon the body, to afford his audience a locus that is an idea, not an actual locus. At the same time, the fact that it is his imagination of her imagination that allows the imagination to embody perversion mandates that the surgeon Giovanni discover the truth behind the other Giovanni. Bianchi continues, "It seems therefore likely that this unfortunate and scandalous creature had her imagination corrupted early in her youth, either by obscene tales that were voluntarily told in her hearing, or by privately listening to the Discourse of the Women, who

are too generally corrupt in that Country. Her head being filled with vicious inclinations, perhaps before she received any incitements from her constitution,
might prompt her to those vile practices, which begun in folly, were continued
through wickedness; nor is it at all unreasonable to believe, that, by Degrees, this
might occasion a preternatural change in the animal spirits, and a s a kind of venereal furor, very remote, and even repugnant to that of her sex" (54). The failure
to find an anatomical explanation leads to blaming the imagination. The imagination, however, is itself corrupted by language, particularly the language of generally corrupt women. Once again the locus of perverse desires is found in language: first, in the structuring principle of the imagination, and then within the
corrupted words of women. I want also to note here that words matter so much
that they can change matter itself: the narrator proposes that even her animal spirits themselves have been altered as a result of hearing these women speak.

Cuvier himself was quite reticent on the functions of the human brain. In his
article on the human brain, he uncharacteristically dwells upon structure and dissection technique rather than function. This is especially curious in light of fact
that his treatment of the brain follows a section on the action and functions of the
nervous system. Cuvier argues that "it is a question of pure anatomy to know to
what point of the body the physical agents which occasion sensations must arrive"
(cited in Figlio 184). Conversely, when Cuvier acknowledges that habit and
imagination shape sexuality, he must turn to the imagination as a structuring
principle for sexuality in order to localize sexuality in the body. Cuvier writes,
"The susceptibility of the nervous system to be thus governed by the imagination, may be more varied than the capacity it possesses for receiving external impressions. The age, sex, and health of the individual; the manner in which a person has been educated, either with respect to his body or moral principles; the
empire which reason holds over his imagination, and the temporary state of his
mind, all produce in this respect astonishing differences; which may be compared
to those that disease, sleep, medicines, and may occasion in the susceptibility of
the nerves for external impressions" (*CA* 2:120). If "astonishing differences" is
some kind of code for perversion, then sexuality has been localized in the imagination. The question of course is where lies the imagination? "Astonishing differences" opens the door to perversion insofar as those differences can interfere
with the functions of the nerves. One can localize "astonishing differences" in the
imagination, but the locus turns out really to be within language, not the body.

In his important *Idea of a New Anatomy of the Brain* (1811), Charles Bell, anatomist and surgeon at Edinburgh, further illustrates the problems that arise once
the brain becomes the locus of sexual sensation. In fact, Bell makes it clear that

sexual pleasure has no necessary function at all insofar as he describes how a man with a phantom penis still experienced sexual excitement of the highest kind. Despite the fact that Bell privately printed only a hundred copies of this work, handing it to friends, he felt the need to record these observations in proper and more scientific Latin. Bell writes, "When a wound on the penis may destroy the glands and there remains nothing but a granulation at the extreme end where it terminates, the sensation of the nerves remains nevertheless and the gratification is the most exquisite of sensations" (11–12). Here, despite the fact that the organ of generation has become a mere "granulation" and thus cannot generate, the sensations of gratification are nonetheless exquisite. Bell adds that "When the nerve of a stump is touched, the pain is as if in the amputated extremity" (11). He would go on to annotate this passage, quoting D. J. Larrey's 1812 *Memoires de chirurgie militaire et campagnes*, which described a soldier who had a subluxation of the eleventh dorsal vertebra, and who was "itched, accompanied by an agreeable sensation which he felt in his genitals; afterwards he stretched out on his bed" (transcribed in Cranefield n.p.; translation mine). Here was a second example of sexual pleasure without function, and Bell felt the need to explain this away by commenting, "This certainly from a pressure or motion in the course of the nerve of the sexual sense" (ibid.). Bell returns to the phantom penis one more time in his annotations, noting once again in proper medical Latin, "When a sore eats up the glans of the penis, unless granulation should appear, at its extreme part, where the chaste tendon ends, sensation appears, and in that part one longs for sensations which are both vivid and exquisite (Cranefield, annotation to leaf 2 recto). What is remarkable about Bell's revision is that in the second instance, Bell is able to take some comfort in the diminishment of felt pleasure: the phantom penis now feels phantom pleasure. With the rise of functional imaging of the brain, whereby we now can see images of parts of the brain being activated while performing certain activities, we now have the technology to prove that sexual pleasure takes place in the brain.

Bell would go on to clarify that the locus of sensation itself was "in the brain more than in the external organ of sense" because, as the phantom penis made clear, "a peculiar sense exist[ed] without its external organ" (11). He further argued that, "if light, pressure, galvanism, or electricity produce vision, we must conclude that the idea in the mind is the result of an action excited in the eye or in the brain, not of anything received, though caused by an impression from without. Excitement is required from without, and an operation produced by the action of things external to rouse our faculties: But that once brought into activity, the organs can be put in exercise by the mind, and be made to minister to the memory and imagination" (12–13). I want to highlight here the terra infirma of localization: impressions are caused from without, without anything being received, but once the mind is activated, it can serve as its own origin. Bell's framing of sensation more in terms of a principle of causality than in terms of an actual clear cause suggests that Kant's purposiveness without purpose may be acquiring a physiology. How do we get from the impression to the idea if nothing is received? To add to all this tenuousness, Bell informs us that the "nerves have double root in cerebellum and cerebrum," mandating at least two origins to sensation (24). Bell concludes that "portions of the brain are distinct organs of different functions" (27).

Bell later contributed a *Bridgewater Treatise on the Power and Wisdom and Goodness of God as Manifested in the Creation,* focusing upon the hand (1833).[13] Although this essay would seem unequivocally to put to rest any possible skepticism about function and its connections to the divine, two features of this later essay are worth noting here. First, Bell takes pleasure completely out of the picture. If the earlier exquisite sensations of the phantom penis caused some doubt as to the function of sexual pleasure, Bell here insists that "pain is necessary to existence; pleasure is not so" (169). He elaborates, "Emotions purely of pleasure would lead to indolence, relaxation, and indifference. To what end should there be an apparatus to protect the eye, since pleasure could never move us to its exercise" (169). I suggest that the phantom penis haunts this later treatise in that Bell now refuses to acknowledge any function to pleasure generally. In fact, he makes pleasure itself perverse because it has no function. "Pain is the necessary contrast to pleasure: it ushers us into existence or consciousness. It alone is capable of exciting organs into activity. It is the companion and guardian of human life" (170). The cost of making pleasure itself perverse was a sadistic deity. One might ask what makes pleasure necessary at all, since it "necessarily" contrasts pain but does nothing. Second, when he returns to the question of phantom limbs, Bell now uses the presence of sensation after the actual limb has been amputated to prove the existence of "muscular sense, without which we could have no guidance of the frame" (199). If even absence can trigger sensation, pleasure can have no necessary function.

Perhaps the most important Romantic neurologist on the subject of the localization of sexual desire was Franz Joseph Gall, who famously argued that the cerebellum was "the organ of sexual love." Daniel N. Robinson in fact credits Gall's concept of "localization of function" with having created the discipline of physiological psychiatry (326). Gall secured his place in the history of neurology by proving the concept of contralateral function, the idea that each side of the brain controlled the opposite side of the body (Goodwin 66). He could do so in part because of his decision to remove brain structures from the brain stem up, rather than as commonly done at the time from the top down. He could thereby trace interconnections with a precision heretofore impossible.

Wordsworth and Coleridge's friend, Henry Crabb Robinson, produced the first major English exposition of Gall's work in 1807, and this later achieved wide diffusion when it was republished in Rees's *Cyclopedia* (Richardson 2001 36). Robinson takes great pains to highlight the fact that for Gall brain organs are the object of the will, and are not autonomous functioning organs. Robinson writes, "The idea of organ is that of an instrument by which a thing may be done, not that of an impulse which necessitates the action" (24), basing this assertion on Gall's insistence that an organ was merely "the material condition which renders the exercise of a faculty possible" (Gall 1835 1:198). Gall is especially key to my argument because despite his materialism and his proliferation of organs of mind, he is actually more interested in the idea of localization than in its actual anatomy (Young 27–28). Moreover, because Gall can only make his case that particular brain functions are localized into his twenty-seven invented organs on the basis of rhetorical figures such as analogy and correlation, not to mention a hypothetical correspondence between skull and underlying organ as well as an imputed causal connection between behavior and faculty (Young 33–36), material body instantaneously and insistently dissolves into rhetoric. This is notwithstanding Gall's own insistence that "nothing whatever in brain physiology has conflicted with an anatomical fact" (cited in Clarke and Jacyna 225). His associate Spurzheim would later expand those twenty-seven organs into thirty-five. If someone as obsessed with localization as Gall allows for so many gaps between the idea of localization and actual locus, then, a concept of sexuality so beholden to localization would seem to be especially resistant to a coherent "style of reasoning" (Davidson). The irony, of course, is that Davidson's notion of sexuality as a coherent style of reasoning is purchased at the expense of not thinking about the incoherence of localization.

Gall would eventually admit that "this beautiful idea of localization is then only a fine and presumptuous chimera," because parts of the brain are "very materially complicated, which renders any localization absolutely impossible" (Gall 1835 6:156, 158).[14] The fact that Gall separates the "organ of parental and filial love" from the "organ of sexual love" meant that sexual love may indeed be perverse, a problem further compounded by the fact that women had larger organs of parental and filial love than men whereas men had larger cerebellums. Thus, in the separate sexes, there was no necessary correlation between sexual desire and reproduction. Gall would later insist that sexual appetite was not a reliable predictor of fecundity (see Sha 2001 23). He would also insist that perverts did exist, though he carefully framed them as exceptions to "any general rule" of his phrenological system because, like libertines, they "artificially stimulate" their cerebellums (Gall *Manual* 157). Gall continues, there are "individuals who are tormented with a singular predilection for their own sex, whilst at the same time they entertain the strongest aversion to the other." He observes, "that men who are afflicted with this species of alienation, as Nero, for instance, have in general a small head, delicate features, dimpled hands, and developed breasts; whilst females, on the contrary, are masculine in appearance and manners" (Gall *Manual* 157–58). In much the same way as Cuvier brackets nonfunctionality outside of epistemology, Gall can only purify his phrenology at the expense of exiling the pervert from the realm of science, while simultaneously inverting the pervert.

We can find Gall's ambivalence about localization recurring in Freud, who in the *Interpretation of Dreams* "entirely disregarded the fact that the mental apparatus with which we are concerned, . . . is also known to us in the form of an anatomical preparation, and I shall carefully avoid the temptation to determine psychical locality in any anatomical fashion" (cited in Fancher 380). Nonetheless, the trace of anatomy was too tempting to reject completely: In *The Ego and the Id*, Freud argues that "consciousness is the superfices of the mental apparatus . . . the topographical terminology does not merely serve to describe the nature of the function, but actually corresponds to the anatomical facts. Our investigations too must take this surface organ of perception as a starting point" (20). While it is certainly true that Freud distrusted topography, noting that one must not take the "spatial or topographical conception of mental life too seriously" (20), my point here is that his study of the sexual instincts begins with the "starting point" of anatomical facts and remains haunted at very least by the idea of anatomical location. In fact, his treatment of the sexual instincts takes pains to "support" his "theoretical considerations . . . by biology" (55). When Freud defined the instincts in terms of "psychical localities" like the id and ego, he made it clear that the legacy of anatomical localization lived on even in psychoanalysis.[15] What were these localities if they had no basis in the human body? To wit, Freud must locate repression, cathexis, and instinct within the "deepest strata of the mental apparatus," even though he cannot specify an actual locus for them outside of language (24).[16]

Again and again we find Freud returning to the idea of anatomy if not the practice of it. Freud writes that percipient consciousness "forms its surface, more or less as the germinal layer rests upon the ovum" (28) and that the "ego wears an auditory lobe—on one side only, as we learn from cerebral anatomy" (29). And he initially searches for an "anatomical analogy" for the ego and finds one in the "cortical homunculus" of the anatomists (31), only to end up "localiz[ing] the ego" in a constitutionally bisexual body (48, 40). Thinking of the erotic instincts in terms of "special physiological process[es]," moreover, enables him to endow "every particle of living substance with Eros" (56). Like Gall before him, Freud uses the idea of anatomical localization when it is convenient, when it can materialize for him his concepts, and jettisons it the moment that it facilitates comprehension of his ideas.

I have shown how the Romantic period witnessed the rise of function in the biological sciences. I have also argued that the rise of function made it more difficult to conceive of a perverted identity. Yet, because localization relied upon tenuous connections between functions and structures, the gaps between structure and function and the increasing proliferation of organs of the mind are the places where we can look for the pervert. Cuvier implies that the absence of sexuality before sexology is a calculated absence as opposed to actual absence because science resisted perverted identity. The skepticisms and problems endemic to the localization of sexuality within the body that I have traced in Morgagni, Cuvier, Geoffroy, Bell, and Gall, however, suggest that sexuality was emerging long before Davidson allows it to have emerged. Davidson's claim that, before Victorianism, sex was anatomy and destiny prevents Romanticists from accounting for why Blake, Byron, and the Shelley's turned to sexuality as a site for thinking about liberation. Gall's "organ of sexual love," Bell's phantom penis, Geoffroy's monsters, and Cuvier's taxonomy based on function together anticipate the concept of physiologic localization, a locus that has no defined locus, whereby "loss of function occurs without structural damage to the neurons . . . as a result of the metabolic changes due to vascular insufficiency" (Waxman 33). I can only speculate that the turn to psychiatric identity as the container for sexuality in sexology was the logical outcome of a century of struggling to locate sexual function in the body and that this struggle forms a crucial if neglected chapter in the formation of heteronormativity. Finally, despite the Foucauldian argument that localization shifted from organs to instinct, an epistemic shift that is taken as evidence for the Victorian birth of sexuality, my reading of Freud shows the trace of anatomical localization, a trace that suggests a neglected continuity between Romantic sexuality and ours.

# CHAPTER THREE

# One Sex or Two?

Nervous Bodies, Romantic Puberty, and the Natural Origins
of Perverse Desires

I now turn from situating perversion in the Romantic period within the context
of the rise of function in the biological sciences. The growing importance of
function made it difficult to conceive of a perverted identity, and this transformation made the absence of the pervert a calculated absence. Thomas Laqueur's
claim that the Romantic period was one in which a two-sex model based on complementarity between the sexes begins to replace a one-sex model of hierarchy,
whereby the female was simply an inferior or inverted version of the male, has
important implications for this argument.[1] Not only does the instability of sex
allows writers such as Mary Wollstonecraft and Mary Robinson to drive a
wedge in between the two ways of thinking about sex and to use this gap to pry
apart sexual difference and political inequality, but also the relation between
sexual desire and sexed bodies in Romanticism was much more complex than either the gap between acts and identities or modern notions of sexual orientation
would have it.[2] Combined, the two models make it difficult for human beings to
turn to sex for coherence and intelligible identities and undermine any single
stable sexed norm against which one can measure perversion. Personal bodily
experience, moreover, resists co-optation into political systems, and this made
perversion especially rife for deployment.

The unrationalized coexistence of contradictory models of sex has key consequences for both the Romantic period and the concept of perversion.[3] Under the one-sex model, differences between the sexes are of degree, not kind. Under complementarity, differences are of kind, not degree. That difference hovers between kind and degree suggests that, far from being a given, the meanings based on sexual difference are open to debate. The very presence of a one-sex model mandated skepticism about complementarity. Two, to the extent that two incommensurate sexes are founded upon a one-sexed body, difference is erected upon the ground of similitude. Because the French Revolution made it possible to question any naturalized hierarchies, the one-sex model no longer could deliver hierarchy as nature; indeed, the revolutionary ideal of equality called into question fundamental notions of family organization and relations between the sexes (Offen 50).[4] Whereas the one-sex model used sex to represent gender, the two-sex model enabled sex to become the foundation for gender. In either case, the legacy of the one-sex theory meant that scientists still very commonly bridged the sexes and gender through analogy; the figure of analogy haunts sexual difference even when the sexes are understood as categorically different. Hence, Coleridge frames sexual difference in terms of "opposites & correspondences" (*SW* 1:286), a framing that explicitly places difference and similitude in dialogue with one another. It is thus not surprising that the Romantics reimagined social relations from the ground up. They had to. The two models of sex do not allow it to reach the critical mass of a stable essence.

It is unclear, moreover, under a model that recognized only one sex what homosexuality would mean. In this view, women were inverted men—men with genitals turned inward as opposed to outward.[5] How does the fact that inversion originates as a way to think about women's anatomical relation to men complicate the use of inversion as a way to make human sexual desire essentially heterosexual? That is, inversion now usually describes the way in which some forms of sexual deviance are conflated with gender deviance; a lesbian woman desires another because she is really a masculinized female. But if women are thought of as inverted men to begin with, how can one tell whether deviance resides in sex or in gender? Nor is it clear how inversion moved from a normative way of thinking about men and women as one sex to a dominant pathological model for framing homosexuality. Bearing the full legacy of the idea of inversion in mind, it would seem that homosexual inversion was indebted to heterosexual inversion and that the drive to explain sodomy or homosexuality in terms of gender inversion obscures an earlier sexual inversion. Rather than seeing a great paradigm shift from gender difference in the one-sex model to sexual difference in the two-sex model, we should be alert to how sex and gender work simultaneously to make difference and inferiority open to debate. Because sex and gender are confused from the outset, perversion has considerable leverage as a result of its incoherence.

Finally, the charge of perversion is only as strong as its rhetorical persuasiveness or its ability to manage incoherence. The key here is to mobilize features of identity (a taste for luxury, effeminacy, violations of certain gender norms) to make the charge of perversion stick. Until perversion sticks, acts will not cohere with identity and the idea of orientation becomes difficult to imagine. This incoherence nonetheless could be politically useful insofar as one could manipulate perversion to work for rather than against oneself.

The simultaneous presence of the one-sex and two-sex models further explains the complicated understanding of puberty in the period. In brief, in Romanticism scientists considered that there was only one feminized sex until the moment of puberty, whereas after puberty full sexual differentiation was achieved. One sex became two in puberty as males gained strength and departed from their original feminized bodies: sexual difference unfolds diachronically, and thus both sexes are grounded upon one. Genitals did not stand in for difference in the way they do now, and this meant that biological sex was more elastic and thus could become a ground for liberation. If one sex became two, difference itself became even more vexed. Hence the period's fascination with a common nervous system, hermaphrodites, and men and women who failed to develop properly. Together, these concerns made it necessary to both question whether difference could be grounded in the body and disrupt essentializing claims of sex and gender.

Although the fairly recent turn to gender in Romantic studies has had a profound impact upon Romantic criticism, we still have few nuanced reevaluations of how biological sex was understood in this period. If sex indeed hovered between essence and representation, it was rife for political deployment. On the one hand, the shift from representation to essence meant that one could challenge representation and question essence; on the other hand, one could turn to biology's newfound essence to ground political differences in the body. Such a reevaluation will help us to see why sex could become the basis for liberation and why perversions of the sexual appetite could be understood as natural. Two ways of reading sex not only pertain generally, but also within one single body there was a metamorphosis from one sex into two during puberty. This meant that the materiality of the body and of sex were quite elastic. The body could both endow Romantic idealism with consequence as well as negotiate those consequences within limits.

This point further refutes Arnold Davidson's claim that sex was exhausted by anatomy before the advent of psychology because such a claim blinds us to the complexities of sex and science in the Romantic period. That eighteenth-century physicians increasingly understood sex and its relation to the nerves and the nervous system, the organs of pleasure, made it impossible to conceive of sex as being exhausted by anatomy, because sexuality now encompassed the entire essentially nervous body, which in turn, under William Cullen's nosology, encompassed "almost the whole of the diseases of the human body" (1786 3:121). By making the basis for all diseases nervous disorders, Cullen and his followers "were, in effect, suspending judgment about their origins" (Oppenheim 8) because an anatomical basis for disease in the nerves had not yet been located. Thomas Trotter, the famous nerve doctor, boasted that "nothing could be discovered by the knife" (194). Nonetheless, his entire framework for understanding disease was grounded in the organs of pleasure. The brain further made anatomy seemingly inexhaustible; not even Gall and Spurzheim's new midline brain dissection techniques could reveal all of the brain's depths. The claim that sex could be exhausted by anatomy is belied by anatomy's ability to function as a black box; because one knew only the output but not the workings of the body, one could ground claims within a body without having to specify how exactly it worked.[6]

The fact that there was only one feminized sex before puberty and two complementary sexes afterward means that biological sex was fluid, developmental, and that anatomy itself was not a destiny but a process. Because puberty reminded the Romantics of the gap between anatomical part and desire, desire could neither be limited to the genitals nor be intrinsically heterosexual. After all, the presence of genitalia could not predict object choice. The shift from one sex to two during puberty meant that one could account for same-sex desire as a form of natural desire because during the window of puberty, one feminized male could certainly be attracted to or by another. Puberty allows for a universalizing narrative about perverse desires, rendering perversity proximate to the norm, even as it pathologizes that desire. Homophobia thereby acquires enormous leverage since sameness as well as difference lurks within. At the same time, those who never developed heterosexual desire could be explained in terms of arrested development, immaturity. This accounts for the proximity of effeminacy to sodomy in this period: all males begin as effeminate males and thus have sodomitic potential. Sodomy and effeminacy[7] are really sexual states that are supposed to remain suspended between childhood and adulthood, but it was the perversity of nature herself that was so traumatic for British medicine: the problem was that, because sex was a process and because everyone went through puberty, everyone was vulnerable to missteps on the way to heterosexuality. The Romantics can also remind us of the steep price we have paid to have sex subsume existence. As Arnold Davidson puts it, post-1869, existence has become "sexistence." That is, we have forgotten how sex is a complex biological process, one that resists the neat binary opposition between male and female. That women are the original inverts, too, suggests that homosexuality and heterosexuality have more common ground that usually acknowledged.

But there is more to this story. Like Jonathan Dollimore, I want to recover the lost histories of subversion within perversion.[8] The inextricability of perversion from nature meant that perversion was central to the maintenance of culture; moreover, because perversion—"turning the wrong way" (*OED*)—requires one stable ground of nature against which to measure the wrongness of the turn and because competing models of understanding sex meant that there was no such stability, perversion and political subversion were inseparable. Studying Romanticism through the lens of perversion, then, allows us to grasp the politics of Romanticism, how Romantic artists went after the nature of biological sex itself, not just culture. They could do so because sexual complementarity was open to debate, particularly because neurology sought to heal the Cartesian divide between mind and body and all bodies made the transition from one to two sexes. To put the case more forcefully, I argue that, without paying attention to the various perversions within the period, one cannot truly grasp the politics of Romanticism since writers such as Robinson, Blake, and the Shelleys knew that the battle had to be fought on the slippery ground of nature. Only our need to separate nature and culture so that one can be the enemy of the other has kept apart the common histories of perversion—turning the wrong way—and of subversion—turning upside down. I want, by contrast, to value both kinds of turning and to insist upon the etymological and historical connections between the two. Such revaluing of perversion will help restore a more radical Romanticism to our view.

## The Nervous Body and Sexual Difference

The Romantic period was dominated by a neurological understanding of the body. Neurology replaced a vascular approach to the body, one solidified by William Harvey's work on the circulation of the blood: Harvey's Romantic legacy is seen in the theory that the nerves were hollow and therefore worked like blood vessels, circulating fluids or animal spirits. This essentially neurological body, a body which stressed sympathy and consent between an increasingly vast and intricate system of neural networks, offered the possibility of bridging the Cartesian divide between mind and body, and connection potentially had enormous positive implications for gender. It also offered a republican model of body politics insofar as the nerves lack any clear unitary command center. No royalty needed apply. Even the brain was broken into separate organs. At very least, with its mind-body reciprocity, neurology undermined any absolute gap between male and female because men and women alike had both minds and bodies. Gall, we recall, considered sex a difference of degree, not kind. Without an absolute gap, the idea of complementarity between the sexes threatened to become a perverse fiction.

Whereas Thomas Laqueur rushes to connect neurology with a newly discovered difference between men's and women's genitals (*MS* 157), I explore the positive implications of neurology for gender because this science at least initially suggested that the differences between men and women—different genitals aside—were essentially differences of degree, not kind. That nervous diseases began as a sign of class distinction rather than as a mode of gender differentiation reminds us why neurology was and could be exploited for feminist causes. Although we tend to think of genital difference as an insurmountable difference, the Romantic period did not view it as such because it relied much more heavily on what we would call secondary sexual differentiation to police the borders between the sexes. Common ground between the sexes or sex meant that sexual equality could take on a life of its own.

It is because neurology had the potential to emphasize an essential similarity of men and women that so many doctors and scientists would later start to look for and emphasize differences. Difference grows out of commonness. Indeed, alienists themselves eventually began to locate female weakness in the lack of tonic vigor or delicacy in women's nerves, or in the fact that women menstruated and therefore were weakened by the loss of blood. Furthermore, craniologists later tried to prove that women had smaller brains. Yet, because so many earlier medical writers on nerves linked weakened nerves to such ubiquitous causes as urbanization, weather, climate, a sedentary lifestyle, heightened sensibility, a taste for luxuries, an addiction to pleasure, and too much thinking, many of the gendered distinctions between male and female nervous systems were the product of culture, not nature, and this meant that later gendered distinctions could be undone.[9] Both Wollstonecraft and Robinson were alert to how urbanization, luxury, and a sedentary lifestyle could disfigure the nervous systems of men and women alike.

Neurology's potential to break down and not reify gender distinctions can be seen even in works that ostensibly support them. Peter Logan's perceptive comment that "although the predisposition [to nervous diseases] is hidden, those conditions that create it are accessible to the physician" (22) is helpful to understanding why. Although predispositions can be grounded in nature, the problem is that the nerves are not yet localizable anatomical signs of disease: the differences between diseased nerves and healthy ones were invisible. For this reason, physicians of the time emphasize conditions, hoping that visible conditions can substitute for the body's invisible nervous ground. To emphasize conditions, of course, is to make culture the ground of biology, even if one admits some connection between condition and predisposition. Once again, the ontology of perversion hovers between nature and culture, not to mention between male and female, and paying attention to it helps identify the gaps between them. These gaps could be and were exploited to further the cause of equality, even gender equality. Logan underestimates the implications of the fact that Trotter's predispositions are both hereditary and acquired. If both men and women acquire the disease, women are not essentially the only sex predisposed to disease.

Because we now tend simply to accept the feminization of nervous diseases, I will now offer numerous examples to make my case that nerves did not necessarily contribute to the idea of sexual complementarity. George Cheyne's *English Malady* ([1784] first published in 1733) aligned nervous diseases with England's wealth and trade, which gave the English an unfortunate taste for "French cookery" and "Eastern pickles and sauces" (51). Neither sex was immune to luxury, and all the English of a certain class were predisposed to nervous diseases. Cheyne shrewdly claimed that the only classes he could not reach were the "unthinking" and the "voluptuous" (xii). With the exception of diseases of men of genius and men of gluttony, John Hill's *The Construction of the Nerves, and Causes of Nervous Disorders* (1758) allows nerves to speak to a common humanity that transcends gender. That nervous diseases "attended with an over exquisite sensibility" (37) do not yet refer to women, points to the fact that neurologists were not necessary hell-bent on refining sexual difference. The famous Swiss doctor Samuel Tissot, moreover, emphasized in his *Three Essays* (1773) that all people of rank were disposed to nervous disorders. Even when he discussed women's nerves specifically, he placed equal emphasis on the social and biological causes of women's nervous illnesses. On the one hand, miscarriages, difficult labors, and the overflow of milk weakened women's nerves. On the other hand, "high life" explained the violent, irregular, and "white menstruations" of the upper classes (57). Tissot implies that, at least until pregnancy, there is simply no biological basis for women's essential nervousness and that luxury had a larger role in shaping the nerves than did gender.

Like Cheyne and Tissot, the Methodist preacher John Wesley singled out neither gender in his *Primitive Physic* (1820), recommending the medical use of electricity, good air, thyme tea, a diet sparing of vegetables, and cold bathing as remedies for nervous diseases (61). And T. M. Caton, surgeon, argued in 1815 that even women's "hysterical diseases" were "attributable to their abstraction from active pursuits [rather] than [to] any organic delicacy of structure" (25). Although Caton does accept the necessary restriction upon the range of women's actions (38), he laments the fact that the absence of activity in women leads their minds to "doubt [their] own resources, [and] becom[e] the slave of every imaginary phantom that moves around it" (38), so he attributes hysteria not to any "organic delicacy of structure" but to cultural notions that make it necessary for women to be inactive. Grounded in neither a wandering uterus nor in the nerves themselves, hysteria has become a disease of acculturation, and the danger is that both sexes might fall victim to it. In fact, men had their own special brand of hysteria, hypochondria.

A close look at works on nervous disease like Tissot's or Caton's reminds us that the connections between weak nerves and femininity are more tenuous and more complex than we tend to remember. William Cullen, an extremely influential medical teacher of the period, in his *Treatise of the Materia Medica* (1789), also argued that strength of body depends on the state of the nervous system (1:76) and that this force depends upon the "force with which the energy of the brain can be exerted" (1:77). Cullen here anchors strength in something as tenuously gendered as the force of brain energy. In 1788, Joseph Johnson published John Brown's *Elements of Medicine*, a work which became the talk of the town (Todd 131). *Elements of Medicine* sought to synergize body and mind and ascribed debility to a sedentary middle-class lifestyle, not to women's nerves (Todd 131–32).[10] In 1796, Sayer Walker published *A Treatise on Nervous Diseases*, in which he, on the one hand, claimed that women's delicacy and habits made them especially vulnerable to nervous diseases (91). On the other hand, "those of the other sex, who approach the nearest to the temperament of females, are the most liable to them [nervous diseases]," thus allowing the nerves to blur the lines between sexual difference rather than refine them (92). If "other sex" walls one sex off from the other, males "with female temperaments" blurs the categories. More to the point, Walker rehearses the medical commonplace that menstruation caused nervousness only to reverse cause and effect. He argues, by contrast, that irregular menstruation is the effect of nervousness, not its cause, and this important reversal makes gender ancillary to nervous diseases rather than an explanation for it. He then proceeds to connect nervous diseases with both sexes and with every class of life. "These diseases," he writes, "are not the exclusive evil of the rich: they visit the cottage as well as the mansion" (96). Who could blame him? And why should a medical man restrict his pool of patients to only one sex or class?

Some doubt concerning the validity of complementarity crops up even in Trotter's *View of the Nervous Temperament* (1807), a work usually construed as hardening differences. Trotter is one of the authors Percy Shelley requests Thomas Hookham to send (Ruston 88). Although Peter Logan insists that in Trotter "the nervous temperament is thus indivisible from the female body" (24), Trotter's complicated etiology of nervousness—heredity, poor air, a lack of exercise, rich food, inappropriate cloathing [sic], novel reading, a passion for drugs, passions of mind, climate, medicine, and a general effeminacy of custom (151)—unravels the already tenuous connections between the female body and this disease. Thus, Trotter lists "literary men" and "men of business" as the top two classes of urban inhabitants who will likely fall prey to nervous illness (37), whereas the female sex is confined to the seventh and last class. And while Logan claims that the "nervous temperament forms a constituent part of Trotter's gender construct" because of women's more delicate nerves (24), the fact that Trotter dwells on the societal conditions that make men and women delicate blurs the line between predisposition and condition. Thus, women's essential nervousness, not to mention Logan's claim that they are given narratives where the bodies of healthy men are not, seem like fictions. True, Trotter does state that the female body is "furnished by nature with peculiar delicacy and feeling" (51) and that "the diseases of which we now treat are in a manner the inheritance of the fair sex" (51–52). But his phrase "in a manner" points to how "inheritance" is really a figure of speech, not a biological marker. His emphasis throughout on environment threatens to overwhelm any innate predisposition. Logan further presumes a necessary gap between male and female bodies—female bodies can only constitute nervous disease to the extent that male bodies and female bodies can be separated—a gap that nervousness forecloses with its emphasis upon "degrees of delicacy" (Trotter 49) as opposed to kinds. With the rise of nervous diseases came a resurgence of the one-sex model.

Trotter would later explicitly describe some predispositions as hereditary and others as acquired (166–75). The predispositions of "literary men" certainly show these confusions, confusions that once again undermine any essential connection between women's bodies and nervousness. "Literary men's" bodies constitute disease as much as women's bodies. Because of sedentary lives, literary men's lungs lose their vigor. Trotter thereby sought to explain why literary men were predisposed for consumption (38). He elaborates, "All men who possess genius, and those mental qualifications which prompt them to literary attainments and pursuits are endued by nature with more than the usual sensibility of the nervous system" (39). If some men have greater sensibility, why must women have sole purchase on delicacy and nervous weakness? Hence, he extends the category "literary men" to include "all the learned professions; and all those who cultivate the fine arts" (40). That Trotter goes after lower-class wet nurses who infect others with nervous weakness through their milk (96, 172–74) supports Logan's argument that nervous temperament was a female contagion. At the same time, however, it raises the issue of class as contagion. "Few mothers, among the decent orders of women, can be supposed to leave their offspring without regret" (95), he admonishes. Due to the general decline of physical labor, everyone was open to nervous disease. Because men were thought to be able to lose their manhood through excessive devotion to pleasure, or "unlawful pleasure," and because the specter of male impotence loomed large in this period, even healthy men had narratives to tell.[11] When Trotter mentions that "persons returned from the colonies . . . bring with them to Britain, indelible marks of the effect of the [hot] climates they have lived in" (48), he makes colonization as well potentially a constitutive factor in nervous disease.

Especially because of its emphasis on sympathy and consent, neurology had the potential to heal the rift between body and mind—a rift that metonymically rehearses the differences between the sexes—and writers such as Wollstonecraft and Robinson took advantage of this potential. Tissot insisted that "so close is the connection between mind and body, that we cannot well conceive the operations of the one independent of some correspondence with the other" (*Essay* 2, 13). In his *Nervous System of the Human Body*, the influential neurologist Charles Bell emphasized that "[bodily] sensation and [mental] volition are combined in every action of the frame" and that these actions are "conjoined" and "in union" (239). If the body could not be sundered from the mind, how could the mind be gendered as masculine and the body remain feminine? Hence, Mary Robinson pointedly asks, "Is woman not a human being, gifted with all the feelings that inhabit the bosom of man? Has not woman affections, susceptibility, fortitude, and an acute sense of injuries received?" (8). Of course, the very integration of mind and body had its price: as Alan Richardson argues, integration could undermine the stability of the self, which changed with changes in the body and its brain (2001 22).

This fundamentally neurological understanding of the body, one that insisted upon a mind/brain reciprocity, helps explain how both Mary Wollstonecraft in the *Vindications of the Rights of Woman* (1792) and Mary Robinson in *A Letter to the Women of England* (1799) could redefine strength from mere physical strength to a kind of strength that was both bodily and mental.[12] Wollstonecraft asked whether men really did have both superior mental and bodily strength.[13] Because superior masculine bodily strength was the very basis for the social contract, the stakes of this redefinition were the ground of patriarchy itself. By redefining the constitution of the female body in terms of intelligence, she seeks to redefine the British Constitution, which is "founded on the nature of man" (92). Wollstonecraft's pun on "constitution" reminds us that the English have no written document even as it makes the political stakes of her notions of the female nervous body clear. If one constitution is the ground for the other, female mental strength demands full political participation, full citizenship.

Whereas feminist critics like Janet Todd have argued that Wollstonecraft underestimated the power of complementarity and "physical difference" (186), I argue that she contested the ground of physical difference and that she did so partly because neurology had the potential to undermine sexual difference. Perversion requires a stable grounding of nature and thus, unsurprisingly, sexologists would later confine sexual desire to identity. More to the point, because complementarity was itself in flux in the period, Wollstonecraft cannot logically be seen as "underestimating" it. She likely was impressed by Brown's work (Todd 132) because it undermined sexual complementarity. Neurology so cemented the connectedness of body and mind that Wollstonecraft's redefinition of strength seems perfectly logical. Wollstonecraft in fact reminded her readers of the "nerveless limbs" of royalty (96), precisely to delegitimize their right to rule. In much the same way as pleasure made kings effeminate, society acculturates women to be weak and slaves to pleasure. Wollstonecraft thus takes advantage of the nascent illegitimacy of royal absolute authority to bolster her arguments against female subordination. As society had wrongly given too much power to royalty and made them weak, it now subjects women, making them useless. Her insistent parallel between the plight of women and royalty further implies that just as royalty must "return to nature and equality" (103), so too must women be made equal.

Not wanting to appear to be arguing for the "invert[ed] order of things" (109), Wollstonecraft grants that "from the constitution of their bodies, men seemed to be designed by Providence to attain a greater degree of virtue" (109). She looks as if she accepts as fact that "nature has given women a weaker frame than man" (112). "Virtue," with its etymological links to manly strength, grounds itself in nerves. Her choice of "seems," however, hints that appearances aside, Wollstonecraft wants to redefine the ground of difference. That "virtue" had already begun to slide into a female province of morality begins to contest the connections of gender to the sexed body. So too does her choice of "degree," which insinuates the falsity of complementarity. She again emphasizes "seems" when she claims, "I will allow that bodily strength seems to give man a natural superiority over woman; and this is the only solid basis on which the superiority of the sex can be built" (124). To the extent that solidity is based on appearance, male strength becomes a Lacanian lack.

If Wollstonecraft gives with one hand, she takes away with the other. Her seeming concession to superior masculine physical strength is undermined by the fact that she wonders what will happen to women's bodies if they are permitted exercise. The "most perfect education," Wollstonecraft opines, "is best calculated to strengthen the body and form the heart" (103). More to the point, she urges that mothers and wives be "allowed [their] constitution[s] to retain [their] natural strength" and "her nerves a healthy tone" (112). By underscoring a causal connection between mental weakness and bodily weakness—"dependence of body naturally produces dependence of mind" (130)—she insinuates that if women are mentally inferior, they were made so by men. Immediately following her alleged concession to superior male physical strength, she writes, "but I still insist that not only the virtue but the knowledge of the two sexes should be the same in nature, if not in degree, and that women, considered not only as moral but rational creatures, ought to endeavour to acquire human virtues (or perfections) by the same means as men" (124). Her insistence that virtue and knowledge "should be the same in nature" begins to redefine sexual difference in terms of degree, not kind. Because complementarity demanded that sexual difference be a difference of kind and not degree, this redefinition must be seen as a challenge to the idea of complementarity, not an underestimation of it. To wit, she insists on *human* virtues and introduces the category of knowledge precisely to suggest that virtue is epistemological not ontological. Thus, she lumps together soldiers and women so that she can ask, "Where is then the sexual difference, when the education has been the same" (105)? The only difference she can "discern" stems from the greater liberty afforded to soldiers (106).

Her concession seems even less of one when she speculates "how much superior mental is to bodily strength" (133). She also wonders, "Should it be proved that woman is naturally weaker than man" (127). She not only doubts his superior physical strength, but also never concedes superior masculine mental strength.[14] Quite the contrary; in fact, she lambastes men for denying women the possibility of "genius and judgment" (141–42).

Once she has unsexed strength, she sets her sights against the gendering of spirit itself as masculine: "I have been led to imagine that the few extraordinary women who have rushed in eccentrical directions out of the orbit prescribed to their sex, were *male* spirits, confined by mistake in female frames" (119). "Spirit" here obliquely refers to the animal spirits, the agents of nervous action. Where some neurologists had emphasized an essentially spermatic economy, whereby there was a homology between the penis and brain, Wollstonecraft sunders any natural or necessary connection between spirit, intellect, and masculinity.[15] Her astronomical metaphor reminds us that "eccentric" can only be gauged by where one locates the proper center. (The *OED* highlights the fact that eccentricity shifts as Ptolemaic gives way to Copernican astronomy.) Moreover, her use of "prescribed" hints at her skepticism at this outdated astronomical view of the world where men are the center and women must orbit around them. This implication is made more explicit when she points out that men fail to see "intellectual beauty" in women, because they want to gratify their libidinal appetites (134). Perhaps Percy Shelley's "Hymn to Intellectual Beauty" has its origins in Wollstonecraft, his mother-in-law, a source that enables him to refute Plato's claim that only men can embody intellectual beauty. Not lost on Wollstonecraft is the fact that male lasciviousness and devotion to pleasure actually weakens them physically, a theory that she would have gleaned from nerve doctors of the time. Adding insult to injury, where fathers have the luxury of "forgetting" the "purpose for which . . . the call of appetite was implanted" (6), women have no such luxury. Nonetheless, whatever superior strength men may have had is now merely an illusion: "thanks to debauchery, [men are] scarcely men in their outward form" (104).[16] Women, by contrast, are "more chaste than men" (231), so they will not be so disfigured. Although "more chaste" would seem to push Wollstonecraft into sexual complementarity, it is a statement of difference in terms of degree rather than kind.

Wollstonecraft's enemy is not the nervous body, but rather the cultural construction of women's bodies in terms of nervous sensibility.[17] For Wollstonecraft, female nerves are not ontologically different than men's. In fact, she makes it clear that, "whilst boys frolic in the open air, women are made sedentary and this "weakens the muscles and relaxes the nerves" (128). She implores that women be allowed to maintain their nerves in a healthy tone (112). Simply changing the ways in which girls are raised will begin to change any seemingly inherent differences of sex. Hence, women do not have weaker nerves; rather, their nerves are insistently "enervated" by a lack of exercise, pleasure (156), luxury and sloth (131), education (219), voluptuousness (249), and false notions of modesty and confinement (105), and female sensibility. "Wealth enervates men" too, she reminds us (253). When she refers to the "enervating indulgences" of luxury (130), she demonstrates that she has absorbed the teachings of such nerve experts as Brown and Tissot. Her preference for the verbal form—enervate—rather than the noun, nerves, deftly transforms any biological ground into cultural process. As she writes, "That woman is naturally weak *or* degraded by a circumstances," her "or" becomes the pivot around which biology slides into culture (141; emphasis mine). And hence she repeatedly unhooks sensibility from any biological basis and makes it clear what men have to gain from encouraging sensibility as women's highest ambition. As she says about Dr. Gregory's advice to daughters, "it is not natural; but arises . . . from a love of power" (111). Her skepticism about the biological bases of feminine sensibility is all the more remarkable because she herself was subject to nervous spasms, and as a governess, saw her employer's physician to treat them (see Todd 100). Yet perhaps this skepticism is what would lead her to implore that "women might certainly study the art of healing and be physicians as well as nurses. And midwi[ves]" (261).

In the end, Wollstonecraft is not content to harness the nerves in order to undermine the notion of sexual complementarity. She will settle for nothing less than overturning what Rousseau called the "perverseness and ill nature of women" (cited in *VRW* 180), arguing implicitly that male encouragement of female sensibility is the true origin of the perverse. Where Rousseau means to pathologize an unobliging wife by noting her "perverseness," the author of the *Vindications* insists that it is Rousseau who has "debauched his imagination" (189). His licentiousness has made him the pervert, an effeminate male. "Nature never dictated such insincerity," she wryly retorts. Hence, she remarks that "the patient endurance of injustice" will result in the "inability to judge right from wrong" (180). Having dispatched Rousseau, and having also insinuated that heterosexual passion is "corrupt beyond recovery,"[18] Wollstonecraft takes on the "perversity of self love" of parental affection (264), maintaining that such affection is really an excuse for tyranny. But perhaps her real coup de grace occurs when she comments that an "unhappy marriage is often very advantageous to a family, and that the neglected wife is, in general, the best mother" (114). At once undermining the sacredness of the middle-class family and the idea that motherhood is compatible with being a wife, Wollstonecraft places adulterous sex right in the heart of the middle-class family. She also blames male licentiousness for it and then perversely insists that it makes women better mothers.

Wollstonecraft considers the extent to which motherhood can be compatible with being a wife, and this line of questioning has potentially devastating implications for normative notions of the family and the denial of women's political citizenship. Both roles are based on biological sex, yet, whereas wifehood could be and was used to deny women citizenship, motherhood "offered an incontrovertible basis for claiming the right to intervene in public affairs" (Offen 60). This split between women's supposed natural roles revealed an incoherence in notions of sex; this incoherence was starting to be addressed in France during the early years of the Revolution, when unwed mothers were no longer to be shamed and divorce was to be easily and sensibly arranged (Tomalin 168).[19] It is therefore not surprising that Wollstonecraft splits the two roles, insisting instead that friendship between the sexes provides a firmer basis for societal happiness. Wollstonecraft's reading of parental love as tyranny further threatens the norm with the taint of the perverse. In the same way she calls attention to how one cannot gauge eccentricity without thinking about what counts as the center, Wollstonecraft takes advantage of the shifting ground of nature to reorient perversion/normalcy so that men are using sensibility to pervert women into their objects of lust. Her tendency to triangulate desire between two women and one man in her novels, moreover, allows her to elevate "purposive, kindred affection between two mothers" over the crude purpose of reproduction (Johnson "Radical Maternity" 170). When she lists female geniuses who have had a masculine education and includes such women as Sappho, famous for loving other women, along with Madame d'Eon, a male-to-female transvestite (*VRW* 172), we can see more fully how she equates genius with sexual and gender deviance (perversion) and thereby argues that one must contest societal notions of sex and gender when they operate to the detriment of women.[20]

In much the same way as her mother sought to undermine the legitimacy of patriarchy through the nerves, Mary Shelley shows in *Frankenstein* that, claims to superior male strength aside, Victor not only succumbs to nervous disease, but also uses his newfound victimhood to excuse his inaction. Just at the nerve doctor Thomas Trotter predicted, Victor begins to suffer from nervousness the moment he concentrates on thought, the discovery of the animating principle of life. "Every night I was oppressed by a slow fever, and I became nervous to a most painful degree; <a disease that I regretted the more because I hitherto had enjoyed most excellent health, and had always boasted of my firmness of nerves.>" (Rieger 51). Too much focus on a single pursuit leads Frankenstein to lose all other "soul or sensation" (50), so much so that once firm and manly nerves soften into girlishness. "I became as timid as a love-sick girl" (51), Victor confesses. When confined to a Scottish hut so that he can make a female monster, Victor again becomes "nervous" (162). Nervous fevers strip his powers of invention, activity, and even language, reducing Victor to victim. He sees himself in terms of a conventional passive and silent woman. Fear that he will be perceived as mad or hysterical enables him to justify doing nothing, as when he explains his silence at the trial of Justine. On seeing Elizabeth's lifeless body, he faints (193). Nervous sensibility not only feminizes men, but also turns what sensitivity they have completely inward as when Victor hears the monster's threat that he will be with him on his wedding night. Despite the monster's pattern to the contrary, Victor interprets this to mean a threat to his own life. Even worse, he sends Elizabeth to bed and, ultimately, to her death because he imagines the future impact that his combat with the monster will have on her (192).

Unlike Victor who "wishe[s] to fly from reflection" (64), Shelley herself turned to "literary labor and the improvement of my mind," as a cure from nervous depression. Thinking was not the cause of her disease but rather its incipient cure (*Journals* 431). And although Victor sees himself as a girl, Shelley insists that the girls in the novel are far more capable than Victor. Whereas he is rendered mute at Justine's trial, Justine offers what defense she can of herself. And whereas Victor sheds tears at the prospect of his own death, Elizabeth's last thoughts are about him. "What is it that agitates you, my dear Victor?" she inquires (192).

Like Mary Wollstonecraft and Mary Shelley, Mary Robinson too concedes that "in some instances, but not always," women are inferior in "corporeal strength" (17).[21] Indeed, Robinson invokes the "genius" of Wollstonecraft in her opening pages (2). Also like Wollstonecraft, Robinson refuses to cede any superiority of mental strength because "in activity of mind, she is his equal" (17). If the former insisted that the mind has no sex, the latter argued that the "immortality of the soul springs from causes that are not merely sexual" (15). Alluding to the common nervous system in both sexes, Robinson points to "a resisting nerve in the heart of both man and woman, which repels compulsion" (70).[22] It is this "resisting nerve" linking body and mind that "will establish her claims to the participation of power, mentally and corporeally" (2). Moreover, it is "custom" that has "decreed her passive," not nature (8).

Warning, however, that one cannot "pretend to estimate mental by corporeal powers," Robinson argues that "if strength or weakness are not allowed to originate in the faculty of thought, Charles Fox, or William Pitt, labouring under the debilitating ravages of a fever, is a weaker animal than the thrice-essenced poppinjay" (54). Robinson could not have chosen better examples: Fox was known as a libertine and thus was—and Tissot, Cullen, Brown, and Wollstonecraft among others would insist—weakened by his love of pleasure, and Pitt, because "he never married or had affairs," was considered by many to be a sodomite (A. Clark *Scandal* 72). Her choice of "poppinjay"—uniting "poppin," a word that refers to a pretty little woman or doll, and "jay," which can suggest a "showy or flashy woman" (*OED*)—thus twice insinuates that, fever or no fever, Fox and Pitt, are really the effeminate "shadows of mankind."[23] Noteworthy too is the fact that Robinson transforms the noun "essence" into an adjectival verb, a syntactical disfiguration that mirrors their sexual disfiguration. That the "Lord of the Creation" was now whittled down to a "puny frame" because of luxury enables her to mock the necessary obedience of women to men, who were now mere "shadows of mankind who exhibit the effeminacy of women" (17–18). As did Wollstonecraft, Robinson recognizes that nervous debility worked against men and the fact that both the manly libertine and the effeminate sodomite were now really only shadows meant that male strength was a chimera. How could there be real male strength if the gamut from the gallant Fox to the sodomitic Pitt led to the same puniness? Robinson's ability to collapse gallantry—conspicuous male heterosexuality effeminized by pleasure—with sodomy was a legacy of a one-sex model that envisioned women as an inferior version of a man.

Yet Robinson will have her cake and eat it, too. On the one hand, she uses a common nervous body to undermine complementarity from within. She thus asks if it is just that a woman strong in "all the powers of the intellect" must be the "obedient slave" of a weaker man (4). This slavery means that she will be "perverted, and debased, by such a help-mate" (4). For Robinson and Wollstonecraft, the seemingly natural argument of woman's weakness was the true perversion of nature, since it valued physical over mental strength, and since it altered women's very bodies for the worse. She also asks whether vice can have a sex (10), only to reply that, "till the passions of the mind in man and woman are separate and distinct, till the sex of vital animation, denominated soul, be ascertained, on what pretext is woman deprived of those amusements which man is permitted to enjoy?" (10). Here she insists that the nervous body has no sex insofar as the nerves are the seat of vital animation, and the passions of the mind must be connected to the body by that common nervous system.

On the other hand, Robinson ascribes to women a superior sensibility: "she is by nature organized to feel every wrong more" (8). And when Robinson insists that "the passions of men originate in sensuality; those of women, in sentiment: man loves corporeally, women mentally: which is the nobler creature?" (10), she thereby endows men with sex (their sexual desire does not transcend mere bodily desire or anatomy) and women with sexuality (sex as personality and taste, and therefore part of the mind). Given neurology's emphasis on the reciprocity between body and mind, she implies that men are perverting sex by limiting its influence to the body.

Whereas Wollstonecraft tries to level the distinctions between men and women, pointing out that sensibility falsely makes women into the complement of the man, Robinson suggests that women have a kind of fortitude that men will never have. She argues, as we have seen, that while men are unsexed by luxury, "education cannot unsex a woman" (55). And she displays her own fortitude when she makes Madame Du Barry and Marie Antoinette heroes for their "Spartan fortitude," "genuine strength of soul," and "sublime effort of heroism" (27). Refuting Burke's rendering of Marie Antoinette into a victim of French revolutionary violence—and thus the poster girl for the return of male chivalry—Robinson urges instead that we "let the strength of her mind, [and] the intrepidity of her soul, put to shame the vaunted superiority of man" (27).[24] Robinson's concluding list of "British Female Literary Characters Living in the Eighteenth Century" made it clear that women artists like Macaulay, More, Hays, painter in miniatures, Cosway, and the sculptor Damer were gaining considerable strength: with it, she hoped to "silence the tongue of prejudice" and to "excite emulation" (96).

## Wandering Testicles: Castration, Eunuchs, and the Descent of the Testicle

I have highlighted how neurology could be used to further feminist causes because it potentially undermined the ground of sexual complementarity even from within. This undermining of complementarity worked insofar as it could persuade readers that sensibility was itself a perversion of nature because it emphasized differences between men and women rather than a common ground. I now turn to the enormous medical fascination with castration, eunuchs, and the descent of the testicle. I do so because they too paradoxically chip away at the notion of absolute difference between two incommensurate sexes by showing bodily sex to be either unstable or a mobile essence. This mobility allowed perversion to be in the eye of the beholder. In the Romantic period, it was not so much the wandering uterus that was the object of medical attention (the wandering uterus was no longer understood to be the given ground of hysteria), but it was the wandering testicle. In addition, the popular medical belief that unused sperm was absorbed back into the body and was necessary to maintain the outward signs of masculinity (beard, strength) meant that sex itself was far from a stable essence: the problem was that men especially could lose their sex. Far from being a fixed essence, then, sex could be harnessed to liberating and repressive ends.

Surgery manuals in the Romantic period regularly described the operation of castration, implying that castration was quite common. The fact that castration was sometimes applicable to both men and women further indicates the lasting power of the one-sex model, even as castration itself returned men to their original feminized bodies. Coleridge, for instance, in his review of two books on uterine disorders casually mentions "the castration of women," meaning the extirpation of their ovaries, but he crossed out this phrase, cloaking it in Latin: *de feminis castratis* (*Shorter Works* 2:880). For the removal of the ovaries to be considered castration, the ovaries have to be thought of as female stones, or testicles.[25] Whereas the doctor he was reviewing thought it immoral to extirpate the female womb even if it was cancerous, Coleridge was in favor of this operation if it could save the life of the woman. The prevalence of castration perhaps then helps explain how sex could be considered a mobile essence, how anatomy could not fully explain sex.

Samuel Sharpe devotes a chapter of his *Treatise on the Operations of Surgery* (1769) to castration, describing it as "one of the most melancholy Operations in the Practice of Surgery" (51). Sharpe's exact language is echoed in the 1771 *En-*

*cyclopedia Britannica* entry under "Surgery." Sharpe sought to restrict the operation of castration, noting that, "although others think it is a necessary operation for Hydrocele, Abcess of the Testis, and Sarcocele," "it is absolutely improper to perform the operation for those diseases" (s.v. Surgery 3:655). Surgeon to the King and the most eminent one of his time, Astley Cooper likewise admitted that a "multitude of testes have been unnecessarily and precipitately removed" (*Observations on the Structure and Diseases of the Testis* 5). John Hunter in 1784–85 opened his surgical lectures by informing his students that he had watched a man die from castration (National Library of Medicine MS 1:3). In his published writings, Hunter comments that the testicles "are so often concerned in some of the most important diseases and operations of surgery" (*Observations* 14). Cooper agreed, urging his students to learn the anatomy of the male organs "more so than any other part of the body" because "nine tenths of surgical diseases we meet with, are in the Male Organs of Generation" (Wellcome Library MS 7096, 6).[26] Women, by contrast, "sometimes render themselves the subjects of lithotomy from perverse and unnatural propensities. I have known a woman put a pebble into the meatus urinanus" (*Lectures* 2:299). One might ask why Cooper doesn't explain male diseases in terms of perverse propensities, especially since he knew that venereal disease was a major cause of testicular diseases. Henry Cline, appointed lecturer in anatomy at St. Thomas's Hospital in London in 1781 and connected through John Thelwall to a radical Paris medical circle (Almeida 6), devoted almost 10 percent of his lectures on surgery to castration, noting that "the diseases of the Testes are very various" (National Library of Medicine MS B400, n.p.).[27] Benjamin Gooch, moreover, describes six cases of castration in his *Chirurgical Lectures* and mentions that cases of castration of chimney sweeps are frequent in London (2:236). The *New Medical Dictionary* quotes a doctor saying that out of a hundred patients, only three survive three years after surgery.[28] Buffon, in fact, argued that castration could be accomplished without surgery, using only hot water and various plant concoctions, though he did not specify which (*HN* 2:483). Buffon did not think castration was terribly dangerous.

Medical writers of the period were fascinated by eunuchs, castrati, partly because they had the potential to reveal the secrets of biological sex, the role that the testicles and ovaries play in secondary sexual differentiation. Castrati in the Romantic period proved that men and women were one sex, since males deprived of testicles became feminized.[29] In a section of his *Essays and Observations on Natural History* entitled "Of the effects that Castration and Spaying have on Animals," John Hunter wrote, "The testes in the male and ovaria in the female . . . influence the whole body and also the mind" (235). Males deprived of testicles when young not only grow like females, but in fact "exceed her in many particulars. . . . And if the male has arrived at full age before the testes are removed, he remains nearly in that state, and does not fall back into the female [state or form]" (235). Two points are of interest here. First, what does it mean that castrated men can exceed the female? It is as if testicles transform the essentially feminine human body into masculinity: how else to explain how castrated males can become more female than females? Second, Hunter expects castrated males to fall back into the "female state": falling back reminds us of a reversion to a single feminized sex. They don't so long as they were past puberty when castrated. Hunter elaborates, "In the human species the shape of the whole body is altered, or rather takes another form, when the male is deprived of the testes he becomes larger in body; a greater quantity of fat is spread over the surface of the body under the skin. The muscles do not swell so much, which produces a softness and delicacy of look" (235–36).

Despite Hunter's claim that the eunuch "takes another form," the castrated male is virtually the same feminized male before puberty. Hence, Hunter catalogues the fact that "the shoulders do not spread out so broadly" and "the voice continues soft and sweet, [and] does not break at the time of puberty" (236). To the extent that the sexes originate as one, sexual difference and the gendered uses to which they are put threaten to collapse.

Hunter offers important clues as to why secondary sexual differentiation had as much, if not more, resonance than genital difference. Because the mind has consciousness over bodily superiority, the failure to gain corporeal strength in puberty means that the male mind will fail to develop superiority as well. Here's how Hunter puts it: "The mind, like the body, has a superiority; as the body is capable of greater execution, so the mind seems to be conscious of the superiority that the body has, by which means its views become more extensive" (234–35). Although he claims "consciousness . . . makes heroes of them all," and although that consciousness is predicated upon the superior strength of the body that develops in puberty only in males, Hunter concludes that bodily superiority "is most likely an original formation of mind, but is capable of being improved or increased by this consciousness" (235). The problem, of course, is that without puberty, one cannot have consciousness of physical superiority, and so it is not clear how the mind could intrinsically have that consciousness. Nor is it clear what the relationship is between original formation of mind and consciousness. The localization of sexual difference between the testicles and ovaria and consciousness, and the fact that consciousness could either be intrinsically different or made different in puberty, meant that the ground of sexual difference was highly volatile, so much so that one had to be very careful when attempting to correlate gender to sex.

Surgeon and friend to the Shelleys, William Lawrence, wrote that "an imperfect original formation of the sexual organs, or the removal of some of them modifies the whole character of the individual, changes the physical constitution in a very remarkable manner, and influences in a no less striking degree the moral habits and dispositions" (s.v. "Generation," n.p.). In Lawrence, biological sex is taking on the essence of the person: his or her habits, dispositions, and very character. Yet as we shall see below, puberty meant that absolute difference had to be at least at the outset, relative. T. Bell wrote in *Kalogynomia; Or, the Laws of Female Beauty* (1821) that eunuchs were capable of erections and coition (144–45). "Perfect eunuchism induces immense changes in the human constitution. The beard and hair of the pubis do not grow: . . . the feminine form is, in some measure assumed. . . . Narses is almost the only eunuch who, in ancient times, exhibited great energy of mind" (146). Bell's point that eunuchs were capable of coition, for example, meant that although literally unsexed, they could assume the role of virility nonetheless.[30] Because virility was at some distance from anatomy, just exactly what was it based upon?

Even when men had their testicles intact, there could be problems. Just because one had testicles did not mean they worked or were in the right place. In 1756, John Hunter made the "exciting anatomical discovery" (Moore 115) while treating patients with congenital hernias that the original seat of the male testicle was in the abdominal cavity and that the testicle usually descends into the scrotum sometime in between the seventh and ninth month of gestation (*Observations* 1786 9). Haller had erroneously concluded that the testicles dropped when the baby took his first breath. My use of "male testicle" reflects the fairly recent shift from seeing the ovaries as the female testicles: we can again see the imprint of the one-sex model when Hunter, for example, lumped the testicle and ovarium together because they are parts "whose uses are equally similar" (*Observations* 47). "Until the approach of birth, the testes of the foetus are lodged within the cavity of the abdomen, and may therefore be reckoned among the abdominal viscera," Hunter notes (*Observations* 2).

Because he knew that the "sex characters" depend "upon the effects that the ovaria and testicles have upon the constitution" (*EO* 1:184), and that the failure

# P L A T E  I.

THE firft figure reprefents the teftes within the abdomen, in an abortive
fœtus of about fix months. All the inteftines, except the rectum,
are removed; and the peritonæum in moft places is left upon the furfaces
which it covers, fo that the parts have not that fharpnefs and diftinct appearance which might have been given to them by diffection.

A  The upper part of the object, covered with a cloth.

BB  The thighs.

C  The penis.

D  The fcrotum.

E  The flap of the integuments, abdominal mufcles, and peritonæum,
turned back over the right os ilium to bring the teftis into view.

F  The flap of the fkin and cellular membrane of the left fide difpofed in
the fame manner.

G  The flap of the abdominal mufcles and of the peritonæum of the left
fide turned back over the fpine of the os ilium. The lower part of
this flap is cut away, in order to fhew the ligament of the teftis
paffing down through the ring into the fcrotum.

HH  The lower part of each kidney.

I  The projection formed by the lower vertebræ lumborum, and by the
bifurcation of the aorta and vena cava.

K  The rectum filled with meconium, and tied at its upper part where the
colon was cut away.

L  That branch of the inferior mefenteric artery which was going to the
colon.

M  The lower branch of the fame artery, which went down into the pelvis behind the rectum.

N  The lower part of the bladder, that part of it which is higher than
the offa pubis in fo young a fœtus being cut away.

OO  The hypogaftric or umbilical arteries cut through, where they were
turning up by the fides of the bladder in their way to the navel.

PP  The ureter of each fide paffing down before the pfoas mufcle and iliac
veffels, in its courfe to the lower part of the bladder.

QQ  The

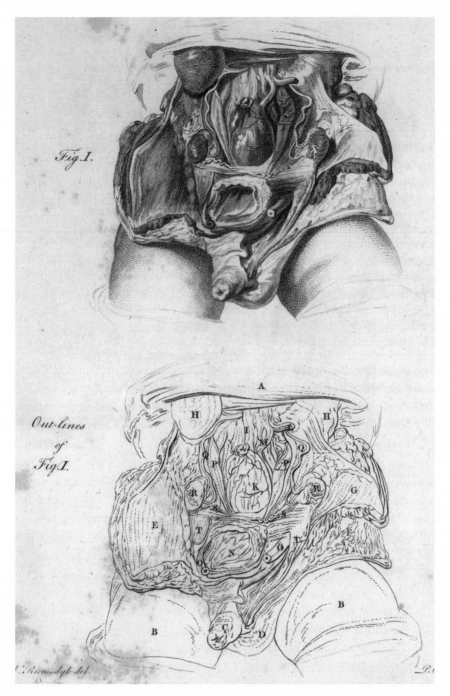

P. C. Canot, Engraver. John Hunter, *Observations on Certain Parts of the Animal Economy*, 1786. Plate 1, "Descent of the Testicle." Courtesy of the National Library of Medicine, Bethesda, Maryland.

of the testicles to descend might lead to effeminacy, what Hunter calls a "tendency towards an hermaphrodite, the testicle seldom being well formed" (*Observations* 18). This discovery implied that sex itself was an unfolding biological process, an implication strengthened by Hunter's admission that the location of the testis may be "variable" (*Observations* 3). By "hermaphrodite," Hunter means a person of ambiguous genitalia. Hunter warns that "sometimes in the human body, . . . the testes do not descend from the cavity of the abdomen until late in life, or never at all" (*Observations* 7). In William Cruickshank's and Matthew Baillie's "Lectures on the Male Organs of Generation," these anatomists worried about the beholdeness of the testicles to gravity. "Gravity can have its share in bringing the testicles from the loins into the scrotum," they lectured, "as it happens before birth, when the head being downward, consequently the testicles must ascend" (National Library of Medicine MS B967 vol. 1). Hunter knew that their descent was sometimes after birth. When both testicles fail to descend, this can have devastating effects upon the manifestations of biological sex. Such deviations were not uncommon: "We see more men who have one testis, or both, lodged immediately within the tendon of that muscle [oblique]," Hunter writes (*Observations* 9). It was perhaps this article on the testicle's descent that led him to remove a testis from a cock and transplant it back into the abdomen of a hen, "where it has adhered and nourished" (cited in Jorgensen 16). Certainly experiments like this one proved that culture could manipulate bodies, that nature and culture were far from mutually exclusive categories.

In his lavishly illustrated *Observations on the Structure and Diseases of the Testis* (1830), Cooper informed his readers that sometimes the testicle waits until puberty to descend, and sometimes that descent can take until the age of twenty-one or even longer (44). After apologizing for the expense of this book and expressing the hope that in future editions readers would be able to purchase groups of plates if they couldn't afford the whole thing, Cooper elaborates on the testicle's descent: "When the testis remains in the abdomen, it makes a strong impression upon the patient's mind, as a suspicion arises that his virility is lessened or destroyed. In a case of this kind I have known the unfortunate subject committed suicide" (45).

Cooper then reassures his readers that although "a testis late in its descent . . . is often lessened in its bulk," "the testis on the other side, with this diminished organ, is sufficient for the procreation of children" (46). I raise this example to show that a psychological understanding of one's anatomy is at odds with the physiological fact of one's actual virility, despite the fact that Cooper tries to correlate the static testicle with a mental impression. The problem is that, even if the testicle's failure to descend causes the mind's impression of diminished virility, the actual fact of the matter is that the man's virility is not necessarily thus compromised. Thus, anatomy is here caught between a foundational explanation of the man's psychological state and the error of that state: the static testicle does not explain the man's psychological error. This developing gap between anatomical fact and the mind's apprehension of one's anatomy makes sex the potential groundwork of liberation in that sex can be about choices rather than destiny. Of course, for this to happen, the gap between anatomy and psychology must not seem threatening.

Cooper moved immediately from the testicle's failure to descend to a description of what happened to a man who had both testicles removed. What is especially interesting about his account of a castrated male is that, even after the operation in 1801, the man "still ha[d] emissions at night" and would continue to do so for one full year. Once again, anatomical fact fails to capture what Cooper thinks is the biological reality of sex. "For nearly the first twelve months, he stated he had emissions *in coitu*, or that he had sensations of emission. That then he had erections and coitus at distinct intervals," Cooper writes, "but without the sensation of emission. After two years he had erections very rarely and very imperfectly" (53). He does not speculate as to the causes of the time lag between the loss of virility and the operation, but the fact that almost two years went by before the man lost his powers of erection meant once again that there was no one-to-one correlation between anatomy and sexual desire. Of course, Cooper attempts to close this lag by pointedly suggesting that he may have sensed emission but did not necessarily have an emission. Even this finessing, however, doesn't quite work because the sensation has no clear origin. What is the empirical basis for this sensation? Cooper ends his treatment of this man's case by the simple statement that "imperfect erectile power remained for . . . months" (53). Not only did the presence of erectile power in spite of castration undermine anatomy's ability to explain sex, but this also meant that virility did not necessarily have a function.

The removal of the testicles was particularly traumatic in light of the widely accepted medical theory that reabsorption of sperm from the testicles was necessary to maintain male secondary sexual characteristics. Writers inveighing against masturbation, for example, regularly warned boys that the practice of onanism would ruin their constitutions. And writers on male impotence warned that too much loss of semen would cause the "impossibility of exercising the venereal act" (Ryan 6). But even more respected medical doctors such as William Cullen believed that without the regular stimulus from the genitals during puberty "flaccidity takes place" in the male body (Wellcome MS 6036).[31] T. Bell held fast to the idea that "when the liquid which in man is secreted in certain vessels for the purposes of generation, is re-absorbed into the system, it communicates a general excitement and activity to the character" (*Kalogynomia* 66). Robert Couper went so far as to marvel that, if the reabsorption of semen into the male body at puberty could authorize such profound changes, imagine what its effects on the female body must be: "How powerful must it be when suddenly mingled . . . with the circulating fluids of the delicate female!" (152). William Hunter, however, disagreed, stating, "I cannot think Semen can be absorbed for any useful purpose, and that anything is naturally absorbed without its being useful is a folly to conceive" (Wellcome MS 7062 2:70). Notwithstanding their differences, these medical writers together anticipate the localization of sex onto the endocrine system, a localization that introduces another important variable in the mapping of sex onto the body. The line between sex and destiny was more convoluted than the genitals alone suggested.

## When Is the Clitoris a Penis?

If castration implied an original and universal feminine body for both sexes—indeed, we now know the masculine Y chromosome to be an add-on to an otherwise female body—the homology between the clitoris and penis provoked a crisis in sexual complementarity. In "An Account of the Free-Martin" (freemartins are sterile cows that are born alongside a bull-calf), published originally in the Royal Society's *Philosophical Transactions* in 1779, John Hunter further showed how a one-sex model and two-sex model could inhabit the same body. Hunter argued, "There is one part common to both the male and female organs of generation in all animals which have the sexes distinct; in the one sex it is called the penis, in the other the clitoris; its specific use in both is to continue, by its sensibility, the action excited in coition till the paroxysm alters the sensation. In the female it probably answers no other purpose; but in the male it is more complicated to adapt it for the purpose of expelling and conducting the semen that has been secreted in consequence of the actions so excited" (*Observations* 46).

Hunter refers to the penis and clitoris in all animals as one part with two different names—they are essentially similar but are named differently. Sexual difference begins as mere nominalism. Yet this tension between similitude and difference, between one sex and two sexes, grows more vexed as function enters the picture. Whereas the penis functions as both an organ of sensibility and an organ of function (it expels the semen), the only function of the clitoris is sensibility or pleasure. This again raises the question: is pleasure connected to function? Hunter seems to suggest it is by having pleasure "continue the action excited in coition," though he never specifies what that action accomplishes.

Because the science of physiology mandated that form betoken function, something which the clitoris seems to violate because it looks like a penis but doesn't fully function like one, the difference of name threatens to take on real functional difference. Under anatomy, the visual similarity between the clitoris and penis was enough to cement their analogousness. Haunting analogy was the legacy of the one-sex model. This violation, I suggest, helps explain how the clitoris gets demonized in medical discourse of the period in terms of the uterine furor, lesbianism, racial difference, and pathology. Either the physiological law that form correlates to function must be wrong or the clitoris must be made monstrous. Hence, Blumenbach referred to the clitoris as an "obscene organ of brute pleasure . . . given to beasts" (*Anthropological Treatises* 90). John's brother, William, the famous anatomist and man-midwife, worried so much about the similarity of the penis to the clitoris that he felt compelled in a medical lecture to state that "it is impossible for a woman with a large clitoris can copulate with another, because the skin does not go around the clitoris as it does around the penis, but ties it down so that it can never be detached like the penis."[32] Alluding to the theory that Sapphic women had large clitorises that made them want to penetrate other women, William Hunter denies that female-female penetration is even possible. As a supplement to the penis that is not quite a supplement, the clitoris threatens the very notion of a visible sign of sexual difference in that it makes some women look like, if not act like, men. If even a large clitoris cannot penetrate like a penis, this leaves open the question why some women want to have erotic relations with other women. To the extent that "penis" and "clitoris" could stand in for the same organ, just how much actual difference was there between the sexes?

Yet the clitoris could also provide an opportunity for the man-midwife to assert his superior professional scientific knowledge over that of the (female) midwife. Professionalization was widely held to be a serious concern in the various branches of medicine, as standards for training and licensing bodies were codified and expanded. In *On the Generative System* (1817), John Roberton sniggers, "It is by no means uncommon for a midwife to be in doubt to which of the

sexes the child, at birth, belongs, but this is completely removed when, on examination, we find whether or not there is a urethra—in the clitoris there is
none" (44). Coleridge too catalogued the "frightful blunder of an ignorant midwife" in one of his reviews of medical literature (*Shorter Works* 2:887), and he
castigated women medical practitioners as being "often notorious poisoners"
(*Shorter Works* 2:1088). Because the man-midwife hovered between the two
sexes, the stakes of his superior scientific and professional knowledge could not
have been higher.[33] This superior knowledge would have to justify his need to
manage women in labor, and his management was legitimated by figuring pregnancy as a disease (see Denham 169–70) and women's natural labors as "imperfect actions" (Denham 168). Of course, it was those "imperfect actions" that
sometimes mandated the masculine intrusion of technology in terms of forceps,
vectis, and other obstetrical implements as well as male scientific knowledge. Indeed, William Osborn went so far as to insist that God had ordained human
labor to be difficult—the human pelvis, he insisted was not designed for labor
and delivery, and thus "inevitable but superior difficulty" and necessary "danger"
lurked behind human parturition as opposed to the easy births of animals—and
it was this difficulty that "rescued the art of midwifery from the charge of inutil-
ity" (3).[34] Not only were both his professional status and right to manage
women at stake, but also, because his very sex was ambiguous, the man-midwife
could not afford not to know how to distinguish a large clitoris from a penis.
The man-midwife Thomas Denham admitted on the one hand that the "clitoris
is little concerned with the practice of midwifery, on account of its size and situation" (45). On the other hand, this did not prevent him from unceremoni-
ously stating, "Should the clitoris increase to such a size as to occasion much in-
convenience, it may be extirpated either with a knife or ligature" (45).[35] Perhaps
the most influential man-midwife, William Hunter, agreed: "The clitoris becomes so much elongated as to be obliged to be cut off " (Glasgow MS Gen 775,
39–40). Mutilation thus was preferable to ambiguity: the clitoris becomes the
object of cathexis because it undermines complementarity at the same time as it
becomes the severed badge of the man-midwife's masculinity (his professional
knowledge). In sum, because the clitoris threatened to the very idea of complementarity, it had to go when its elongation obscured the differences. Perhaps
this is what led Blake to remark, "And while the Sons of Albion by severe War
and Judgment bonify/The Hermaphroditic Condensations are divided by the
Knife/The obdurate Forms are cut asunder by Jealousy and Pity" (*Jerusalem*
58:10–12 E 207). The knife was the anatomist's weapon of choice.

# Romantic Puberty

If a common neurological body, castration, and the clitoris all together suggest fundamental doubts about the two sexes, the problem was exacerbated by puberty.[36] Until this point, the problem has been historical in that the Romantic period was a key moment of transition in thinking about sex. With puberty, however, the historical problem becomes even more coextensive with the body insofar as the body literally undergoes a transition from one feminized sex to two. Now that both models of sex inhered in the body, the crises could not be ignored. Given that puberty so often went awry, not even the basic facts about sex were unarguable.

First, a legal definition of puberty as it was understood in the Romantic period. According to the *Encyclopedia Britannica* (1771) puberty is defined as the age when a child is capable of procreation (3:517). Immediately following this terse definition, the writer of this entry sends the reader to the entry under law. Legally, puberty is designated the age of minority, and this was from the age of fourteen, if male, and the age of twelve, if female, until the age of twenty-one. Because puberty then lasted at least seven years—Buffon's claim that males did not arrive at perfection until thirty made puberty an astounding sixteen years long—puberty was a significant period of transition in the Romantic period. William Cullen bested Buffon, arguing that full manhood was not achieved until thirty-five years of age. This meant that puberty lasted for twenty-one years (*Materia Medica* 16)! The legal stakes of this transition were that minors were ineligible for political rights. If it were true that women did not really undergo secondary sexual differentiation as Hunter claimed, women could not, in fact, participate in politics. Of course to make this claim, one had to ignore menstruation and the growth of breasts during puberty.

I focus on puberty because it shows how sex was considered a biological process in Romanticism, a lengthy process that could go dreadfully wrong. Once again, the body provides a kind of materiality that is open to change. Premature puberty could be particularly traumatic, especially when it frustrated both the one-sex and two-sex theories. Dr. Cookson, of Lincoln, described the case of Charlotte Mawer, a girl who at age three and a half menstruated and had breasts and pubic hair. Cookson remarked that she was a "strong-built womanly kind of child," and he did "not find this girl has exhibited any particular marks of attachment to the other sex; but I have thought it right to caution the mother on this head; though I am apprehensive she will not survive many years. It may be a matter of curious speculation, whether this child can be impregnated, conceive, and produce her kind—I am inclined to think in the affirmative" (118). Because her body bore the signs of being ready to reproduce, yet she did not experience sexual desire, Cookson attempts to close the gap between anatomy and desire through speculation. In Keatsian fashion, he imagines her to be a ravished bride. Astley Cooper writes in the *Medico-Chirurgical Transactions* a year later that at four and a half Mawer "is quite a little woman in her appearance, except as to her countenance, which is childish. [She] does not seem to have any sexual feelings, or an uncommon degree of modesty." Not quite a believer, Cooper went to the parish register to confirm her age and he reported that she was indeed the age reported. By April 1812, Cooper notes that she has "become modest." Mawer again shows a gap between desire and anatomy: though she is anatomically sexually mature, she seems to have no desires. Cooper tries to correlate modesty with puberty, and with that he has more success.

Not just women were vulnerable to errors of puberty. John Hunter cites five cases of men whose breasts enlarged during puberty; moreover, in one of these cases the father "applied his left nipple to the infant's mouth, who sucked and drew milk from it in such quantity as to be nursed by it in perfect good health" (*EO* 238). These cases attest to what sexual dimorphism attempts to finesse: the gaps between bodies and sexual dimorphism. His genitals were inspected and not found to be any different from any other man's (*EO* 238). John Flint South considered another case of premature puberty in John Sparrow, who was five years of age, muscular, and had seminal emissions at night. According to his mother's narrative, the boy's linen was stained two or three times a week. Because her son was faint and pallid on the next morning, "she was induced to watch him, and thus ascertained the real cause, which, alarming her very much, she applied to her medical attendant, who recommended cold bathing of the whole body, three times a day" (78). His nocturnal emissions then became less frequent (once a week). Writing in his own voice, the doctor then meticulously catalogued the boy's size, including the length and width of his erect penis, and he noted that his "occiput [was] extremely prominent" (79). Dr. South tried to pin the cause of it on "the enormous size of the cerebellum, which Drs. Gall and Spurzheim state is always the case when the genital organs are developed in a great degree" (80). Here, the body's sex is explained by the brain, an explanation that undermines the need to make his erect penis an object of medical knowledge.

Sparrow later captured the attention of John Gordon Smith, who added in the *London Medical Repository*, "I was assured that he is an entire stranger to sexual ideas and impression; the company of females exerting no influence upon him" (358). Yet perhaps the most interesting feature of Smith's account of Sparrow is that he feels the need to begin the article with a long disquisition concerning "the regularity of bodies"—human and planetary (353–56). He then introduces the case as an anomaly, bringing it to a close by remarking upon the "peculiarities of this monstrosity, to account for which would perplex the most intelligent among philosophers" (358). He concludes with a highly unscientific observation that "while such as are distinguished by exceptions, analogous to those in the present instance, must be objects of curiosity to the naturalist, but, in all probability, of pity, at the best, to those who are socially connected with them" (358). This startling and uneasy conclusion more than undermines the equanimity of Smith's opening pages, leaving Smith unable to account for deviation and monstrosity in the midst of all the supposed regularity he initially celebrates. These valiant attempts to frame this case within the argument from design wind up frustrating that argument, forcing Smith to turn from science to pity.

While the descent of the testicle and premature puberty begin to complicate the ontological solidity of sex, suggesting that the work of sexual differentiation was an ongoing biological process sometimes uncompleted until thirteen years of age or not at all, Hunter's work on secondary sexual characteristics undermines the unquestioned priority of the genitals as the marker of sex. Hunter lays out the distinction between primary and secondary sexual characteristics in his "Account of an Extraordinary Pheasant" (originally published in the Royal Society's *Philosophical Transactions*) when he claims,

> It is well known, that there are many orders of animals which have the two parts designed for the purpose of generation different in the same species, by which they are distinguished into male and female: but this is not the only mark of distinction in many genera of animals; in the greatest part the male being distinguished from the female by various marks. The differences which are found in the parts of generation themselves, I shall call the first, or principle; and all others depending upon these I shall call secondary. The first belong equally to both; but the secondary will be found principally, although not entirely, in the male. (4:73)

Although this passage insists upon sexual differentiation and the importance of genital difference, I highlight ambiguities that begin to undermine the solidity of sex and the primacy of genital difference. Especially curious is that Hunter would call attention to a sex change in birds as "extraordinary" when this was a known scientific fact (Quist 97). Once again, both one-sex and two-sex models compete for attention. Hunter makes genital difference one of the many "marks of distinction" of sex: note how "mark" becomes "marks" in the above passage. Elsewhere, Hunter gives more definition to these marks when he writes that, "the male may be always distinguished from the female by his noble, masculine, and beautiful figure" (*EO* 1:184). Hunter claims, moreover, that secondary sexual differentiation is largely confined to males: it is "principally" in the male. This suggests that until secondary differentiation takes place in puberty, the sexes are more alike than they are different and that both sexes are feminine until puberty.[37] After all, at puberty, the male "los[es] that resemblance he had to the female in various secondary properties" (*Observations* 65): "he . . . leaves the female state and undergoes a kind of change or metamorphosis like the moth" (*EO* 184). Lest we imagine that Hunter's remarks on sex do not so much pertain to human beings, at the end of his essay on female pheasants, Hunter draws attention to how "even in the human species, . . . that increase of hair observable on the faces of many women in advanced life, is an approach towards the beard, which is one of the most distinguishing secondary properties of man" (*Observations* 68). If males before puberty are feminized, and if females after menopause were masculinized, the biology of sexual difference refused to provide much of a foundation for complementarity and gave precious little stability for cultural notions of difference. Wollstonecraft and Robinson show how this instability could prove liberatory even for women.

We can witness the legacy of the one-sex model along with the diminished role of genital difference in a key anatomical text of the period, Andrew Bell's 1798 *Anatomia Britannica*. Bell was engraver to the Prince of Wales. The first two parts of Bell's work ignore sexual differentiation: even the depicted penis does not need to refer to difference if women have an analogous clitoris or if women's organs were simply inside the body, not outside. That the first two parts contain plates taken from Albinus (1697–1770) perhaps explains the absence of attention to sexual differentiation. For Albinus, there was clearly one sex, not two. Bell does not feel the need to update these images; his reproduction of them in an emphatically British anatomy insists that they still embody knowledge good enough for the British Empire. That is to say, the idea of incommensurate sexual difference did not hold so much sway as to make these plates seem like misinformation or error or even antiquarian knowledge.

The third part of Bell's grand *Anatomia Britannica*, however, foregrounds sexual difference but emphasizes difference of proportions between the sexes, showcasing the proportions as understood by the Ancient Greeks, before turning to anatomy itself. These engravings are adapted from the famous anatomist William Cowper. Cowper's drawings may have influenced Blake (Connolly 46–

58). Of course, proportional differences only became truly visible post-puberty. Bell uses statues of Apollo and Venus to prove that men have larger shoulders, longer sternums, and smaller pelvises (3:12–16). Three pages of tables list all of the proportional differences. Accordingly, the texts to the anatomical plates of man and woman emphasize proportional differences rather than different genitals. The illustrations depict difference in such a way as to allow the genitals to be swallowed up by proportion. To wit, the engraving of the man insists on the proportions between various features, labeled from *a* to *v* along with *y* and *z*, leaving his dwarfed penis and testicles the letters *w* and *x*. Of course, the man's genitals are placed at the very center of his body and thus prefigure Blake's rendering of Orc's genitals.

The textual commentary for the illustration of woman states, "Woman, in whom the symmetry or proportion differs from that of a man . . . nor will any action, in which a woman uses her utmost strength, occasion such a swelling or rising of the muscles and other parts to appear as is the case in men; the great quantity of fat placed under the skin of Women, covering their muscles, &c, so as to prevent any such appearance" (part 3, plate 43). Her breasts and genitals are dwarfed by proportional difference (part 3, plate 43).[38] Again proportional changes and muscular development are the result of puberty: genitals are neither a clear nor persuasive marker of difference, but, in this case, her proportions are not inscribed onto the body: the only two features on her body that are labeled are her mammae and pudendum. Her pudendum, however, is engulfed by the width of her large hips, and the drapery she holds draws our attention away from her breasts. Whereas the other two books allowed the male skeleton to stand in for both genders, the third part has engravings of both male and female skeletons.[39]

Hunter and Bell were by far *not* the only medical adherents to this notion of one-sex before puberty, two sexes thereafter. We can see it in John Bostock's *Elementary System of Physiology:*

> The generative organs . . . exercise a peculiar and specific influence over the system at large, affecting its general form and its powers, both mental and corporeal, causing the growth and development of particular parts, and giving to the individual, in a more remarkable degree, those characters which constitute the peculiarity of sex. The constitutional difference of the two sexes during infancy is not very considerable, but at the period of puberty, when the generative organs are developed and their functions established, the difference is very much increased, and continues during the remainder of life. (1824 3:22)

# THE

## First Anatomical Table

### OF THE

# HUMAN BODY

## EXPLAINED.

BEFORE we enter upon the Anatomical Defcription of the Human Body, it may not be improper to take a view of the Proportions of the different Parts of a well-formed Man, and of the relative Proportions of the Male and Female, in the living State.

From the crown of the head 1, which is covered with the hair, to the upper part of the forehead A, is the third part of a face.

The face B, begins at the roots of the loweft hairs, which are upon the forehead A C, and ends at the bottom of the chin K.

The face is divided into three proportionable parts; the firft contains the forehead A C; the fecond, the nofe G; and the third, the mouth and the chin H I K.

From the chin to the upper part of the fternum, or breaft bone,—two lengths of a nofe.

From the top of the fternum to the bottom of the breaft, called fcrobiculus cordis, O,—one face.

From the pit of the ftomach to the umbilicus or navel R, one face ;—the Apollo has half a nofe more.

From the umbilicus to the pudendum U, one face.

From the pudendum to the fmall of the thigh above the patella or knee-pan Z,—two faces.

From the lower part of the knee to the fmall of the leg above the ankle D, two faces.

From the ankle, or malleolus internus, to the bottom of the heel,—half a face.

A man, when his arms are ftretched out, is, from the extremity of the longeft finger of his right-hand to the extremity of the longeft of his left, as broad as he is long.

From one fide of the breafts to the other below the nipples N N, two faces.

From the pit of the throat to the top of the fhoulder, or extremity of the fpine of the fcapula,—one face ; from thence to the bending of the cubit or elbow,—one face and a half; thence again to the wrift, one face and a nofe. The hand with the fingers extended, contain one face : So that four faces, a nofe, and half a face, is the diftance between the pit of the throat and extremity of the middle finger ; which, upon extenfion of the whole arm, &c. will amount to five faces, rather more than lefs.

The foot, a face and a nofe in length.

As to the breadth of the limbs, no precife meafure can be given, becaufe the meafures themfelves not only vary according to the quality of the perfons, but according to the motion of the mufcles.

A man is two lengths or faces from the point of each fhoulder; that is to fay, from the upper part of the fternum between the clavicles, called the pit of the throat, to the extremity of the fpine of the fcapula, called the top of the fhoulder, one length ; and fo, on the other fide.

The breadth of the hips of a man is one length and a half; that is, from the great trochanter of the thigh-bone of one fide to that of the other ; the precife places of which bones are interfected by an horizontal line drawn from the pubes on each fide.

L The pomum adami, or protuberant part of the larynx, which is much larger in men than in women.

M The fternum or breaft-bone appearing under the fkin, &c. between the two pectoral mufcles.

O The fcorbiculus cordis, commonly called the pit of the ftomach, under the fkin, &c. Precifely in this place is the cartilago enfiformis.

P The epigaftrium.

Q Q The hypochondria, or fpaces under the fhort ribs.

R The region of the umbilicus.

S The hypogaftrium.

T One of the ilia.

U The pubes.

V One of the inguina, or groins.

W The penis.

X The fcrotum

Y Y The thighs.

Z Z The knees.

a a The legs.

b b The tarfus, or bending of the foot.

c c The metatarfus, or fore-foot.

d d The toes.

e e The fhoulders.

f f The arms.

g g The fore and back parts of the elbows.

h h The fore-arms.

i i The carpus or wrift.

k k The metacarpus.

l l The fingers.

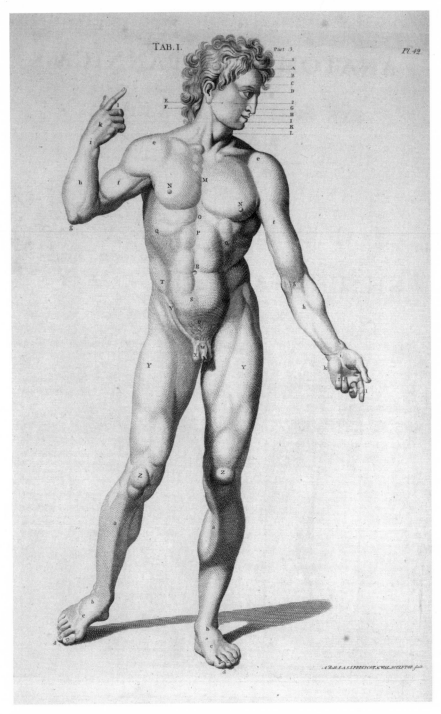

Andrew Bell, *Anatomia Britannica*, "First Anatomical Table of the Human Body." Courtesy of the National Library of Medicine, Bethesda, Maryland.

T H E

# Second Anatomical Table

OF THE

# HUMAN BODY

E X P L A I N E D.

———————

R EPRESENTS the fore-part of a Woman, in whom the fymmetry or proportion differs from that of a Man : Firft, Moft remarkably in this, that the fhoulders are narrower; the Man having two lengths or faces in the breadth of his fhoulders, and one and a half in his hips; whereas a Woman, on the contrary, has but one face and a half in her fhoulders, and two in her hips. Secondly, The clavicles, or collar-bones, and mufcles in general, do not appear in Women as in Men; whence it is that the outline of the one, as painters exprefs it, differs very much from that of the other. Nor will any action, in which a Woman ufes her utmoft ftrength, occafion fuch a fwelling or rifing of the mufcles and other parts to appear, as is the cafe in Men; the great quantity of fat placed under the fkin of Women, covering their mufcles, &c. , fo as to prevent any fuch appearance.

A A The mammæ:                                      B The pudendum.

T H E

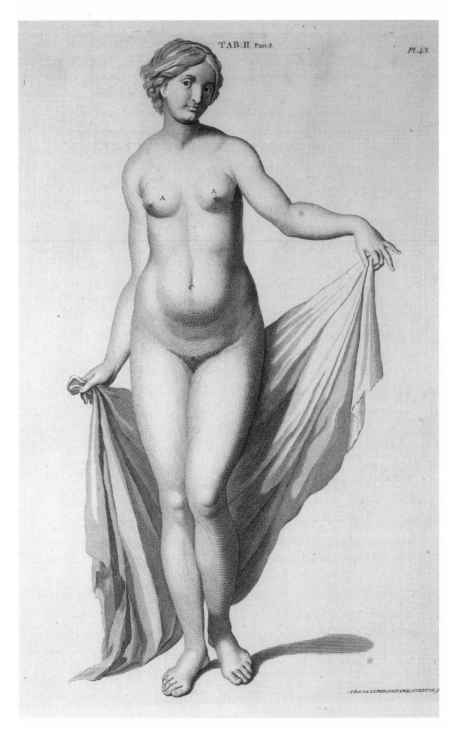

Andrew Bell, *Anatomia Britannica*, "Second Anatomical Table of the Human Body."
Courtesy of the National Library of Medicine, Bethesda, Maryland.

Like Hunter, Bostock downplays genital difference—there is not a great difference between infants of both sexes—preferring instead to read the "characters which constitute the peculiarity of sex" at puberty. Bostock then localizes sexual difference in "the anatomical structure of the body" and in the body's "chemical constitution" (2:22). The movement of body from anatomy to chemistry allowed chemistry's newfound explanations for the attractions of one particle over others to replace the visible body as explanation.[40] Speaking of boys and girls, John Roberton, a member of the Royal College of Surgeons, wrote in his *Observations on the Mortality and Physical Management of Children* (1827) that "if the sexes differ but little in their physical structure: if they breathe the same air, digest the same food, have duties and difficulties before them equally arduous, how comes it that, while the one is encouraged to strengthen the frame by exposure and exercise, the other is trained in seclusion, stigmatized as a romp for every exhibition of vivacity; . . . her occupations and amusements tending to produce indolence and muscular debility" (244). Because he so limits the differences of physical structure between boys and girls, Roberton questions how cultural differences can be based on so little.

The French approach to puberty provides a startling contrast to the English. Montpelier physician P. M. Ferrier wrote in "De la pubérté considerer comme crise des maladies de l'enfance" ("Of Puberty Considered as a Crisis of Illness") that "the signs particular to puberty are more characterized by men than women. His limbs up till then have been soft and delicate, begin to become pronounced, his chin becomes covered with hair, his voice changes, and the seminal liquor secretes itself, and his body presents the complete energy that characterizes the male" (7, translation mine). On the subject of puberty in women, Ferrier defers to Rousseau, citing that their eyes, the organs of the soul, find their language of expression, they learn how to blush (6). Insofar as Rousseau's fictions are taken to bolster scientific fact, Wollstonecraft was right to go after him. Unlike his English counterparts, however, Ferrier described puberty as a natural revolution: "the revolution of puberty is a work of nature" (23). If Ferrier sought thereby to naturalize revolution, to give it a historical precedent in every (mostly male) human body, he also helped to pathologize revolution insofar as he connected puberty with a health crisis. If puberty were a revolution that required the careful management of doctors, it nonetheless helped to naturalize revolution.[41]

Wollstonecraft supports the notion of one sex before puberty when she argues that "girls and boys, in short, would play harmlessly together, if the distinction of sex was not inculcated long before nature makes any difference" (*VRW* 129). She insists that societal notions of sexual difference inscribe themselves onto bodies long before nature can conform to what we now call gender. The fact that there was originally only one sex means that all claims grounded upon nature—especially Rousseau's attempt to give the mind a sex and to naturalize female sensibility—must be given especial scrutiny. To the extent that, as Hunter argues, primary sexual difference (genitals) are the cause of secondary difference and differences in the sex organs do not lead to further sexual differentiation in women, sexual differentiation becomes contingent upon both an absence and a presence, with women's genitals as presence causing a secondary absence of differentiation. Because Romantic medicine did not simply accept the primacy of genital difference, sex itself was a precarious ground of difference, a *terra infirma* rendered even more unstable because it is tied to both presence and absence. Read in this light, Wollstonecraft harnesses the idea of one original sex to undermine the legitimacy of complementary constructions of gender while rejecting the necessary hierarchy of the one-sex model.[42] Of course, Hunter's inability to see female sexual differentiation in puberty, especially his blindness to menstruation, points to how the male puberty could stand in for female puberty.

In fact, Wollstonecraft alludes to the work of naturalists and their work on puberty when she argues,

> It has also been asserted, by some naturalists, that men do not attain their full growth and strength till thirty; but that women arrive at maturity by twenty. I apprehend that they reason on false ground, led astray by the male prejudice, which deems beauty the perfection of woman—mere beauty of features and complexion, the vulgar acceptation of the word, whilst male beauty is allowed to have some connection with the mind. Strength of body and that character of countenance which the French term *physionomie*, women do not acquire before thirty, any more than men. (162–63)

It was Buffon who insisted in his famous discussion of puberty in *Histoire Naturelle* that men did not arrive at the state of perfection until thirty, since their strength required more intense work on the part of nature. Women, by contrast, were rendered perfect by age twenty (518). By refuting Buffon, and by calling attention to the sexism inherent in a female notion of beauty that did not include the mind, Wollstonecraft once again downplays the role of physical strength and refuses to accept an inferior notion of maturity for women.

Women's beauty, like men's, is essentially an intellectual beauty. Her reference to physiognomy, which she would have gotten from her reading of Lavater and Buffon, further cemented the body/soul connection insofar as features of the face were read as windows into the soul/mind. And because both men and women come to maturity at the same time, Wollstonecraft insinuates, one cannot deny women political rights on the basis of immaturity without also denying men's.

Buffon, however, was not entirely an enemy to Wollstonecraft's cause. His bold statement that the hymen and caruncles were merely imaginary signs of virginity (*HN* 490–92) might have been what emboldened Wollstonecraft to "throw down the gauntlet and deny the existence of sexual virtues, not excepting modesty" (139). If there is no physical sign of virginity, the morals that are grounded upon it also evaporate.[43] Blumenbach would agree, commenting that "this little appendage to the female body is all the more remarkable, because I cannot imagine any physical utility attaches to it" (*Anthropological Treatises* 170).

Hunter elaborates on the relative insignificance of genital difference, "Thus we see the sexes which at an early period had little to distinguish them from each other. . . . The male at this time [puberty] recedes from the female, and assumes the secondary properties of his sex" (*Observations* 68). Elsewhere he comments that "the distinction of the sex, exclusive of the parts of generation, is but very small in childhood and youth. Boys and girls are very similar in all their features when first formed; even the parts peculiar to each are similar to one another [in the embryo]; both seeming to shoot out from one point, but each on a different plan; therefore they become very different by the time they arrive at perfection" (*EO* 1:186). Again, I note Hunter's insistence that the sexes *become* different and in so doing he downplays the role of genital difference. These secondary characteristics show that sex is not an achieved state, a fact all the more compelling once we recall that the average life span in the 1750s was thirty-six (Porter 1995, 440). Indeed, if the male "recedes from the female" in puberty, then sex is, at least for roughly the first third of life, less an opposition than a continuum, a fact that once again suggests the one-sex model has much truth to it. To make matters worse, women in menopause begin to acquire some secondary characteristics of men: namely, facial hair. By figuring even mature women as children—as arrested males—Hunter makes it virtually impossible for women to acquire the maturity that is so necessary for poetic authorship in this period (Ross 155–60). As we have seen, Wollstonecraft vehemently contested the separation of male maturity from female maturity.

When Hunter remarks that "there is often a change of the secondary properties of one sex into those of the other" (*Observations* 64), he underscores the fluidity of biological sex. He adds, "The female, at a much later time of life, when the powers of propagation cease, loses many of her peculiar properties; and may be said, except from mere structure of parts, to be of no sex; and even recedes from the original character of the animal, approaching in appearance towards the male, or perhaps more properly towards the hermaphrodite" (*Observations* 49). In no way then is sex in the living human being a stable essence. And, when Hunter marvels that the "testicles [are] the cause of the inclinations, yet they do not direct these inclinations: the inclinations become an operation of the mind, after the mind is once stimulated by the testicle" (*EO* 1:19), he adds still another gap between anatomy and sexual desire, although he does insist that the testicle must stimulate the mind to take over. The fact that this anatomical cause does not direct the inclinations introduces a potentially insurmountable gap between sexual aim and sexual object, opening the door to the universality of perversion.

All of this instability in sexual differentiation is further troubling, given the fact that Hunter ascribes congenital malformations to the existing primordial germ. Hunter frames his essay on the extraordinary pheasant with the remark that "every deviation from that original form and structure which gives the distinguishing character to the productions of nature, may not improperly be called monstrous. . . . As far as my knowledge has extended, there is not one species of animals, nay there is not one single part of an animal body which is not subject to extraordinary formation. Nor does this appear to be a matter of mere chance; for it may be observed, that every one has a disposition to deviate from nature in a manner peculiar to itself. . . . Each part of each species ha[s] its monstrous form, as it were, originally impressed on it by the hand of nature" (*Observations* 63). If every species has a disposition to monstrosity, and if each part has its "monstrous form originally impressed on it," monstrosity is eradicable from nature herself. To make matters worse, nature directs the progress of monstrosity. If nature herself is at once normal and monstrous, and if nature has a disposition to the monstrous, then the distinctions between the norm and the perverted will not hold up; nor will the social distinctions that are based on them stand. By logical extension, sexual complementarity is thus rendered perverse because it partakes in an innate propensity to monstrosity.

John Hunter was so fascinated by the role played by the testicles in puberty that he went so far as to transplant a cock testis to a hen.[44] The operation was a qualified success in that the transplant took. Hunter did "in all probability consider the possible effect of the cock testis, transplanted to the hen, on secondary sex characters and on sex behavior" (Jorgensen 15). Because Hunter did not detail these remarkable experiments himself, we must turn to the notes of his students to get a sense of what Hunter thought he was doing. The student writes, "Here is the testicle of a cock, separated from the animal, and put through a wound, made for that purpose, into the belly of a hen; which mode of turning hens into cocks is much such an improvement for utility as that of Dean Swift when he proposed to obtain a breed of sheep without wool" (cited in Jorgensen 15–16). Two points can be made here: one, Hunter imagines the possibility of a sex-change; and two, he fantasizes biological sex can bend easily to the will of a surgeon. In fact, hens bearing functional testicular grafts develop combs and wattles like a normal cock, but retain their female plumage and spurs (Jorgensen 15). This is perhaps why Hunter claimed that his experiment did not attain perfection.

In his *Physiological Lectures* of 1817, John Abernethy, president of London's Royal College of Surgeons and Hunter's former pupil, was still mulling over Hunter's pheasant, even though thirty-seven years had elapsed since Hunter's first publication of the essay in the Royal Society's *Philosophical Transactions*. Abernethy dwelled on the fact that Hunter had observed the "sexual character to have been annulled by age, the appropriate external signs were not only discontinued, but some times opposite ones were exhibited" (77–78). Sex, it would seem, refuses to become an essence. Abernethy continued, "He really seems interested in observing, that old women sometimes are bearded, and the old hen pheasant forms and displays the beautiful plumage of the male bird" (77). What Hunter discovered, though he did not know it, was that human beings have both "sex" hormones—testosterone and estrogen—and the balance of the two can shift as we age. Hunter's pupil concludes, "According to Mr. Hunter's notions of life, those occurrences which denote sexual character are to be considered as the effects of sympathies existing between remote parts of the body; which, like other instances of sympathy, are liable to occasional failure and considerable variation" (78–79). Abernethy's insistence that sexual character is the effect of sympathy between remote parts of the body highlights the centrality of sex to the body as well as its essentially fluid and variable nature. It is this variability that allows it to support arguments for equality and democracy. Once again, anatomy does not imply destiny.

This tenuousness of sexual differentiation thus is captured in the phrase that

William Lawrence, the surgeon, friend, and physician of the Shelleys, used to describe the sexes before puberty: an "equivocal state" ("Generation," n.p.).[45] Lawrence's emphasis on the tenuousness of puberty is especially surprising in light of the fact that Lawrence ascribes to the two-sex model: the "generative organs [of men and women] are different in kind; and their whole constitution has in each its particular type." Consequently, he dismisses out of hand unfounded analogies between the clitoris and penis. Nonetheless when he broaches the subject of puberty, Lawrence remarks, "it is however only at the epocha of puberty, . . . that the assemblage of all the sexual traits is exhibited to our observation . . . the particular differences . . . are not equally remarkable, and at one time cannot be distinctly traced." He continues, man's "equivocal state does not last long: man speedily assumes the features and character which mark his destination; his limbs lose their softness and the gentle forms which he partook with the female." Although it is true that Lawrence allows for the fact that the differences could have been there from the start—the problem is that we cannot see or recognize them—his attention to perceptual difference goes away when he describes the "equivocal state" of the male. These features are unequivocally grounded in his gentle limbs and originary softness. Once again, before puberty, the male is imagined as a feminized male, and, once again, biology will not quite underwrite complementarity. If the two sexes were originally one, sexual difference is potentially bridgeable, relational rather than incommensurate, and if the state of puberty could last as long as twenty-one years, the differences between ontological beings and states begin to evaporate. Conceiving of ontology both in terms of being and states allows ontology material plasticity, and perhaps explains Blake's interest in states of being.

This is not to say that the medical understanding of puberty was always necessarily helpful to equality. William Lawrence uses female puberty as evidence of her inferiority. Woman, by contrast to man, "departs from her primitive constitution less sensibly than man" ("Generation," n.p.). Lawrence's choice of "primitive" relegates women to an earlier evolutionary state even as it denies and discounts the actual transformations in women during puberty. If that weren't bad enough, Lawrence adds, "delicate and tender, she even retains something of the temperament belonging to children. The texture of her organs does not lose all its original softness." Yet the idea that the two sexes were originally one undermines the complementarity that he upholds. Likewise, if he, on the one hand, claims that the influence of "education and habits . . . is not sufficiently powerful to induce us to overlook the existence of a radical innate difference in the physical structure of the sexes," he, on the other hand, insists that "the influence of education, habits and customs, is so extensive, that it is difficult to distinguish between the results of these causes, and of the supposed original distinctions in organization." His emphasis on "supposed" undermines the radical innateness he sought to essentialize, as does his lack of clarity in the difference between what is innate and what belongs to culture.

Nonetheless, I want to develop the positive implications of Lawrence's term for capturing puberty, "equivocal state," particularly because "equivocal" itself slides from normality to perversion. Claudia Johnson has helped us to see the nuances of this term in *Equivocal Beings*, calling attention to how Wollstonecraft especially employed this term to distinguish real republican manhood over acculturated sentimentalized foppery, but Johnson misses the fact that "equivocal" referred both to a natural biological state, a state before puberty, and a kind of perverted being, a castrated male or hermaphrodite. That is to say, if prepubescent males are naturally effeminate, republican manhood is not so much an embodied ideal as it is a useful rhetorical device. Certainly, I am suggesting that Wollstonecraft was more aware of the costs of promoting republican manhood than Johnson credits her as being; indeed, Wollstonecraft's systematic unhooking of gender and strength, along with her collapse of mental and bodily strength, indicates the extent to which she sought to undermine the very foundation of patriarchy. Lawrence himself moves from the "equivocal state of puberty" to describing "equivocal individuals," beings who "have an acute voice, weak muscles, [and] a softness and laxity in the general organization." This missed fact of "equivocal's" slide from normal to pathological accounts for the rampant homophobia[46] of the period: all men went through puberty, so all men had the potential to stay in the "equivocal state." "Equivocal state," moreover, threatens to collapse difference between the sexes, especially if there were a connection between "equivocal states" and "equivocal beings." If both sexes went through the "equivocal state" of puberty, the sexed body could serve as a ground of similitude and difference, an instability that could prove useful to the discrediting of complementarity.

"Equivocal" further threatens the normative claims of heterosexual desire insofar as it destabilizes the sexed body itself. What would prevent, for example, one equivocal being for having desire for another equivocal being? This threat is especially dire given that Cullen suggested puberty could last as long as twenty-one years. The fine line between the effeminate sodomite and the prepubescent male not only underscores Eve Kosofsky Sedgwick's point that homophobia in the eighteenth century was not so much about the oppression of homosexual men as a means of organizing the entire spectrum of male relations (*Between Men* 88–91), but it also implies that perverse desires have their origins in normality. Indeed, perverse desires begin with a general skepticism in the very idea of absolute sexual difference, itself a contested site of normality.

In the context of these widespread medical debates about sexual difference, William Blake's ambiguously sexed figures, his muscular females, become a means of interrogating human relationships generally, rather than, as Anne Mellor suggests, a stylistic tic taken from Michelangelo.[47] Just as Mary Wollstonecraft and Mary Robinson suggest, superior male strength can no longer ground patriarchy; nor can male activeness justify male domination over female passivity. And just as these women ground their assertions of female strength in a common nervous body, Blake's poetry teems with allusions to nerves and nervous fibers.[48] Against a cultural backdrop that envisioned the human body as feminine at least before puberty, Blake masculinizes the human body and one outcome of this masculinization is that strength can no longer ground patriarchy. In the poet's most feminist work, *Visions of the Daughters of Albion*, Blake not only echoes Wollstonecraft's *Vindications of the Rights of Women* in his very title, suggesting that an echo does not have to be feckless, but also Oothoon refuses to accept a mind/body split and is open to the "moment of desire"(7:3 E 50). Blake scholars have long wrestled over identifying the sex of such figures as in Blake's *Jerusalem*, plate 28, copy D, not to mention various figures in the *Four Zoas* manuscript. The male and female chained together in the frontispiece to the *Visions* are depicted in such a way as to emphasize their anatomical similarities, not differences. By making it difficult for his readers to correlate gender and sex to his drawn bodies, Blake demands a reexamination of how gender/sex get mapped onto bodies.[49]

And if Blake saw sex not as an essence but as a biological process, the moths on the title-page to *Jerusalem* thus potentially refer to the bodily transformation into puberty—recalling John Hunter's likening of puberty to a mothlike metamorphosis. Hunter also pointed out that moths "are a long time in copulation. The large moth is some days" (*EO* 224), making them Blakean symbols of gratified desire. If the body could undergo such major changes as puberty and sexual differentiation, then the dynamic body could serve as a basis for the overall awakening into liberty that Blake's *Jerusalem* demands. That is to say, utopia can be grounded in a flexible and changeable body, one that does not restrain desire. To underscore this potential, Blake depicts the large female moth at the bottom of the title page in such a way as to suggest her wings already contain Los's globe of light found on the frontispiece to *Jerusalem* (notice the two orange circles around both sides of the moth's hair [Paley, plate 2]).The globes within her left wings are, at least in the Yale copy, the same color as Los's globe. This link between the moth and Los's light is heightened when the poet depicts the moth as translucent, rendering it with a light watercolor wash (plate 14) underneath God's rainbow. Moreover, by having "a moth of gold & silver mock[s] [Los's] anxious grasp" (*Jerusalem* 91:49), Blake puts bodily metamorphosis at odds with Los's "Ratio of Reason" (ibid.).

This makes all the more sense given that the goal of *Jerusalem* is to unite the fallen human body into the divine, a unification that cannot take place without a revolution in the ways in which people think about sexuality. Blake, of course, would have no truck with chastity as a virtue, and getting rid of fallen sexuality was critical to the human attainment of the divine. When we can see Los even in the wings of a moth, Blake suggests that we are steps closer to liberty. John Hunter's and William Lawrence's references to biological sex in terms of a state as opposed to in terms of being would also have been suggestive to the poet, whose figures insistently shift between states, classes, and beings.

In the *Book of Urizen*, Blake perhaps further questioned sex as an essence when he depicted the globe of life blood developing nervous fibers first. Only after "eternity on eternity," "At length in tears & cries imbodied/A female form trembling and pale/Waves before hid deadly face" (Plate 18:6–8 E 78). In the poet's view, nerves would seem to be the essential groundwork of the human body and only much later does he depict the "imbodiment" into female form. The poet's acute awareness of how sexual difference prevented fourfold vision opens the door to the possibility of his skeptical examination of sexual complementarity.

## From Puberty to Pederasty

Thus far I have shown how two ways of thinking about sex helped to make perversion an especially powerful form of leverage. It is because we have lost sight of the volatility of biological sex in the Romantic period that we have yet to understand fully how and why Voltaire, Jeremy Bentham, and Percy Shelley linked pederasty with puberty. Bentham in his manuscript "On Paederasty" sought to explain the "prevalence" of the homoerotic "taste": he did so by first ascribing it to "not an indifference to the proper object but of the difficulty of coming to the proper object" (92). Homoeroticism was the consequence of a homosocial boarding-school culture that made heterosexual relations difficult, but Bentham then proceeds to quote Voltaire, linking such desire with puberty.

As did Bentham, Shelley very probably got the connection between puberty and pederasty initially from Voltaire's very popular *Dictionnaire Philosophique*, a book that Shelley owned.[50] In the entry entitled "Amour Socratique," Voltaire wrote, "Young males of our species, raised together, and feeling the force of nature begin in them, and not finding any natural object for their instinct, fall back on what resembles them. Often a young boy, resembles for two or three years a beautiful girl, with the freshness of his complexion, the brilliance of his coloring, and the sweetness of his eyes; if he is loved it is because nature makes a mistake; one pays homage to the fair sex by attachment to one who owns its beauties, and when the years of resemblance disappear, the mistake ends" (17:180; translation mine). Crompton notes that "the earliest version of this essay began by asking, 'how did it come about that a vice which would destroy mankind if it were general, that a sordid outrage against nature, is still so natural? It seems the highest degree of deliberate corruption, and yet it is the ordinary lot of those who have not yet had the time to be corrupted'" (*Homosexuality and Civilization* 516).

Voltaire here raises a number of important issues for us to consider. He cannot avail himself of the excuse that boys who profess Socratic love are corrupted; consequently, he is forced into pitting nature against nature. But how can an "outrage against nature" be natural? The origin of perversion is thus in nature herself, a collapse that means deviation comes from within, and one that destabilizes the binary oppositions that legitimate social order. Voltaire's point that boys in puberty "fall back on resemblance" runs the danger of making desire itself homoerotic: sameness is the ground for desire as puberty shifts one sex into two. In fact, the very slipperiness of "resemblance," which after all contains difference within similitude, helps to insinuate homoeroticism into the natural process of puberty. Although the passage above makes clear that "resemblance" refers to the similarity of one feminized male to a female, resemblance can also refer to the resemblance of one feminized male to another feminized male. If homoeroticism is veiled by the feminization of the male—his androgynousness makes it possible to believe that desire is still intrinsically heterosexual—the ability of resemblance to straddle the homo/hetero divide hints that desire itself may not be based completely on difference.[51] The kind of thinking that understood the clitoris to be an analogous penis meant that resemblance could actually bridge the two sexes. In theory, then, heterosexual desire could resemble same-sex desire. Such instability is further heightened by the fact that biological sex moves from sameness to difference in puberty. For this reason, Voltaire insists that resemblance is merely a fallback position. Nonetheless, as the fallback position, resemblance as same-sex desire becomes ontologically prior to heterosexuality, a positioning that undermines the very naturalness of heterosexual desire.

"Homage is paid to the sex by attachment to one who owns its beauties," continues Voltaire. The original French reads: "On rend hommage au sèxe, en s'attachant à ce qui en à les beautés" (17:180). Lost in the translation is the reflexive verb, which implies that the work of attachment is being done by itself. (Imagine the denials that would be possible if English had reflexive verbs!) The problem, of course, is that at puberty females have no necessary monopoly on beauty, and *sèxe* here resists stabilization into biological sex. If males are feminine, then they can be beautiful, too. Here, we should recall Percy Shelley's insistence in his preface to his translation of Plato's *Symposium* that objects of erotic interest be first and foremost "as perfect and beautiful as possible" (D. Clark 222); almost as an afterthought, he will insist that erotic objects be natural. That the object of erotic attraction be natural comes in third, following temperance, hints that nature may be Shelley's afterthought.

The transition into puberty makes the materiality of the body no less slippery than language is; textualization refuses to liberate materiality into language just as materialization does so much more than constrain.[52] Recognition of this problem perhaps accounts for Voltaire's syntax: his stretching of pronouns and prepositions in *à ce qui en à* harnesses syntactical circumlocution to distance the objects, which passively become attached to each other. Voltaire's pronouns refer to ambiguous referents. Compounding the sexual confusions, Voltaire refers to this as *cette méprise de nature*, a phrase that either means a mistake by human beings about nature or the mistake (feminine gender) of (female) nature. In French, the feminine gender of nature and of mistake elides the two into one. To the extent that even nature may herself make this mistake, how are humans supposed to avoid it? Linguistic nuances coupled with nature's mistake further the naturalness of perversion.

All is not lost, however. At the end of puberty, which Voltaire limits to only a few years, "the resemblance disappears and the mistake ends" (17:180). Here, naturalizing the mistake complicates the ontology of mistake and, thus, the consequences for it. The resemblance of the feminized male to the female is so strong that even nature herself allows herself to be fooled. If even nature loses track of sex, how can man be blamed for same sex desire?

In his "Discourse on the Manners of the Antient Greeks," Percy Shelley, too, connects homoeroticism with puberty. Shelley cannot imagine sex between a man and an adolescent to be consensual, and thus he refers to it in terms of "so detestable a violation" (D. Clark 222). That sodomy is a crime punished by hanging in this period perhaps explains why Shelley's makes a show of his disgust.[53] The fact that he cannot imagine anal intercourse to be pleasurable—recall Erasmus Darwin's linking of the nerves of the anus with the penis—intensifies his disgust. Like Voltaire, Shelley figures homoeroticism in men as a particularly passive form of desire: the agent of sexuality is not really an agent. Here, however, is Shelley's reference to puberty:

> If we consider the facility with which certain phenomena connected with sleep, at the age of puberty, associate themselves with those images which are the objects of our waking desires; and even that in some persons of an exalted state of sensibility that a similar process can take place in reverie, it will not be difficult to conceive the almost involuntary consequences of a state of abandonment in the society of a person of surpassing attractions, when the sexual connection cannot exist, to be such as to preclude the necessity of so operose and diabolical machination as that usually described. (222)

Until now, critics have not understood why Shelley would connect pederasty to puberty.[54] Shelley seems to do so because he can thus understand homoeroticism as a prepubescent form of desire, and he can make that desire seem passive rather than active. In making homoeroticism essentially passive, Shelley asks why it results in the death penalty. Much in the same way that sexologists like Iwan Bloch, Havelock Ellis, and Magnus Hirschfeld made homosexuality a congenital form of identity to excuse it from criminal punishment, Shelley, Voltaire, and Bentham intimate that homosexual acts are involuntary and are, therefore, implicitly natural.[55] Hence how can they be punished?

Like Voltaire, who took refuge in language that displaced the agent behind the desire, Shelley connects sodomitic desire with nocturnal emissions, a natural—if perverse—wasting of sperm. Shelley's choice of "associate themselves" mirrors the work of Voltaire's French reflexive verb. Shelley needs to make this desire "involuntary," and to do so he obliquely refers to the fact that males before puberty are feminized males. What would prevent a female from seeking erotic relations with another female if the ground of difference were so vulnerable? But to align homoeroticism/pederasty with the natural process of puberty is to insist that such desire is part and parcel of a natural biological process and that the purported waste of sperm is likewise natural. If this is the case, Shelley's main point that homoeroticism would never have gained ground in Ancient Greece if women could have been considered objects of beauty, not to mention his claim that such male-male desire is "unnatural," falls away. The fact that Shelley finds contemporary Italian women no less ugly than Ancient Greek women potentially explains the prevalence of sodomy in current Venice.

Lending even further weight to this universalizing narrative about perverse desires is the fact that Shelley includes "persons of an exalted state of sensibility" like himself in the group of those who might have been led astray. Although Shelley in this essay tries to insulate contemporary Britain from pederasty, his connection of it to puberty, a connection that he could have gotten as well from his friend, William Lawrence, insists on a universalizing narrative of sodomitic desire. That universalizing narrative was further strengthened by the poet's later admission in his prose fragment on friendship that male-male friendship must be "wholly divested of the smallest alloy of sensuality" (D. Clark 338). His choice of "divest" leaves open the possibility that male-male friendships are inherently sensual: after all, one cannot divest a thing of what it does not have. The fact that this desire is passive—that the subject never actively seeks it—heightens a universalizing vulnerability to it. Such universal vulnerability suggests that Shelley is thinking in terms of homoeroticism generally and that he is not limiting homosexual desire to a specific kind of relations between a boy and a man. Perhaps for this reason, the poet refers to pederasty as an "operose and diabolical machination" (D. Clark 222). The danger of course is that heterosexual desire will revert to its homoerotic origins: homoerotic here stands in for same sex and the possibility that there is really only one sex. Desire is based on "resemblance."

## We Are All Potential Hermaphrodites

Romantic puberty shows not only the tenuous ground of sexual difference, but also the instability of heterosexual desire in the Romantic period.[56] Medical interest in hermaphrodites was another key symptom of that instability. This is even the case as surgeons, men-midwives, and doctors sought to shift the ground of the discussion on hermaphrodites from ontology to epistemology: medical writers in this period grow increasingly skeptical of the existence of human hermaphrodites and begin to insist that hermaphrodites are really a mistake of judgment rather than an ontological ambiguity. This skepticism was the logical result of the raising of the stakes in the definition of a hermaphrodite: a hermaphrodite now had to have two sets of functioning genitals to be considered a true hermaphrodite. Notwithstanding this shift of uncertainty from being to issues of professional competence, medical understanding of hermaphrodites demonstrates once again that sex resists bifurcation. Moreover, the biologist Joan Roughgarden speculates that "hermaphroditism is more common in the world than species who maintain separate sexes in separate bodies" (31). There is simply no getting around the ambiguities of sexed bodies and sexual desire. Even wishing away of the possibility of human hermaphroditism did nothing to refute the existence of what we now call intersexed individuals, people with ambiguous genitalia.

To wit, M. Vacherie, surgeon from Brussels, comments on Michael-Anne Drouart, as she/he was being shown in Carnaby Street, London, that "when it was born, it was so strongly marked with the Types or Characters of both the Male and Female Sex, . . . they gave it the two Christian names of Michael and of Anne" (4). Vacherie continues, "As it grew up, the Predominion which they imagined observed of the Female part, determined them to call it a girl" (4). By distancing himself from *their* imagined sense of a predominion, Vacherie hopes to enable a medical perspective to unravel this conundrum, this grammatical it. He therefore looks closely at Michael-Anne's genitals and determines it to be imperforate penis, one tied down by a frenum, which prevents penetration. When the eye fails, Vacherie inserts a probing finger into the subject's "vulva" and finds no clitoris. "There is no appearance of that round and glanduous body in this subject, which is doubtless absorbed, and supplemented by the penis" (10). Two problems arise: first, how can he be sure this is a penis, especially when it does not have a "proper passage or conduit for the seed" (8)? Second, whereas other medical writers would have argued this to be a clitoris since an imperforate penis was considered to be a clitoris, how can Vacherie know that the clitoris was absorbed and supplemented by the penis? The word "doubtless" is perhaps a key symptom of Vacherie's epistemological panic, a panic intensified by the penis's origin as a clitoris.

Vacherie, it turns out, must rely upon the subject's declaration of sexual "inclination towards the female sex" to call this organ a penis (17), a reliance that not only demonstrates that the patient has greater purchase upon sexual knowledge than a surgeon, but also undermines Vacherie's authority to name this organ a penis. In keeping with his need to arrest ambivalence, Vacherie decides that the "vulva" must really be a "passage designed to do the office of the urethra" (16–17). Notwithstanding his minute visual and physical examination of the body, Vacherie can only conclude, "ambiguity of sex diffused through the whole body. And upon the whole, it is plain to the Public, is possest of such exterior distinct marks of the male and female sexes; as make it doubtful to which this equivocal being belongs" (17). Despite his knowledge of the bodily interior, Vacherie is reduced to the public common knowledge of bodily surfaces and the manipulation of language. Forcing ambiguity to testify to the male sex, Vacherie must bend the body's intransigence to his categories to his will.

Like Vacherie, George Arnauld, surgeon of London, opens his 1750 *Dissertation on Hermaphrodites*, perhaps inauspiciously by announcing that "whatever degree of accuracy and wisdom nature employs in the composition and frame of the human body, we have oftener seen her swerve from these, and as it were, forget herself" (9). If nature "swerves" from wisdom and accuracy as she composes the human body in much the same way that perversion marks a turning the wrong way, and if she does so more often than not, then what is the ontology of perversion? Perversion's very grounding in nature allows artists of the period to destabilize this opposition even further to their own benefit. In trying to account for variations among human beings, Arnauld implies that nature becomes bored—she is "tired out and spent with producing every day the same things over and over"—and thus she "throw[s] into her productions a variety but little conformable to her laws" (9–10).

Elaborating upon the very fickleness of nature, Arnauld claims that she

> sometimes withholds from the body the parts the most necessary; in another subject, she is pleased to multiply them, often allots them situations, connections, and dimensions, the most extraordinary and fantastical; she separates what, according her own laws, should be joined, and joins what ought to remain separate: hence arise those deformities in the strokes or features, those members ill-articulated, those disproportions, those imperfections of organical parts, and those combinations, so monstrous and out of the common road, that it is with difficulty we discover nature even in nature herself.

What began as a list of innocuous varieties soon sprawls into deformities and monstrosities. If nature cannot be found even in nature, and if even nature violates the very laws she presumably creates, the origin of perversion must be found in nature herself. Arnaud pushes this point to its logical conclusion when he coyly adds that "some affirm Adam was a hermaphrodite before the fall" (14). This reminds us that even God thought of the two sexes and sexual differentiation only as an afterthought. Arnauld does, however, insist that one can "with difficulty" find nature within nature. A true medical specialist can do it, he hopes.

Even more perplexing are Arnaud's categories for thinking about hermaphrodites. After defining "hermaphrodites" as "him or her, in whom the parts, which form the essential difference between the two sexes, are found together, either perfectly or imperfectly" (11), Arnauld divides hermaphrodites into four categories: male hermaphrodites, female hermaphrodites, perfect hermaphrodites, and imperfect hermaphrodites (14). While his definition already begs the question that if the two parts can be found together, how can they speak to an essential difference, the fact that Arnaud states that the "bad formation of parts of generation cannot be a hermaphrodite" rubs against his categories of imperfect and perfect because the imperfect hermaphrodite is categorically not a hermaphrodite.

Fanning the flames of confusion, Arnauld then describes beings "with a penis of the man, yet without being perforated like it, makes them almost resemble eunuchs, who can enjoy coition without the perfect consummation of the venereal act" (18). Lumping these under "a subject ill organized which can not [*sic*] properly be called an Hermaphrodite," Arnaud once again threatens to empty out the signifier of hermaphrodite, launching instead into a chain of signifiers: hermaphrodite, eunuch, tribade. Materiality of the body becomes the materiality of medical language. Yet, since they almost resemble eunuchs, they cannot properly be called eunuchs either. As a result, Arnauld then labels them tribades, those who "have the impudence to act the part of a man with your own sex, and make yourself pass for one" (18).

Seeking to reassure his European readers, Arnauld then informs them that "these sort of women are pretty rare in Europe, but formerly were common in Egypt" (19), though he does remind his readers of the very recent example of Anne Grand-Jean. By the end of what begins as a seemingly clear *Dissertation on Hermaphrodites*, hermaphrodites have become ontological oxymorons who can only be embodied in a chain of signifiers insofar as the hermaphrodite's body is always exceeding language. Yet it is their ability to straddle even the most deliberate of categories that makes them testify to the ambiguities of biological sex in the Romantic period and the inability of medical science to arrest biological sex, no matter how elaborate the taxonomic schemes. At the heart of the eighteenth-century hermaphrodite, then, was a resemblance between material-

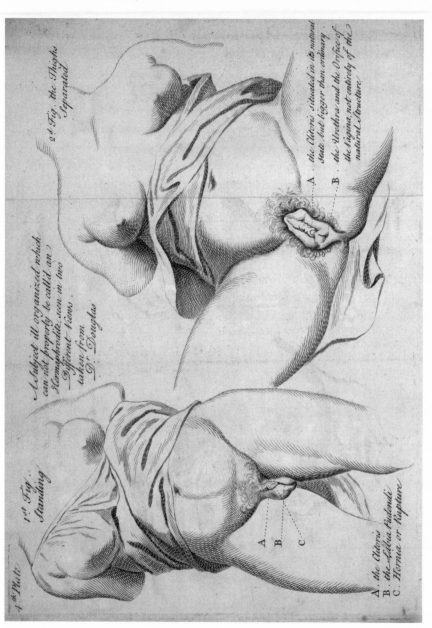

George Arnaud de Ronsil, from *A Dissertation on Hermaphrodites*, 1750. Courtesy of the National Library of Medicine, Bethesda, Maryland.

ity and language, a kind of textualized body that manifested the ambiguities of sex itself.

The great John Hunter did not think of hermaphroditism as a matter of key concern in animals at least; it took "no great effort or uncommon play in nature to unite them in those animals in which they are commonly separated" (*Observations* 46). Hunter even looked to hermaphrodites to solve the problem of evolution: what triggered the dimorphism of sex? In a footnote, Hunter remarked, "Is there ever in the genera of animals, that are natural hermaphrodites, a separation of the two parts forming distinct sexes? If there is, it may account for the distinction of sexes ever having happened" (*Observations* 46). The very fact that he can think beyond human sexual dimorphism, even imagine hermaphrodites to be an evolutionary link between sexual monism and dimorphism, suggests why complementarity did not automatically become law.

Hunter's thinking about hermaphrodites grows more interesting and more vexed as he contemplates human forms of this monstrosity. Because he thought of the clitoris and penis as essentially the same part, as we have seen, he thought it "impossible for one animal to have both a penis and a clitoris; the part which they have must of course partake of both sexes" (*Observations* 47). Hunter's ability to read sameness onto difference prevents him from imagining a human hermaphrodite with both a clitoris and penis.

But, as in medical treatments of hermaphrodites generally, any promised clarity quickly dissolves. Hunter divided hermaphrodites into two classes: the first, "a union of the two sexes, . . . which is the most common; and the parts of the one [sex being] formed like those of the other" (*EO* 1:249). The sexual parts "are as subject to malformation as is any other part of an animal, and they are subject to a monstrosity [to which] no other part can be well subject" (*EO* 249). Why does Hunter need a distinction between malformation and monstrosity, especially given that he has just made "bad formation" one of the classes of monsters (*EO* 248)? Hunter then labels the former, the common hermaphroditism, "natural hermaphrodites," but even they can "admit of monstrosity" (*EO* 249). Now the categories blur further: natural hermaphrodites are not necessarily monsters. Once again perversions of nature are partly natural. He elaborates,

> We can make out the different parts of the sexes in a monstrous hermaphrodite much better than in the natural one; because we are perfectly well acquainted with the parts in the instances of their perfect division, as in the distinct sexes; but we are not so well acquainted with the distinct parts in the natural hermaphrodite; be-

cause they are not so similar to those in the distinct sexes. If we could have a monster from a natural hermaphrodite, in which the parts of one of other of the two sexes only were formed, then we might make out the parts, as they are combined, in the natural hermaphrodite. There are all degrees of monstrous hermaphroditical formations. It may be in a small degree or great degree in every part peculiar to the distinction of the sexes; or it may be only in one of the parts which distinguishes the one sex from the other. The occurrence in one sex of a peculiarity of the other, may be of three kinds. The first is a similarity of a whole that is common to both sexes, such as the body generally, but which has, naturally a shape peculiar to each: for example, when a woman is shaped like a man, or a man shaped like a woman. The second is a similarity of a part which is common to both sexes, but which has naturally a size peculiar to each; as where the (clitoris) of the female imitates in size the penis of the male; the breast of a male imitating that of the female; . . . The third is where the peculiarity of one sex is added to another; as an ovarium added to a male, or a testis added to a female. (249–50)

Among the interesting paradoxes here are the fact that monstrous hermaphrodites make normal sexual distinctions more visible than natural hermaphrodites; as the categories of monstrous hermaphrodites explode, hermaphroditism threatens to become more common than natural sexual development, and the shift to degrees of monstrosity leads to a treatment of degrees of sexual shape of men and women along with the common part that men and women share, one that is only distinguished by size. If hermaphroditism is too common, how do we know what is natural? That hermaphroditism can be tricky to localize exacerbates the situation, because it points out that sexual difference itself is not easily localized. Note, for example, how sexual difference has become linguistic simile: "shaped like a man." Hunter's insistence upon a language of mimesis whereby the clitoris "imitates" the penis and the breast of the male "imitates" the female's runs the danger of reducing sexual difference to mimicry.

Finally, if sexual difference is really about differences of degree and not kind in that a penis is just a bigger clitoris and that a woman is shaped "like" a man and vice versa, the very perceptual differences between the sexes that Hunter seems to take for granted threaten to dissolve away. Thus, it is hardly surprising that Hunter himself ends his discussion of hermaphroditism in uncertainty. Describing a child, born at Brownlow Street Hospital, Hunter wrote that he "had what I should have called a divided scrotum, and the penis lying beneath the divisions; but it turned out to be a female. The external parts were the two labia, which were corrugated . . . transversely" (*EO* 1:250). When Hunter insists that he "should have called" the parts a scrotum—when in fact he claims they are labia—sexual difference has again returned to nominalism, and refuses to be grounded securely in the body. The net gain, however, is a sense of materiality—perhaps a surgeon's sense of materiality—that is open to rather than resistant to change.

Matthew Baillie's *The Morbid Anatomy of Some of the Most Important Parts of the Human Body* (1793), one of the very first books on pathological anatomy published originally in English, also sought to make hermaphrodites a mistake of medical judgment, rather than an ontological ambiguity.[57] Baillie's work reached eight editions (Rodin 23). Although Baillie acknowledges at the outset that there many diseases with "morbid actions only" that do not "produce any change in the structure of parts" of the body (i), pathological anatomy must confine itself to diseases that have altered structures, ones that can be localized, or else anatomy has nothing to add to our knowledge of disease. Baillie shrewdly added a list of symptoms to each chapter in the second edition (Rodin v), an addition that sought to bridge the gap between dead bodies and live ones, but one that threatened to confuse subjectively felt symptoms with scientific localized diseased structures. But once again hermaphrodites raise unanticipated problems: for example, while commenting on mistaken hermaphrodites, Baillie defines an enlarged clitoris as a natural defect, yet if the defect is natural, what separates pathological anatomy from anatomy itself? Baillie writes,

> An enlarged clitoris is also a natural defect. At birth, the clitoris in such a case is often larger than the penis of a male child of the same age. It has a well formed prepuce and glans, together with a fissure at its extremity, so as to resemble almost exactly the external appearance of the male organs. These cases have given rise to a mistake, with regard to the sex, and females have been often baptized for males. On most, however, where there is an enlarged clitoris, the sex may be determined by the following circumstances. The labia are well formed, and when handled, no round bodies are felt in them, like the testicles. The fissure at the extremity of the glans does not lead to any canal of the urethra, but under the glans, and at the posterior extremity of the fissure, there is an opening which leads immediately to the bladder. I should believe, that by putting a small straight probe into this orifice, and passing it into the bladder, it could be at once determined on most occasions, whether the child was male or female. If the child should live to grow up, the clitoris enlarges, but, I believe, not in the same proportion as the penis would do. It

is a most unfortunate monstrosity, because it depresses the mind, by a consciousness of imperfect formation in a very important part of the body. Such cases have
often been mistaken for hermaphrodites. (283–85)

Baillie tellingly classifies the mistaken hermaphrodite under "diseased appearances of the external parts" (283), firmly rooting the elongated clitoris within
pathology. Notwithstanding the discipline of pathological anatomy, the trou-
bling ontological issues that Baillie sought to extirpate will not quite go away.
For example, if an enlarged clitoris is a "natural defect," how does one use the
enlarged clitoris to explain the possibility of unnatural Sapphic desire? And how
does one know an enlarged clitoris from a normal one? How large is too large?
Baillie must make sure that the hermaphroditic patients he describes had no desire for either sex. "Natural defect," I might add, merely substitutes one ontological confusion—how can defects be mistakes of nature?—for another, how
can one sex look like another? If one needs to physically probe the body to determine its sex, sexual difference cannot be a visual difference. Also, why does
Baillie limit himself to "most cases": what does it mean when the scientific
probe can't invariably penetrate to the truth? Finally, I note the shift from scientific probing of the body to belief: the doctor believes that the woman's clitoris will not continue to grow as a man's penis does. What beyond clitoris envy
might allow him to ground this claim in mere belief? Once again, the two sexes
threaten to dissolve into one.

In his appendix to the *Morbid Anatomy*, Baillie treats a second and perhaps
even more disturbing example of hermaphroditism, lumping this one under
"diseased appearances of the vagina" (Appendix 138). Despite admitting that
she is a real hermaphrodite, Baillie seeks through classification under diseases
of the vagina to do away with ambiguous ontology and to locate hermaphroditism firmly within the female sex and within pathology. "Appearance," however, threatens to undermine the authority of pathology. He writes, "She wears
the apparel of a woman. She has a remarkably masculine look, with plain features, but no beard. She had never menstruated; and on this account she was de-
sired by the lady with whom she lived as a servant, to become an out patient at
the Nottingham Hospital. . . . The vagina was found to terminate in a cul-de-
sac, two inches from the external surface of the labia. The head of the clitoris,
and the external orifice of the meatus urinae, appeared as in the natural structure of a female, but there were no nymphae. The labia were more pendulous
than usual, and contained each of them a body resembling a testicle of a mod-

erate size, with its chord. The mammae resembled those of a woman. The person had no desire or partiality whatever for either sex" (Appendix 139–40). Here, masculine look collides with feminine dress, and natural structures of the female collide with labia that are really scrotums. Baillie elides the appearance of disease in the female vagina with her physical look of masculinity, an elision that attempts to make appearance have scientific weight. Yet, whereas in the first example, Baillie's medical knowledge could arrest the mystery at least provisionally—that hermaphrodite was really a mistaken perception—here the doctor can only speak the language of resemblance and appearances, a language that commits to perception but not to claims of ontology. It turns out that both the mistaken and real hermaphrodite only lead to claims about perception. Baillie's very insistence upon resemblances raises the question if sex is more about appearance or ontology.

Like Baillie and Hunter, Everard Home tries to make hermaphrodites an epistemological problem in his "Account of the Dissection of an Hermaphrodite Dog," published in the Royal Society's *Philosophical Transactions* (1799). Not surprisingly, he comments that, "in the female, there are two malformations of the organs of generation, which give an appearance to the external parts, tending to *mislead the judgment* respecting sex" (162; emphasis mine). The first is a large clitoris, which he attributes to a hot climate. Home believes the accounts of large clitorises are wholly exaggerated, except in the case of Mandigo women, one of whom had a clitoris of three inches in length (163). That is to say, he hopes that British women do not suffer so. "The large clitoris is very common among Mandingo." The second is a prolapsed uterus, which can resemble a penis (164). Baillie had also argued that an inverted vagina "has sometimes been mistaken for that species of monstrous formation called hermaphrodite" (280).[58]

Lapsed judgment, though, cannot account for all hermaphrodites. To wit, Home cites Baillie's second example of a person with a pendulous labia containing a testicle. He also cites the example of a man who gave suck to a child of two months (171). Home then speculates why such examples can occur. He writes,

> In considering the influence of the testicles upon the constitution of the male, which is rendered so evident by contrasting it with those cases in which the testicles are imperfect, it leads to a supposition, that the ovaria may have a similar influence upon the constitution of the female; and that when the ovaria are imperfectly formed, or when the testicles are substituted for them, although the external parts are decidedly female, the person may grow up, deprived of that feminine

character which the constitution would have acquired, if the ovaria had been capable of producing their influence upon the body. To this cause may be attributed the unnatural bias which some women have shewn, to pass through life in the character of men. The circumstance of some women, after the time of breeding is over, (at which period the influence of the ovaria may be considered as lost to the constitution,) approaching nearer to the male in appearance, and acquiring a beard. (172–73)

I have quoted this passage at some length because it is much more complicated than it might seem. Although sex looks anatomical given that testicles and ovaries influence the body, there are a number of strange features to this discussion that anatomy does not quite explain. First, Home thinks about ovaries and testicles as interchangeable rather than as incommensurate organs. Second, he is quite comfortable analogizing from the male to the female: analogy bridges the gaps between the sexes, a point that undermines complementarity. Ovaries have similar influence as the testicles. Third, Home opens the door to bodies "with decidedly female parts" that nevertheless lack a female character, a gap that insists that gender does not necessarily coincide with sex. The presence of such a gap should undermine the idea that the Romantics understood sex as gender. Fourth, when women undergo menopause and begin to look like men, if the ovaries no longer influence the woman, what accounts for her transformation into masculinity? This masculinization suggests that the sexes are really one masculine sex until the ovaries take over. If not, what anatomical feature accounts for this masculinization? And how can an arrested ovary explain an increased masculinization if it is the testicle that performs the office of masculinization? In any event, this 1799 article should put definitively to bed the idea that until sexology and the rise of psychiatric knowledge, anatomy exhausted sex. Sex in this period was unusually recalcitrant to material fixity.

All of this conjecture leads to a stunning conclusion. Home suggests that all human beings at the outset have hermaphroditic potential insofar as the "ovum, previous to impregnation, [has] no distinction of sex, but [is] formed as to be equally fitted to become a male or a female foetus; and that it is the process of impregnation which marks the distinction, and conduces to produce wither testicles or ovaria, out of the same materials" (175). Home did not know how close to the truth he was: that the clitoris and penis begin from the same embryonic structure and until about the eighth week coexist in the fetus (Laqueur 1990 169). His conclusion nonetheless undermines the notion of complementarity inasmuch as all fetuses are potential hermaphrodites: they all have the capacity to grow both sets of genitals. He adds further that "the clitoris, originally, appears therefore equally fitted to be a clitoris or penis" (Home 176). Because ovaries and testes are made out of the very same material, sex and bodily materiality are understood as flexible rather than as given. Moreover, if ovaria can substitute for the testes, this implies that hermaphroditic potential is not necessarily limited to the fetus. Although he began by linking hermaphrodites with "errors of judgment," then Home cannot wish away hermaphrodites by stronger professionalization, greater knowledge. The ambiguities of sex are here to stay because we all have hermaphroditic potential. Such potential suggests that the division of sexes into complementarity can be undone and that the human body, as Blake imagined, can be reunited into a whole in spite of its sexual divisions.

We still argue today over what the Romantics understood about biological sex. Anne Fausto-Sterling has sought to destabilize and dismantle the two-sex model, which has become ontology, doxa. Focusing on intersexual births (estimated as 1.7% of all births), Fausto-Sterling proposes instead that there are really five sexes: males, females, herms (hermaphrodites), merms (pseudo-male hermaphrodites), and ferms (female pseudo-hermaphrodites) (78). By acknowledging the ontology of the intersexed as legitimate and natural, Fausto-Sterling hopes that these new categories will help stop what is for her the barbarous practice of infant genital surgery, which can cause scarring, often requires multiple surgeries, and can eliminate the possibility of having an orgasm. In a larger view, Fausto-Sterling's five sexes are designed to get at how gender and sex become somatic facts (235). Cautioning that sex is a developmental biocultural system and not a static entity, Fausto-Sterling reminds us that anatomic function and how one experiences one's sexual body change over time (242). Like Fausto-Sterling, Joan Roughgarden examines the ways in which biology has understated and pathologized the sexual diversity of the animal kingdom, and she even suggests that hermaphrodism is the norm of the animal kingdom (2004 31). Moreover, she argues that, although biologists understand males as the producers of small gametes while females produce large gametes, they often wrongly assume that the gamete size binary translates into corresponding "binaries in body types, behaviour, and life history" (26). Even this seemingly secure definition of sex in terms of gamete size can be undermined if we consider that although the egg is about a million times the size of a sperm, the totality of sperm (1,000,000) in an ejaculate is roughly equivalent to the size of the egg.[59]

In his study of the neuroanatomy of the libido, Donald Pfaff agrees that sex is part of a developmental biocultural system, and he illustrates this by showing how in arousal the "hormones as internal signals have molecular sequelae that interact with synaptic inputs from the external stimuli to control behavior" (48). Warning that it is incorrect to state that hormones control behavior, Pfaff argues instead that sexual arousal is a complex orchestration of external and internal influences (100) involving, among other actors, the hindbrain, midbrain, and the forebrain, physiological and biochemical processes in the testicles and ovaries, the endocrine glands, and other anatomical pathways.

In sum, because of competing ways of thinking about sex in Romanticism, sexuality was rife for liberation. Not only did a one-sex model undermine the idea that the sexes were both incommensurably different and complementary, but also perversion had the power to undermine ideas of the natural, especially those like feminine sensibility that buttressed patriarchy. To make matters worse, when even nature makes mistakes or swerves from her path, why should human beings be punished for similar errors? Together, such medical concerns as a fundamentally neurological body, castration, eunuchs, the descent of the testicle, and hermaphroditism made it possible to think in terms of sexual equality. If these topics further underscored the legacy of the one-sex model, the French Revolution made it difficult for hierarchy to be naturalized in a sexed body. Insofar as puberty transformed one feminized sex into two, it brought to crisis both sexual difference and the necessary heterosexuality of human desire, and it had the potential to do so within every human body. The body's plasticity and the mobility of sex explain why Voltaire, Bentham, and Percy Shelley would turn to puberty to help explain same-sex desire. By aligning same-sex desire with a natural rite of passage, they helped universalize homosexual desire and suggest that desire was based upon resemblance rather than difference. Read in this light, perversion and normalcy were part of a continuum, not a binary opposition, and thus the trick was to persuade others of this continuum and its consequences. Finally, to the extent that it was possible to see sex as something inscribed upon the body by both biology and culture, one could begin to question whose interests were served by the forms of inscription sex took.

# CHAPTER FOUR

# The Perverse Aesthetics of Romanticism

## Purposiveness with Purpose

Until this point, I have shown the extent to which function became the gold standard of biological knowledge. I have also indicated that this standard was under enormous pressure by virtue of the fact that one could not ascertain function without the "perversity" of nonfunctioning organs. The scientific separation of sexual pleasure from reproductive function did not help. Biology sought to exile the perverse from the domain of knowledge; nonetheless, that exile betrayed indebtedness to the perverse for its knowledge. Such a vexed relation to the perverse explains how scientists could extol function yet recognize the limits of thinking about biological organisms in terms of function. Read under the aegis of function, the body becomes reduced to parts and not wholes, and one loses a holistic sense of how the organism interacts with its environment.

As scientists began to insist upon function as the criterion for biological knowledge, they defined life itself in terms of purposiveness to counter the limitations of limiting the body to function: otherwise will becomes reduced to blind instinct. Scientists of the period needed Kantian purposiveness because it enabled them to do away with final causes and thus limit their work to the empirical. Moreover, Robert Richards has shown the extent to which Romantic biologists found Kantian purposiveness helpful: "The biologist judges an organism to be purposiveness according to a specific plan of which he can become aware—even if he cannot determinatively claim the plan was indeed the cause of the organism" (71). At the same time, as life became understood in terms of purposiveness, aesthetics consolidated itself around a resistance to function and to self-interest. Because purpose, function, and self-interest threatened to reduce art to determinism, mere bodily appetite, or mere subjectivity, aesthetics not only positioned itself against function, but also insisted that aesthetic apprehension was central to freedom and liberation: after all, how could one approach the condition of freedom if one were enslaved by purpose? Yet, in much the same way scientists were beholden to the perverse despite their wariness of it, aestheticians needed purpose despite their declared resistance to it or aesthetics would lose its educative function, its capacity for *Bildung*, aesthetic education.

The inability of aesthetics to actualize an ideal self prompts Marc Redfield to label it a "phantom formation:"[1] one that needs an educative function even when it denounces function. Like scientists, aestheticians turned to purposiveness because it enabled the art critic to judge a painting as purposive, without then having to specify "the plan or rules by which beauty has been produced" (R. Richards 71). As the Romantic cult of genius made it necessary to declare one's flouting of the rules, purposiveness became all the more useful because it offered an account of origin without having to specify it. At the simplest level, the discourses of aesthetics and science could meet because medicine was one of a few career alternatives for educated men. To wit, Winckelmann, Kant, Percy Shelley, and Keats all studied medicine, and Coleridge had long-standing interests in both aesthetics and medicine.

Here I argue that insofar as aesthetic purposiveness suspends function, it is an important form of perversity. In a larger view, this chapter asks why a distrust of interest, purpose, and function can be so valued within aesthetics—marking aesthetics off from other more worldly and interested forms of apprehension—and so anathemized within sexuality.[2] Although rarely seen as such, aesthetics, in other words, has often been another name for perversion—given its usual distrust of function, interest, and purpose—and as such it provides a useful lens for thinking about and revaluing sexuality without function or reproduction. Rather than being simply unnatural, sex without regard to function can lead to freedom: as Kant and Schiller argue, it is only by casting aside purpose that one can approach the condition of freedom. Under the aegis of love, sex can resist purpose, seeking instead the form of purposive mutuality.

Part of the reason why aestheticians take aesthetics and sexuality to be in-commensurate discourses is that sexuality seems antithetical to *Bildung*. Where sexuality is conventionally aligned with reproduction, aesthetics is to stand out-side the immediate demands of purpose while nonetheless leading to *Bildung*. Hegel argued that "art has the capacity and the function of mitigating the fierceness of the desires" and by this he meant "eliminating brutality and tam-ing and educating the impulses, desires, and passions" (53). Instead of thinking about sexuality and aesthetics necessarily in terms of difference and conflict, the Romantics thought that both could lead to *Bildung* as long as sexuality was not necessarily reduced to reproduction and as long as something like aesthetic pur-poselessness kept purpose at bay while allowing aesthetics to educate. To vary-ing degrees, Coleridge, Longinus, Burke, Winckelmann, and Payne Knight wed aesthetics and sexuality by reorienting them both toward purposiveness, which is to say, perversity. They could do so in part because Longinus, Payne-Knight, and Winckelmann demonstrated sexuality, even a perverse sexuality, to be a cornerstone of aesthetic education, at least in Ancient Greek thought. In-deed, the discovery of the ruins of Herculaneum and Pompei cemented connec-tions between a neoclassical aesthetics, the obscene, and a sodomitic culture.[3]

As names for the absence of function, perversion and aesthetics share a mu-tual distrust of function, but this distrust does not do away with the need to have a function. The perverse aesthetics of Romanticism has two distinguishing fea-tures that seem to contradict each other. On the one hand, Romantic writers de-clare their hostility to purpose, and figure Romantic artworks as organic living organisms that have purposiveness. Biology literally informs art. On the other hand, they align themselves with perversity and purposiveness precisely to lib-erate human sexuality from reproduction and aesthetics from the nitty-gritty demands of purpose. Hence, in various ways, Kant, Coleridge, Burke, Longi-nus, Winckelmann, and Payne Knight link aesthetic apprehension with free-dom, connect purposiveness/perversity to liberation and yet, in so doing, grant even sexual perversity a purpose. The scientific separation of sexual pleasure from function meant that sexuality could take the form of purposive mutuality instead of being about what Sade dismissed as the "dull business of population" (201). That purposiveness in Sade's case was for the express purpose of celebrat-ing the anarchy of waste and in the process doing away with such cherished no-tions as motherhood. By separating sexuality from reproduction, and, by think-ing about sexuality as having the form of purposiveness, one could thereby evaluate whether the forms that liberation took actually achieved liberation, and for whom. In a larger view, perversion facilitates the overturning of the standard view that links aesthetics to waste or uselessness and understands that waste to be a "secondary supplement to the utility value of a product" (Zizek 247). It is, rather, the use that is a "'secondary' profit of a useless object whose production cost a lot of energy in order to serve as a fitness indicator" (ibid.).[4] From the standpoint of evolution, then, waste functions as a form of purposiveness.

The solution was to endow aesthetics with a purposiveness with purpose. "Purposiveness with purpose" amounts to a perverse take on Kant who defined beauty as "purposiveness without purpose." Although none of the Romantics ascribed to "purposiveness without purpose," Kant's original formulation does matter because it is about the link between the problem of reading nature as having ends—Is sex for reproduction? Is reproduction its end? If other ends are achieved, are they the ends it was meant for?—and an aesthetic that sees the ends of art as occurring only when one treats art as without purpose. Aesthetic apprehension sees objects without reference to their actual ends. But aesthetic apprehension has a purpose for Kant, regardless of how it apprehends objects: it shows us how to look at the world as ethically meaningful without making the philosophically untenable claim that any transcendent force created that meaning. Kant replaces purpose with the concept of the objective purposiveness of nature. In like manner, one may split sex from its function, engage in it without intended end, and that engagement will take on an ethical or political significance. And in like manner, one may think that the ends of art may only be achieved if one treats art as without end and these issues come together when the art directs itself toward the discussion of sex.

But this purposive aesthetics had an even more insistent purpose. Romantic writers turned perversely toward an insistent sexuality within their aesthetics, creating an eroticized aesthetics that sought to blur the lines separating poet and audience through a common nervous physiology. Shelley thus imagined another "with a frame whose nerves . . . vibrate with the vibrations of our own" (Essay "On Love" Reiman and Fraistat 2002 504): the echo between "vibrate" and "vibration" seeks to enact such intersubjectivity while allowing for difference. In placing so much emphasis on what might be considered sordid sensuality, the Romantics perverted aesthetics by bringing aesthetics dangerously close to the feckless, fleeting, and passive pleasures of the body, what Kant considered mere sensation or agreeableness, not aesthetic judgment, and what the philosopher Jerrold Levinson labels improper pleasure (13–16). They gave

pride of place to the sexual in their aesthetics in order to engage and move readers by appealing to common desires, feelings, and affects because such emotions
make action possible. My emphasis on perversity expands our sense of Romantic aesthetics by acknowledging the swoon of pleasure in Romantic art, one that
is deliberately at odds with the rational force of a stance. By perverse, I also
mean to capture the reasons why so much of Blake's, Byron's, and Percy Shelley's erotic imagery resists reproduction, why they link sex with purposeless
love instead of reproduction.

Of course, this aesthetic strategy had great risk. Shelley and Byron had to re-
tract some of their more risqué remarks; Blake's *Four Zoas* manuscript bears the
traces of censorship. Nonetheless, they realized that even improper aesthetic
pleasure need not automatically entail selfishness, mere physicality, and ephemerality because it could enhance love. Turning away from the necessary selfishness of marriage, Shelley uses sibling incest to embody disinterest, a strategy
that undermines the idea that sexual desire is necessarily about use and interest.
More important, sexual desire without reproduction was not necessarily feckless insofar as it united couples in a bond of mutual purposiveness. If the com-
parison of aesthetic pleasure to sexual pleasure risks ephemerality and mere
bodily sensation, it gains potential physiological impact upon the body, the bite
of materiality. By reminding audiences that aesthetics originates in a sensate
body, a body that is often denied within aesthetics, Romantic writers not only
revalued the physical, but also asked how aesthetics could cut itself off from its
very source of strength in the name of disinterest. Through incarnation, fantas-
matic or actual, historical signification acquires the status of inarticulate but
palpable self-evidence. Insofar as bodily sensation resists the neat schematics of
sex, gender, and desire, the body could be pressed into the service of liberty. Finally, if the swoon of pleasure could purge the body of custom, it could also
move aesthetics away from outright purpose and toward purposiveness, a maneuver that would allow aesthetics to reconcile its educational role—*Bildung*—
with its mandate to further liberty.[5] When sex enhanced love, moreover, it did
lead to the form of purposiveness in mutuality or aesthetic disinterest.

The examples of Romanticism's perverse aesthetics are legion. Even Wordsworth turned to the physiological pleasures of poetry as a panacea to the "savage torpor" caused by industrialism, insisting that the "vital juices" circulate in
poetry and prose alike ("Preface to *Lyrical Ballads*" 249, 254). "We have no sympathy but what is propagated by pleasure," mused the poet (258), and his choice
of "propagate" linked that pleasure to sexual pleasure. Pleasure propagates sym-

pathy, and the figure of sexual intercourse works to make pleasure productive.[6] Nonetheless, his admission that readers sought "outrageous stimulation" (249) hinted that pleasure could be masturbatory. Keats published "La Belle Dame" under the pseudonym of Caviare, parading his sensuous excesses and in the process redefining chastity in terms of "kisses four."

Keats was hardly the only Romantic poet glutting his passions: Rosa Mathilda—a.k.a. Charlotte Dacre—responded to a craze for DellaCruscan poetry by raising the temperature on passionate metaphors. She would go on in *Zofloya* to not only insist that women had intense sexual desires, but also show how desire would not obey any dictates of race. In "The Mother," Charlotte Smith acknowledges that motherhood often went hand in hand with illegitimacy and praises the compassion that led to the creation of the Foundling Hospital (104).[7] Nicknamed the "English Sappho," Mary Robinson in *Sappho and Phaon* dramatized the rapture and fecklessness of heterosexual passion, settling instead for poesy's ability to "calm the miseries of man" (Sonnet Introductory 157). She thus just says no to the obligatory epithalamion that should conclude sonnet sequences. And then there is Blake, for whom sexual pleasure was a key component of his "aesthetics of deliberate engagement" (McGann *SV*). Nor should we forget Hazlitt's *Liber Amoris*, or Hunt's "Story of Rimini," or Burns's erotic lyrics. Through the swoon of erotic energy, many of these writers hoped to move readers to a state of engagement.

Rather than avoiding the taint of the sensory and pleasurable, then, Romantic writers and artists sought to exploit a sexualized aesthetic as a "privileged point of contact between the supersensible and the sensory worlds" (Redfield viii). On the one hand, the tangibility of sex is especially therapeutic to aesthetics, given that aesthetics celebrates nothing less ineffable than human potentiality. On the other hand, Shelley, Blake, and Byron turned to affect and even sexual affect because it "threatens belief frameworks and the forms of self-assurance on which they rely and which they also sustain" (Altieri 44).[8] To wit, Percy Shelley decided to write about the Cenci family for the "deep and breathless interest" it awakened (*HM* 2176), and he made Laon and Cythna incestuous lovers, explicitly to "startle the reader from the trance of ordinary life" (Preface 2:106). Shelley continues, "It was my object to break through the crust of those outworn opinions on which established institutions depend. I have appealed therefore to the most universal of all feelings, and have endeavoured to strengthen the moral sense by forbidding it to waste its energies in seeking to avoid actions which are only crimes of compassion" (ibid.). Shelley turns to affect because only it can

break through the crust that has become synonymous with the lives of his readers. And the breaking through of this crust is necessary before change becomes
possible.

Moments of erotic ecstasy also invite the reader's identification with the text,
and such identification becomes a potential solvent for identity,[9] a solvent that
enables our identifications to set the stage for "eliciting our own passionate investments and clarifying paths they might take beyond the work of art" (Altieri
24). Identity must be dissolved so that desire can become a true agent for change.
Byron emphasizes the mutability of passion in *Don Juan* precisely to promote
philosophical skepticism about marriage and courtship, not to mention the heterosexual family. Hazlitt shows how the voraciousness of erotic desire dissolves
identity in his *Liber Amoris*, a dissolution emblematized in his smashing of the
statue of Napoleon. Hazlitt thereby has no choice but to move beyond a
Napoleonic idea of masculinity. Moreover, as with Juan and Haidee, Manfred
and Astarte, or Laon and Cythna, these moments of erotic ecstasy can show us
what genuine intersubjectivity should look like, a relationship that is based on
mutual consent and mutual caring. Because this mutuality allows each party to
play the roles of subject and object of desire, this complex dynamic shift in subject position not only enables consideration of what genuine consent looks like,
but also enables lovers to limit the role that hierarchy plays in erotic relations.

I do not mean to deny the underside of Romantic eroticism: the sadistic
strain in mostly French authors Mario Praz so ably documented decades ago.
His was a selective view, and he underestimated the role of irony. The British
Romantics were well aware of the price of that sadism and, for example, sought
to confine that tyranny onto Oriental despots like Sardanapalus or Othman or,
in the case of Hazlitt, real despots like Napoleon.

If the Romantics were invested in a perverse aesthetics in the sense that they
were interested in aesthetics and sexuality as Kantian means to apprehension,
and deeply invested in the ability of sexual pleasure to invite rapture, they added
insult to injury when their aesthetics glorified a sexuality without reproduction.
David Hume was in part to blame for their distrust of reason. He famously remarked in his *Treatise on Human Nature* that reason was "utterly impotent" and
that it had "no influence on our passions" (509). If reason could not motivate,
then an aesthetics stressing reason could offer nothing to engage audiences; disinterest, moreover, might invite disengagement. It perhaps becomes easier to
swallow the idea that the Romantics tended to celebrate sexuality without reproduction when we recall that none of the big six, not even sober Wordsworth,

represent poster boys of normative middle-class sexuality.[10] Kant separated sexuality from reproduction when aesthetic judgments were at issue: even though flowers were known to be the reproductive organs of plants, one could apprehend them as "free natural beauties" as long as one "pays no attention to this natural purpose when he judges the flower by taste" (Pluhar 229).[11]

The philosopher Alphonse Lingis can help us unpack the importance of sexual ecstasy without reproduction as a figure for mutuality. Sexual desire cannot have as its teleology reproduction because the act of copulation puts an end to it, and such desire exists both in young children and the old who cannot reproduce (20). Sexual desire, by contrast, does not "desire to terminate itself; it is itself voluptuous, it wishes to intensify itself, to be" (20). The end of the libido is "paradoxically the other's presence no longer teleological" (22). This suspension of teleology brings us close to Kant's purposiveness without purpose, a paradox that mandates that I further unpack the relevance of Kant to my argument.

Kant, of course, did think pleasure was central to aesthetics because it was impervious to the determining force of concepts and because its necessary subjectivity demanded communication in a form of universal assent. Pleasure and feeling are the "determining ground of the aesthetic judgment" (Schaper 371) and the judgment of taste, "connected with the feeling of a pleasure . . . at the same time declares [it] to be valid for everyone" (Pluhar 221). However, he sought to confine aesthetic pleasure to the harmonious balance of the imagination, judgment, and reason, and limited the apprehension of that pleasure to contemplation of the form of beauty as if that form had a conscious intent behind it: works of nature could only be apprehended aesthetically or judged teleologically. Kant argues, "The very consciousness of a merely formal purposiveness in the play of the subject's cognitive powers, accompanying a presentation by which an object is given, is that pleasure" (Pluhar 223). And that harmonious balance could only be achieved to the extent that aesthetic pleasure itself was disinterested, that it did not offer any personal satisfactions. More to the point, in order for beauty to compel universal assent, it had to go beyond the mere agreeableness of empirical sensation. Hence, Kant defined beauty in terms of a purposiveness without purpose.[12]

But what was the ontology of such pleasure, especially within a context of British empiricism? Not only could Kant take advantage of the German language to ward off sensuousness—in German, *Sinnlichkeit* and *Lust* tar both sexual gratification and lower-order sensuousness/pleasure with one brush[13]—but he, from the vantage of the British Romantics who actually read him, threatened to abstract pleasure so much so that it would become empirically unrecognizable. In his critique of teleological judgment, Kant nonetheless allows a very remote analogy between generation and purpose, not for the sake of "knowing nature or its original cause, but rather for 'the same practical power of reason in us' by which he previously analogized the purposiveness of nature" (Shell 239). "Although relative purposiveness points hypothetically to natural purposes, it does not justify any absolute teleological judgment," Kant adds (Pluhar 369). As long as the analogy of living organisms to art was for heuristic purposes, such as opening an avenue for scientific investigation, and not for any actual transcendental claims, generation could analogize purposiveness.[14]

Kant recognized at least a heuristic benefit to thinking about aesthetic purposiveness in terms of generation. To the extent that the British Romantics worried about what they viewed as Kant's dangerous abstractions and his resistance to sensuousness, they sought to harness yet modify his generative purposiveness. I suggest that the British Romantics both envisioned sexuality in terms of a Kantian purposiveness without purpose, for the scientific and political reasons I have outlined in the previous three chapters, yet purposely sought to counter the potential disengagement of an overly abstract aesthetics through an eroticized aesthetics, one that sought to harness the ability of desire to effect change without necessarily predetermining the forms of that change. By separating sexual pleasure from reproduction, sexuality could become a figure for equality, making it purposiveness with purpose. Where Kant thought purposiveness enabled either a means of scientific investigation that could remain scientific so long as transcendent claims were limited to the immanent structure of nature, or a means of apprehending aesthetic forms as if they had been willed, Romantics such as Coleridge and Shelley turned to a purposiveness with purpose to credit art with palpable effects without predetermining the form of those effects in advance. The fact that reproduction frustrates all forms of mechanism and technicity (Krell 12), moreover, made it a powerful ally in reinforcing organicist ways of thinking about the world.

In the Romantic period, the discourses of aesthetics and sexuality were not so far apart in that discussions of love, often a euphemism for sex, regularly upheld the ideal of disinterested love. That is, a kind of aesthetic disinterest is what defined true love. To the extent historians of sexuality have spent so much of their energies on the meanings of sexual acts throughout history, love has been neglected.[15] With the neglect of love comes the neglect of sexual disinterest, or a purposive mode of apprehending eroticism. Hence, David Hume thought that love of beauty mediated between lust and benevolence insofar as one felt momentarily kind to one's object of lust (*Treatise* 443). Even the *Bon Ton Magazine* gave at least lip service to the ideal of disinterest. Although skeptical of claims of disinterested love, it nonetheless defined love as that which subsists after enjoyment or what it called "sordid interest." "There is a love, which seems a contradiction to the power of interest: and that is, when some raw, silly novice takes a passion for an object very much disproportioned to him; but neither does this deserve the name of genuine love. It only supposes a more than ordinary eclipse of reason; a blind rage" (11). Although this statement would seem to deny the very possibility of disinterested love, the magazine returns to the idea of disinterest when it must teach readers how to recognize love over lust. "The test of both is enjoyment. If love subsists unabated after it, the love was real; if not, it was only lust" (11). Without lust, it is impossible to know either love or disinterest. To abject lust is thus to abject the possibility of knowing love. The misogynistic Marquis de Sade railed against marriage laws that made women the sexual property of a particular man: as the upholding of an individual private interest over the interests of all men in all women, marriage was an infringement of male liberty (319). Unlike most social contract theorists, Sade paid heed to the sexual contract that underwrote the social contract.[16] He did so, however, on behalf of male libertinism rather than female liberation.

The bottom line is that Romanticism's perversity has much to teach us about aesthetics and erotics: their perverse interest in the purposive role of sexual pleasure, their need to engage audiences, and their fear that rationality could be an abstracted form of disengagement can help reopen such questions as why sexual pleasure must be antithetical to aesthetic pleasure and whether it is possible to think of sexual pleasure as disinterested pleasure. In much the same way as Isobel Armstrong chides close reading because it does not go close enough to the affective elements of a literary text, aestheticians often downplay the role of sensuality in aesthetic discourse because they wrongly assume that such sensuality can only lead to selfishness. Kant's theory of beauty suggests otherwise. The perversity of Romantic aesthetics thus reminds us of the repressed ground of much aesthetic thinking: erotic pleasure, a pleasure that can neither be subsumed by rhetoric nor by reproduction.

## Coleridge's Kant

This chapter begins with Coleridge's relatively unknown contributions to J. H. Green's lectures on aesthetics because they shed light upon Romanticism's perverse aesthetics, reminding us that physiology, sexuality, and aesthetics are far from opposing discourses. Green was a professor of anatomy at the Royal Academy from 1825 until 1852.[17] Several features of this essay are especially relevant. For one, it begins and ends in physiology and anatomy, suggesting that the body need not be exiled from aesthetics. In point of fact, Coleridge demands that anatomists apprehend body parts aesthetically and uses the anatomist's aesthetic apprehension of body parts to illustrate what an artist should do. Coleridge writes, "The anatomist himself really seeks for an Idea—not to learn what this or that Limb—Hand for instance—is—but to learn what a Hand is—as he seeks beauty for the sake of scientific truth, so will the Artist seek scientific Truth" (*Shorter Works* 2:1311). Coleridge weds science and aesthetics so that he can bracket the determining force of purpose because the idea of the hand must transcend any particular hands. The idea of hands performs an analogous function to Kant's idea of purpose, purposiveness, as it attempts to neutralize the determining force of purpose, as does the idea of beauty for truth.

Coleridge's explicit revision of Kant's purposiveness without purpose takes place in the poet's remarks on fitness: "This fitness to the total subject must not appear as the product of a Design . . . the conclusion is that Design must exist in the equivalence of the result, virtual Design without the Sense of Design" (2:1314).[18] Put another way, Coleridge recognizes that, under the aegis of function, sexuality is reduced to instrumentality and animal instinct. Fitness must not appear as the product of design because this will let the "product . . . then be contemplated as a machine or tool" (2:1314). It must also not appear as designed because "the Will will not appear in its own form, but in the form of the Understanding" (2:1314). Here we must recall Kant's insistence that the beautiful cannot be understood in terms of concepts because concepts are determining. Like purposiveness without purpose, "virtual design without the Sense of Design" is a way of bracketing intent, replacing it with the category of intentionality. Although Kant did place key importance on the perception of beauty because that is what had to be articulated in terms that would compel universal assent, Coleridge seems to devalue the perception of design, preferring instead to collapse result with design. The end result is still that objects are to be perceived as if their results were designed, leaving any actual design out of the equation. Coleridge aligns himself with Kant's need to have the beautiful compel universal assent when he insists that the "Objective Beautiful . . . ha[s] . . . not a fitness to another Object; but a fitness to the Subject, i.e., the Mind" (2: 1313). The object of beauty must not merely be the object of utilitarian ends; moreover, this emphasis on the mind is also Kantian in that the subject who apprehends it is more important than the object of beauty. When Coleridge captures this in the term "Felicity and the power of felicitous production is Artistic Genius" (2:1314), he recalls Kant's definition of genius as "the talent that gives rules to art" (cited in Orsini 164). Like Kant, who locates purposiveness in the apprehending mind that understands form as if it were willed and who understands genius as that which allows the aesthetic faculty to determine for itself the rules, Coleridge insists that felicity is the purposive prerogative of artistic genius.

Second, by linking aesthetics to man's need to seek sympathy for himself in others, Coleridge makes human sociability and sexuality the origin of aesthetics. Coleridge's language merits sustained consideration on this point:

> But it is characteristic of Man to seek when matured to a certain grade of cultivation, i.e., humanization, to perfect himself—and as far as he has succeeded, to seek a sympathy for himself in others of his fellow men. He seeks for something out of himself as in the former instance—but what he seeks, is a reflex of his own inward—he seeks a subject (a soul we say) similarly constituted & affected with his own individual Subject or Soul—and this sympathy must be sought for therefore for that which constitutes the perfection or ultimate end, of his animal frame—as the latter consisted in an harmonious balance of Organs & Organic Powers, so must this consist in a harmony and Balance of his mental powers & faculties.—But to excite this sympathy, he must produce a something which shall represent this balance. Consequently, here too he produces <an external> but an IDEAL product—i.e., a product which has no other purpose but that of representing the Ideas &exciting a similar ideal state in the minds of others sufficiently advanced &c. (2:1310)

Despite the overwhelming homosociality of Coleridge's sympathy—the poet depicts intersubjectivity as between men—Coleridge firmly places the origin of aesthetics in what he would later call man's gregarious instinct, or instinct to sociability. That instinct is loosely based on the sexual instinct. Coleridge writes that the gregarious instinct "began as his sexual instincts," but he made clear that the gregarious instinct was not determined by the sexual (2:1394). It is the very need to excite sympathy in another person that leads to the creation of an ideal product, one that has no purpose other than to represent the ideas and to excite a similar state of harmonious balance in others. Just as the "as if "of Kant's purposiveness permits the universal apprehension of form as willed, Coleridge's "no other purpose" limits the determining force of purpose by insisting upon the ideal of exciting sympathy in another so that "the living balance of all the faculties which constitute the human mind" can be achieved (2:1311) without specifying what that sympathy or balance is ultimately to achieve. "No other purpose" furthermore allows the ideal to limit the contagion of the real.

My key point here, however, is that Coleridge explains how the sexual and the aesthetic have a common origin in the need of man to find something outside himself, an outside that must be beyond both instinct and purpose to be outside the self. Coleridge, we recall, deplored Malthus's reduction of human sexuality to appetite, precisely because that made human sexuality animalistic and denied both free will and the spiritual dimensions of sexuality (P. Edwards 158). Such a common origin further suggests that aesthetics and sexuality are compatible insofar as both seek "the perfection or ultimate end, of his animal frame—as the latter consisted in an harmonious balance of Organs and Organic powers, so must this consist in harmony and Balance of his mental powers & faculties" (2:1310). Kant, of course, would have rejected thinking about perfection in terms of aesthetic judgment because perfection can be a determining concept (Pluhar 228). Above all, where Kant worries about apprehension and limits teleology to the teleological judgment, Coleridge worries about the harmonious effects of the aesthetic while tempering crude purpose. He thus aligns aesthetics and life, all the while insisting that sexuality and aesthetics mature beyond instinct (crude reproductive purpose) into the form of organic perfection.

Third, insofar as Coleridge defines beauty in terms of a harmonious balance between "all the faculties with constitute the human mind" (2:1311), faculties including "the Organs and the Organic powers" (2:1310), the imagination, and the passions, sensuality is necessarily part and parcel of aesthetic discourse. Here Coleridge is perhaps indebted to Longinus, who insisted that vehement and inspired passion was one of the few true sources of the sublime. Kant, too, valued balance of rational faculties, but his need to separate thought from matter—for Kant, *Gedanke*/thought is equal to emptiness (Shell 377–78)—kept him from including sex, except by way of a very distant analogy, and one that only held up so long as it enabled apprehension. Coleridge's anatomic aesthetics equates life and spontaneity and thus becomes a helpful guide to understanding how sexuality and aesthetics could be considered allies in Romanticism. Not only do sexuality and aesthetics have a common origin in man's sociability, but also the beautiful must perversely leave behind questions of design, purpose, or else art remains instinctual and degenerates into a mere tool. Yet this resistance to purpose paradoxically has the purpose of "exciting the ideal state" in the minds of others. Now that Coleridge has suggested the common basis of sexuality and aesthetics, I turn to Longinus because he analogized sublime transport in terms of Sapphic orgasm.

## Longinus and the Sapphic Sublime

If the Romantics needed to authorize their perverse turn to overt sensuality in their aesthetics, they had to look no further than Longinus,[19] who quotes Sappho's famous fragment 31, on love in *On the Sublime*. This popular treatise inaugurated the fad for the sublime in the eighteenth century. Describing the burning love that Sappho has for another woman, fragment 31 is sexually explicit while suspending reproductive function. While Longinus means to praise Sappho for her "skill in selecting the outstanding details and making a unity of them" (14), he is captivated by her ability to capture what all "lovers experience" (15). Sappho tries to capture the state of having been moved by one's desire, and it is this possibility for affect and desire to change the person that both Longinus and the Romantics found so compelling in an eroticized aesthetics. As Sappho knows only too well, the rapture of erotic pleasure takes the self outside of cognition, and breaks it into fragments that must be unified. But that rapture can only work so long as purpose and rhetorical persuasion are suspended: the mere whiff of rhetoric has the capacity to shut down transport. Longinus also could not have chosen a better example for sublime transport, in that such transport invades and takes over the self, rendering it a feminized and passive version of itself, only later to be actively reunified. Longinus speaks of sublime transport as a kind of "amazement and wonder [that] exert invincible power and force and get the better of every hearer" (2). However, because in Greek thinking passivity was thought to invite all kinds of illnesses, it was crucial to enact that unification. The feminization that sublime transport brings thus must be arrested by rhetorical purpose and return the subject to the liberation of self-mastery.

Despite Longinus's insistence on elevated subject matter and elevated diction, Sappho's fragment is also a description of sexual orgasm and, as such, sexual pleasure perversely supplements aesthetic transport. Perversity is on four grounds: one, noble diction is put to use to describe orgasm, and, two, this orgasm is generated by desire of a woman for a woman. Third, as Susan Lanser reminds us, since *trope* is itself "drawn from the Greek *tropein*, to turn, the trope is a perversion, a breaking of rules, a seduction of language from its proper course" (23). All this perversity reminds us of how purpose undermines and threatens liberty. By limiting desire to reproduction, one loses the capacity to think about the aesthetics of desire, how the forms desire takes can enhance self-mastery and freedom. So, too, does it remind us of the costs of that liberty: self-restraint and the need for rhetoric to contain sublime transport. Fourth, to the extent that Sappho reasserts mastery over her feminized body, active and passive are no longer securely gendered.

The first charge of perversity is somewhat mitigated by Longinus's later claim that expression can cancel out vulgarity. Although Herodotus is on the verge of vulgarity when he describes Cleomenes cutting his own flesh into little pieces with a knife, Longinus claims that "these phrases come within an inch of being vulgar, but they are so expressive that they avoid vulgarity" (37). This begs the question of how expressiveness cancels out vulgarity. Of course, Longinus does say that "it is wrong to descend, in a sublime passage, to the filthy and contemptible, unless we are absolutely compelled to do so. . . . We ought to imitate nature, who, in creating man, did not set our private parts or excretions of our body in the face, but concealed them as well as she could" (50). One could argue that he is compelled to invoke Sappho.

The second charge is less easy to duck. Longinus wants to endow the sublime with powers beyond rhetoric: whereas persuasion is subject to rational control, "sublimity, on the other hand, produced at the right moment, tears everything up like a whirlwind" (2). As Longinus imagines it, the sublime effects a corporeal revolution, one embodied in the effects of orgasm that Sappho inimitably describes. Hence, his treatise on the sublime ends with a promissory note for one on emotion, a topic that promises once again to embody language. Felt on the pulses, language acquires the capacity to move and engage readers. The third charge—that tropes are themselves a perversion of language—renders the sublime a perversion of language, taking readers out of ordinary rhetoric. That this perversion can effeminize the audience for the sublime forces Longinus at times to choose rhetoric over and at the expense of his beloved sublime because only rhetoric can arrest that transport and remasculinize the sublime subject since transport as the loss of control is feminizing and renders one passive. Finally, notwithstanding Greek culture's longstanding connection of passivity with feminization, Longinus's use of Sappho in the end troubles gender insofar as it makes sublime feminization necessary for the assertion of masculinity or mastery. He thus renders the sublime as the Lacanian phallus, the feminization that makes masculinity possible even as Sappho's control undercuts any essential connection between masculinity and mastery.

Longinus's sublime whirlwind sheds key light onto Blake's engraving of Dante's *Inferno*, "The Circle of the Lustful: Francesca da Rimini ('The Whirlwind of Lovers')." Together, Blake and Longinus illustrate the power of the erotic sublime. Dante describes the whirlwind in the following stanza: "La bufera infernal, che mai non resta,/mena li spiriti con la sua rapina:/voltando e percotendo li molesta" (*Inferno* 5:32–34). Unlike Dante, who takes considerable pains to remind us that the winds of passion are infernal, rooting up, molesting (*molesta*), and raping (*rapina*) those who let reason serve desire (*Inferno* 5:32–33), Blake transforms this whirlwind into a positive rapturous force, one that threatens to swallow the viewer into its path as it crosses from the top left to the bottom right of the page. Blake taught himself Italian before attempting to illustrate Dante. Not only do Dante's insistent end-stopped lines and disciplined *terza rima* arrest this rapture (note as well the caesuric pressure of his double negative: the wind that never [*mai*] not [*non*] rests), but also his syntax reverses subject and object so that the wind (*la bufera infernal*) is the only agent of this stanza. The purported subjects have been reduced to possessive pronouns that bear the mark of the subject in that they must grammatically agree with the subject who is possessed. But if possessed, they are therefore not true acting subjects (*la sua rapina, li molesta*). Hence, Dante disfigures the subjects grammatically and syntactically.

Blake clues us in to his radical revision of Dante by picturing in the sun two lovers engaged in passionate sexual embrace. In contrast to Dante's formal control, Blake depicts the whirlwind in such a way that it moves beyond the page: the portion of the whirlwind that encapsulates Francesca is somehow connected to the rest of the wind, but that connection must be imagined by the viewer. Moreover, the whiteness in the whirlwind insinuates no end even as it links it to the divine light. Where the dark engraved lines elsewhere insist upon the borders of the plate, the whiteness within the whirlwind encourages the viewer's eye to wander into the margins. The fact that this sun resembles a halo, moreover, transforms the pagan Virgil into the iconography of Christ. Such a transformation reminds us of Christ's links to Blake's Luvah or lust, and this eroti-

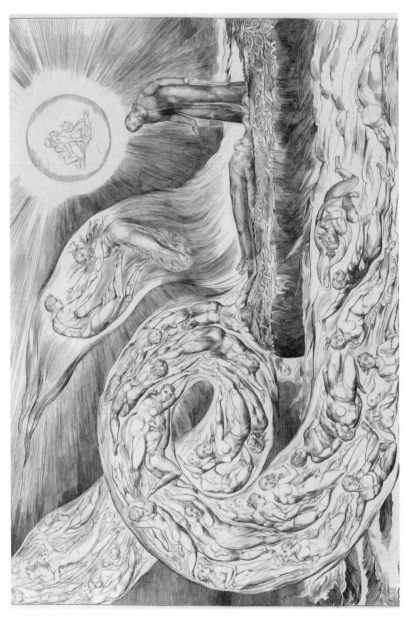

William Blake, "The Circle of the Lustful: Francesca da Rimini" ("The Whirlwind of Lovers"). Courtesy of John Windle, San Francisco.

cism is, for Blake, the path to fourfold vision precisely because it can break down the viewer's predetermined frames. Thus, Blake supplements the holy halo with eroticism, a substitution that belittles Christian distrust of the flesh. In harsher terms, Blake hopes to rape his reader of his or her subjectivity because it is only by giving up that subjectivity that one can see the need for, much less attain, higher vision. Blake's whirlwind of lust is later iconographically repeated in his sketch of the circles of stairs that lead to paradise (see Klonsky, plate 93, 117). In much the same way as Longinus wants the sublime to transport its audience because that transport finesses many of the boundaries established by culture, Blake both argues for the value of passionate rapture and literally embodies it. But this rapture has its costs: the shattering of the self.

Blake helps us to delve more deeply into the costs and benefits of Longinus's investment in Sappho's descriptions of orgasm. Here's Sappho's fragment, the one quoted by Longinus:

> But in silence my tongue is broken, a fine
> fire at once runs under my skin,
> with my eyes I see not one thing, my ears
> buzz,
> Cold sweat covers me, trembling
> Seizes my whole body, I am more moist than grass;
> I seem to be little short of dying. . . .
> But all must be ventured. . . .[20]

Although many translators of Sappho have rendered *chloros* as green, Jane Snyder reminds us that, in early Greek, *chloros* means liquid or moist (33). The fact that the singer describes herself as dying, itself a Greek metaphor for orgasm (Snyder 33), further supports the distinct possibility that she is referring to her vaginal secretions (Snyder 33). In any case, trembling carnality wrests, momentarily, control over the mind's ability to apprehend the body in terms of a unified subject, and fragmentation and momentary passivity of the self are the necessary price to be paid for sublime and sexual transport.

Orgasm thus is an especially powerful if dangerous supplement to sublime transport insofar as the experience of it is not beholden to tropes. While Longinus insists that certain tropes like apostrophe and metaphor and hyperbole are, in the right orator's mouth, the source of the sublime, he also recognizes that tropes once perceived as tropes threaten to puncture transport into mere persuasion. Even worse, once tropes become perceived as tropes, the audience is on its guard and mere persuasion becomes difficult. Noting the outrageousness of hyperbole, Longinus admits that, "As I keep saying, acts and emotions which approach ecstasy provide a justification for, and an antidote to, any linguistic audacity" (45). Here, in much the same way that orgasm instantiates the transport the sublime may or may not provide because it is dependent upon tropes, acts and emotions rescue the trope from itself: they justify and provide the antidote to the trope. We see more of Longinus's ambivalence to tropes in his treatment of metaphor. Longinus's metaphorical examples are insistently tethered to the body through anatomy. The body is a "tabernacle," the neck an "isthmus," and the heart, "a knot of veins" (38). As Neil Hertz observes, "It would seem that the moment itself that fascinates Longinus, [is] the point where the near-fatal stress of passion can be thought of as turning into—as indistinguishable from—the energy that is constituting the poem" (5). Hertz makes clear that such transport renders Longinus and Sappho equal partners in the creation of the sublime. Yet, if tropes are both the antidote and the poison, this explains why Longinus seeks a transport not contingent upon tropes and why he welds metaphor to anatomy in much the same way as Sappho's line, "fire at once runs under my skin," blends metaphor and physiology, fusing them into one. The fact that Longinus is so attuned to the anatomy behind metaphor suggests his awareness of the carnality of Sappho's body and how that carnality resists yet demands mastery.

Longinus's ambivalence toward tropes is further developed in his treatment of the battle of the Gods in Homer's *Iliad* when Homer describes the seemingly human fear of the Gods. Longinus comments, "But terrifying as all this is, it is blasphemous and indecent unless it is interpreted allegorically; in relating the gods's wounds, quarrels, revenges, tears, imprisonments, and manifold misfortunes, Homer, as it seems to me, has done his best to make the men of the Trojan war gods, and the gods men" (11). The power of tropes to transport is deliberately undone by Longinus, who not only counters Homer's metaphors with allegory, but also takes the reader outside of Homer's frame of reference when he addresses the reader through the figure of apostrophe: "Do you see how the earth is torn from its foundations?" he asks. If Longinus initially sides with sublime transport over rhetoric because rhetoric is sublimity interruptus, he in this moment recognizes the need for rhetorical purpose over purposive transport because it prevents indecency, the literal rendering of gods in terms of human beings. Apostrophe and allegory must arrest Homer's sublime transport, lest gods degenerate into men. As long as men become like gods, transport does not seem so objectionable. Without the on/off switch provided by rhetoric, it turns out, sublime transport is not necessarily a good thing.

But Sappho's orgasm offers a supplement within a supplement insofar as lesbian desire replaces penile penetration. For all the brilliance of Hertz's Freudian interpretation of Longinus as having through tropes attempted to domesticate Oedipal conflicts, Hertz misses the boat. I will note that he is not alone: Jane Snyder shows how many twentieth-century readers, even some respected classicists, have interpreted this song as "a wedding song written for performance at the nuptial ceremonies of the groom" (29) and, in the rush to heterosexualize Sappho, have missed or deliberately overlooked Sappho's apostrophe, her turn from the unidentified man to the female "you." By turning perversely to female pleasure, Sappho blithely infers the penis as the lack, while the vagina embodies presence even via synecdoche. In light of the "extraordinary phallicism" of Ancient Greek culture (Halperin *OHY* 102), Sappho's refusal of the penis as telos to some extent liberates the sexuality of women. Seeing orgasm as pleasure rather than as an end allows sex to take on *Bildung:* sex thus becomes part of an aesthetics of the self, one whose self-mastery is necessary for freedom. Because women are in fact capable of self-mastery, discipline can no longer be securely gendered as masculine.

Yet it is crucial to note that even pleasure itself is not the point. Michel Foucault informs us that Galen insisted pleasure must be taken as nothing more than the by-product of the act, it must not become the reason for the act, or else the body might become addicted to its pleasures (*Care of the Self* 139). By emphasizing the speaker's awareness of her own body, Sappho stresses the reestablishment of mastery that must take place during desire. Writes Snyder, "Despite the role played by the woman whom the speaker observes, the song focuses on self-reflective perception; the speaker observes not so much an external object as her own self" (29). The focus is on the active perceiver: the I who sees the eye that is blind. Moreover, the fragment ends with an invitation to mastery; notwithstanding her proximity to death, "all must be ventured."[21] Absent in the translation is Sappho's careful rhetorical balance, the metrical and alliterative symmetry between the phrases, *alla pan tolmaton, epei kai peneta.* The *alla* (but) announces the turn to mastery/courage/daring even as the *pan* gathers together Sappho's fragments, while the syntactical balance and equal number of stresses in each phrase enacts the very mastery she invokes.[22] Though not writing about Sappho, Foucault provides another potentially helpful Sapphic gloss in his *The Care of the Self:* "The medicine of the *chresis aphrodision* did not aim to delimit the pathological forms of sexual behaviour: rather, it uncovered, at the root of sexual acts, an element of passivity that was also a source of illness" (142). It is for this reason that Longinus emphasizes Sappho's having made a unity of details, and not the bodily parts that are splayed across her page. Sappho's enjambment encourages Longinus's unification.[23] Furthermore, in her use of *chloros,* Sappho can be read as refuting the ancient Greek notion that women's bodies were porous, wet, and [therefore] unable to control their own boundaries (Wilson 84). In spite of the wetness of her body, Sappho does not lose sight of her perceiving mind. By focusing upon her skill in making a unity of details (14), Longinus credits Sappho—and, by extension, women—with the power to control their porous bodies.

This perverse turn in Sappho allows Longinus to unify sublime aesthetics and sexuality, notwithstanding the potential of the private parts to "spoil the beauty of the creature as a whole" (50). Of course, not only are Sappho's private parts decorously couched in metaphor and synecdoche, but the meter regularizes and knits together the various fragments. Sapphic sexuality initially has no ostensible function outside of pleasure. Instead of a phallic pleasure that excessively privileges one part, Sappho disperses pleasure throughout her body, thereby underscoring the limits of phallicism (Wilson 85). However, as her *alla*/but makes clear, it is not so much the pleasure than the self-mastery or unification that is at issue. If sexuality embodies sublime transport leaving pleasure as a by-product of self-mastery, it also helps to model a reintegration of the self into a larger whole outside itself. Unlike the persuasive designs of rhetoric, sublime transport fosters an aesthetics of the self whereby identity has become a style of self-actualization, a means of unification of the fragments of the body into a coherent whole. Just as sublime transport has no palpable designs on the subject, no obvious purpose other than the goal of rebuilding of the subject, the sublime trope is purged of rhetoricity, rendered void of obvious purpose outside of self-mastery. Because aesthetic self-mastery is paradoxically necessary for freedom, the determining force of purpose is moved closer to purposiveness, but only as long as phallicism can be rejected.

Hence Longinus must suggest that sublime transport stands outside of rhetoric, and he insistently localizes it within the body of Sappho, in her "mind and body, hearing and tongue, eyes and skin" (15). Furthermore, he introduces Sappho by remarking that "every topic naturally includes certain elements which are inherent in its raw material" (14), and praising her for "draw[ing] on real life at every point" (14), thereby not only substituting the body for language, but also grounding metonymy in the body. And he sums up Sappho's excellence by remarking "lovers experience all this," making her nonphallocentric experience of love stand for all lovers' experience. If the rhetorical purpose behind transport is too clear, then transport risks complete fecklessness even as it defies liberty because it is determined by purpose. And hence he can appreciate the powers of visualization (phantasia) (20–24), a kind of rhetoric that does not seem to be rhetoric insofar as it becomes internalized in the mind of the audience.[24] With that internalization, phantasia exceeds rhetoric and "enslaves the hearer as well as persuad[es] him" (23).

What orgasm lends to the sublime is the power of embodiment to resist the limitations of tropes. Orgasm shows us what transport must look and feel like. What the rhetorical sublime lends to sexual orgasm is the obligation to rebuild the self into a coherent style of mastery, an obligation that Longinus reminds us of at the start of his treatise when he laments Caecilius's failure to teach his audience "how to develop our nature to some degree of greatness" (1). And Longinus hopes his work will become "useful to public men" (1). Foucault suggests why sexuality would acquire such a central place in the Greek aesthetics of the self: "The care of the self . . . is a privilege duty, a gift-obligation that ensures our freedom while forcing us to take ourselves as the object of all our diligence" (47). Through Longinus, Sapphic sexuality therefore offers its own kind of *Bildung*. Only by suppressing the rhetorical intent behind sublime transport can Longinus render this gift/duty. From a Kantian perspective, this suppression is what perverts rhetoric into a kind of purposiveness without purpose, what imparts to rhetoric the power of sublime transport.

It should come as no surprise, then, that Longinus ends his treatise by dwelling upon the evils of slavery to one's desires. "I wonder," he muses, "whether what destroys great minds is not the peace of the world, but the unlimited war which lays hold on our desires, and all the passions which beset and ravage our modern life" (52). Longinus continues, "One might describe all slavery, even the most justified, as a cage for the soul, a universal prison" (52). By rendering slavery into metaphor (unlimited war, cage), Longinus has of course given us a way to free ourselves from it, and by extension the tyranny of desire. His rhetorical phrasing, "one might describe," further alerts us to the coming of a trope, to its potential fictiveness. Indeed, he has trained us to be so alert by enumerating the various figures (24–30) that "generate sublimity" (24). In much the same way as one is merely enslaved to sexual pleasure if one does not allow self-mastery to follow the state of passivity, the feminizing powers of Longinus's

sublime can only bring health if the immediacy of transport leads to a deliberate unification, the task of a suppressed rhetoric. This is the lesson of Sappho.
After all, Longinus insists that "she only *seems* to have lost . . . her mind and
body, hearing and tongue, eyes and skin . . . and to be looking for them as
though they were external to her" (15). And this is what enables Longinus finally
to appreciate the control one has over rhetoric, that perverse trope always already within the sublime that prevents enslavement.

## Winckelmann's Perverse Aesthetics: From Physical Beauty to Aesthetic Apprehension

In a chapter on perverse aesthetics, Winckelmann would certainly number
among the usual suspects. In fact, he is one of its poster boys. Despite his Con-
tinental origins, his influence in England was enormous. Henry Fuseli translated his *Reflections* into English in 1765, and this was reprinted in 1767 (Heyer
and Norton 1). Hume, Blake, and Shelley read him carefully. As Winckelmann
makes clear in his early *Reflections on the Imitation of Greek Works in Painting and
Sculpture*, proper understanding of ancient Greek eroticism is central to his aesthetics because the Greek body beautiful was an allegory for an aesthetics of the
self that understood the mind's role in the creation of beauty. That is, rather
than assuming the reproductive ends of physical beauty, Winckelmann initially
casts aside crude purpose for intellectual apprehension. Understood properly
and allegorically, physical beauty is the means through which we can understand
intellectual beauty. Thus, this early work begins with the nude Greek male body
and culminates in a treatment of allegory. As Plato and Socrates had to ascend
the ladder of beauty in the *Symposium*, so Winckelmann invites his readers
along a similar ascent. Because physical beauty can only become intellectual
through the allegoric apprehension of it, allegory unites both sensation and
reflection, and in the process pits a kind of purposiveness (intellectual beauty)
against crude purpose (mere physical beauty).

Winckelmann begins his *Reflections* by treating natural beauty, and by this he
means largely the natural beauty of Ancient Greek men. Describing the handsome young men in the gymnasia, performing exercises in the nude (11), as well
as the "strong and manly contours" these "exercises gave the bodies of the
Greeks" (7), one senses that it is the philosopher's own blood that briskly flows,
not the swift Indian's he describes (7). The rapture of pleasure allows the work
of art and the connoisseur to meld. Yet Winckelmann ends this treatise with a

discussion of allegory precisely because, as he learned from Plato and Socrates, one can only get to intellectual beauty by first understanding the significance of physical beauty.[25] One must learn to "paint allegorically" because "painting goes beyond the things of the senses" (61). To borrow from my discussion of Sappho's role in Longinus, it is less the physical beauty that matters than the reasons behind that physical beauty: the Greek aesthetic sense of the sexualized self, which legitimates physical sensuousness. That sensuousness, after all, is what invites viewers to ponder its larger aesthetic significances.

Hence, I note that Plato and Socrates appear three times in the opening section on natural beauty: once when Winckelmann highlights the fact that an "ancient interpreter of Plato teaches us" that beautiful images come from the mind alone (7), again when it is Socrates who teaches others "to enrich his art" by watching the naked handsome men in the Gymnasia (11), and yet again when Wincklemann alludes to how "Plato's Dialogues . . . portray to us the noble souls of these youths" in the Gymnasia (13).[26] Even Winckelmann's placement of the first Platonic reference is significant: he alludes to the mind's apprehension of beauty before he indulges in his descriptions of that beauty. Although the sensuousness of his descriptions may later suggest otherwise, Winckelmann's cart is not before his horse, a point underscored by the fact that the *Laocoön* here allegorizes "the perfect rules of art" (5). Immediately following Winckelmann's beautiful descriptions of Greek men in the *Reflections*, he explains carefully what this says about the Greeks. "Everything that was instilled and taught from birth to adulthood about the culture of their bodies and the preservation, development, and refinement of this culture through nature and art was done to enhance the natural beauty of the ancient Greeks" (11), writes Winckelmann. The Greeks lived in a climate that made possible to live out ideal beauty in their physical bodies, but their style of living—their aesthetics—made it possible for physical bodies to remain commensurate with the ideal.

Physical beauty, thus, is an allegory for the Greek aesthetics of self, an aesthetics that embraces the homoeroticism of Ancient Greek culture so long as the self-mastery that is the end goal of that aesthetic is continuously upheld. For this reason, Winckelmann describes their regimen: infants without swaddling clothes,[27] exercise, diet, avoidance of any abuse of the body, learning to draw so one better appreciates beauty, the use of clothing to show off that body, naked appearances before state authorities to ward off any signs of fat, beauty contests, games and festivals as incentives for exercise, and training in how to create beautiful babies (7–11). Yet it is not until the final section of this work entitled allegory that we are prepared to apprehend the allegory within Winckelmann's text, the allegory that imitates the perfection of the Ancient Greeks even as it reminds his readers of how difficult it will be for modern culture to imitate the Greeks successfully. His contemporary audience, after all, has to contend with such physically disfiguring diseases as smallpox and the English malady, nervous diseases (11), not to mention "the emaciated tensions and depressions of our bodies" (19), illnesses Winckelmann would have encountered while he studied to become a doctor.

Having grasped the aesthetics of Winckelmann's *Reflections*, readers are better positioned to understand Winckelmann's somewhat confusing statement on Greek imitation, that "in the masterpieces of Greek Art, connoisseurs and imitators find not only nature at its most beautiful but also something beyond nature, namely certain ideal forms of beauty" (7). How can imitation be simultaneously natural and beyond nature? Yet this double-faced perception is precisely what allegory demands, a constant dance between the other speeches within it. Winckelmann thus understands mimesis allegorically, as being caught between Greek sensuous bodies and the perfection they embody, and between that perfection and a more intellectual ideal, one that apprehends physical perfection as part of the Greek aesthetics of the self. I might add, what wider otherness could allegory straddle than the one between sexed bodies and their apprehension?

In the final analysis, since Greek beauty is precisely what Wincklemann thinks is good taste, it is the reader's responsibility to bridge through allegory the divide between Ancient Greece and Enlightenment Dresden, as well as the divide between sensuous and ideal beauty. He underscores that "sensual beauty provided the artist with all that nature could give; ideal beauty provided him with sublimity—from the one he took the human element, from the other the divine" (17). Indeed, Wincklemann's first paragraph refers to seeds and the fact that Minerva chose Greece because it would be "productive of genius" (3). The reader must now actively and appropriately cultivate those seeds. Winckelmann provides the example of Nicomachus's judging of Zeuxis's Helena, an example that hints at the multifaceted vision necessary to understand beauty. "Behold her with my eyes," Winckelmann quotes, a command that takes us into the body and into language. This is precisely what he demands that readers do with an allegorical understanding of Greek eroticism: one that both swoons and reflects on that swooning. The enormous success of Wincklemann's *Reflections* meant that few in the Enlightenment would have a choice but to do precisely that.[28] By allegorizing Greek sexuality, Winckelmann at once abstracts the delectable Greek body into an aesthetic regime and yet makes that body felt so that it can matter. In Winckelmann, then, desire unhooks itself from reproduction so that purposiveness can reorient physical delectation into an aesthetics of the self.

## Burke's Learned Voluptuary

Burke also, if unwittingly, recognizes the value of perverse desire. Immediately after Burke links the sublime in his *Philosophical Inquiry on the Origin of Our Ideas of the Sublime and the Beautiful* to pain and terror, he announces, "Without all doubt, the torments which we may be made to suffer are much greater in their effect on the body and mind, than the pleasures which the most learned voluptuary could suggest, or than the liveliest imagination, and the most sound and exquisitely sensible body, could enjoy" (1:7).[29] Like Longinus, once the issue becomes the effect of the sublime, eroticism and the sensate body take center stage. Having declared the impossibility of all doubt, however, Burke goes on in the next three sections to dwell on "the passions of generation" as if the modifier "learned" had not sufficiently rationalized his voluptuary. "Those which belong to generation have their origin in gratifications and pleasure; the pleasure most directly belonging to this purpose is of a lively character, rapturous and violent, and confessedly the highest pleasure of sense" (1:8). Although Burke wants to separate aesthetic and sexual pleasure because aesthetic pleasure might take on the sordid sensuality of the body, the danger is that this separation will cut aesthetic pleasure off from empirical sensation, the very ground of his aesthetics. For this reason, Burke turns to the figure of the "learned voluptuary" simultaneously to ground his aesthetics in the sensations of pleasure and to distance his aesthetics from the body. He nonetheless describes the sublime in terms of tumescence (Paulson 69), because his need to distance the sublime from any actual experience of horror threatens to leave his aesthetics hanging in mid air.

Sex therefore plays an important if unappreciated role in Burke's rhetoric of sensation.[30] I will show how sex in Burke provides an important basis for reflection in his empiricism, even when he contemplates the significance of erotic loss, and the extent to which both his sublime and beautiful aesthetics are beholden to this reflection on sex. Moreover, does reflection or sensation make the aesthetic truly aesthetic? Although Burke does his best to empty out pleasure, even noting that "pleasure, when it has run its career, sets us down very nearly where it found us" (1:3), the problem is that sexual pleasure is one of the two basic kinds of passions that human beings can experience—the other being those of society more generally (1:8)—and that sexual passion is really the underlying cause for man's quest for beauty. Moreover, the beautiful has its origins in "the social instincts directed towards the generation of the species" (Potts 115). As long as generation remains the origin of the beautiful, aesthetics cannot escape the orbit of brute instinct.

This humble origin thus creates a need to distinguish between vulgar desire (purpose) and aesthetic beauty (purposiveness), but the problem again is that aesthetic beauty may have no empirical origins.[31] To the extent Burke attempts to ground his aesthetics in our sensations of pain and pleasure, the body is the only ground of his aesthetics. Burke writes, "The passion which belongs to generation, merely as such, is lust only" (1:10). Unlike beasts, man, however, "who is a creature adapted to a greater variety and intricacy of relation, connects with the general passion the idea of some social qualities, which direct and heighten the appetite which he has in common with all other animals; and as he is not designed like them to live at large, it is fit that he should have something to create a preference, and fix his choice; and this in general should be some sensible quality; as no other can so quickly, so powerfully, or so surely produce its effect" (1:10). On the one hand, "something" directs men's passions: the invocation of design suggests that it is God. Burke defers, however, from naming it. His circumlocution "it is fit" begs the question of who or what makes it fit. On the other hand, the real danger is that the "idea of social qualities" may not have the effect that raw undeniable sensation has, because it is a reflection that is once removed from a sensation. Note how once again effect on the body leads the focus back to lust. In the end, Burke admits that beauty is a "mixed passion," one that partakes of both lust and ideas: the former provides the effect, the latter the key criterion that distinguishes the vulgar from the aesthetic. Because humans' control over lust is what distinguishes them from beasts, the stakes of the suppression of lust are high indeed. At the same time if reproductive purpose is quashed entirely, the door is opened to sexual perversion.

Burke thus opens up a perverse gap between the lusty drive toward generation—what he calls "a great purpose" (1.9)—and the purposive idea of beauty—in man, an "idea of some social qualities" (1.10). "To what end," Burke confesses, "this was designed, I am unable to discover" (1.10). The social quality of beauty opens up a gap between purpose and beauty that he hopes to foreclose by having beauty direct the passions between "women and men" (1:10). "Something" and "it" are the symptoms of this gap as they are words that defer referentiality. But what happens if men become objects of aesthetic beauty? What happens if the idea of beauty no longer corresponds to a heterosexual narrative?

Burke writes, "If beauty in our own species was annexed to use, men would be much more lovely than women . . . to call strength by the name of beauty . . . is an abuse of words" (3:6). If beauty weren't perverse or annexed to use, men would become objects of beauty for other men. In theory, the fact that Burke stipulates beauty and lust to be wholly different (3.1) prevents beauty from leading to sexual desire or, in this case, homoeroticism. The problem is that, although Burke begins his discussion of beauty by separating love from desire or lust he winds up conflating the two, admitting that desire may sometimes operate along with it [love] (3:1). "We shall have a strong desire for a woman of no remarkable beauty; whilst the greatest beauty in men, or in other animals, though it causes love, yet excites nothing at all of desire" (3.1), Burke initially writes. To prevent misinterpretation, Burke is careful to define love as "that satisfaction which arises to the mind upon contemplating anything beautiful" (3.1) and lust as "an energy of mind, that hurries us on to the possession of certain objects" (3.1). Although his punctuation and sections attempt to keep apart love and desire, aesthetics and sexuality, the fact that desire operates together with love means that desire will not abide by his philosophical categories. His choice of "satisfaction" collapses lust and love because satisfaction reminds us of the body's needs. Love further shades into lust when Burke admits that "it is to this latter (desire) that we must attribute those violent and tempestuous passions, and the consequent emotions of the body, which attend what is called love in some of its ordinary acceptations" (3.1). As ordinarily understood, love is lust. Indeed, by the time he treats the "physical causes of love," the distinction between love and desire has completely evaporated in the "softened, relaxed, enervated, dissolved, and melted away" body (3:19). Although separating beauty from use in humankind would seem to allow it to remain aesthetic, the danger is that it will have no real connection to the sensate body. Hence, the mere contemplation of purposiveness leads Burke back to purpose.

Perhaps Raimonda Modiano has put it best: "The best description of Burke's concept of love is to call it preferential lust. Unlike the brutes who are satisfied with any mates as long as they are available, men become attached to women through the mediation of the Beautiful which enables a preferential fixation on the objects of desire" (198). Indeed, in the place of lust, man has sexual "preferences"—"it is fit that he should have something to create a preference"—(1:10) and the gap between a preference and an instinct, otherwise known as free will or mind, is what allows for such a perverse turn. Too bad Burke has to admit that beasts have "preferences" too in that they stick to their own species (1:10). All is again well when Burke can distinguish between the preferences of beasts and the preferences of men: theirs do not "arise from any sense of beauty which they find in their species" (1:10). Because beauty is what allows men to form a particular attachment—it makes them monogamous and makes their desire purposive as opposed to crudely purposeful—it is crucial to Burke that men's preferences be different from those of beasts. The fact that he has to use the same word "preference" as well as admit that men are motivated by both lust and love hints that sexual perversion in human beings is inevitable whether it manifests itself in the lack of monogamy or in homoeroticism. Despite the stench of bestial purpose, Burke cannot forsake it completely. In his earlier work, *A Vindication of Natural Society*, Burke had described the mind of man as a perverse organ because it is "too active and restless a Principle ever to settle on the true Point of Quiet. It discovers every day some craving Want in a Body, which really wants but little" (13). The mind thus invents more wants than it actually has, a perversion of nature that may express itself in desire.

That Burke elsewhere tries to cultivate manly chivalry and to direct this manly chivalry toward sympathy for royalty further suggests that perversity could be a real potential problem should custom lose its hold over gender.[32] Of course, as Mary Wollstonecraft recognized, the turn toward chivalric manhood is simultaneously a turn to sentimentalized foppery, a turn that unmans the man even in the name of manhood. The very gap that is the gift of culture—the social marks a turning away from raw lust—is the same gap that opens the door to perversion. Wollstonecraft denounced Burke for his fostering of "equivocal beings," and in 1780, when Burke rose in the House of Commons to protest the pilloring of two sodomites, he based his argument for clemency upon the fact that sodomy, though "detestable," was a crime "of the most equivocal nature and the most difficult to prove" (cited in Kramnick 84). The slide from equivocal sex to equivocal language moves equivocation from ontology to epistemology. Although Burke's point is that because we cannot know if the charge of sodomy is accurate, accused sodomites deserve mercy, his displacement of equivocation onto language and away from sex papers over ontological confusions in the meanings of sex itself.

When Burke considers the ethical implications of his aesthetics, the costs of reflection go even higher. Rather than saving aesthetics from carnality, reflection threatens to be itself perverse insofar as it contradicts natural feeling. Burke notes, "men often act right from their feelings, who afterwards reason but ill on them from principle: but it is impossible to avoid an attempt at such reasoning, and equally impossible to prevent its having some influence on our practice, surely it is worth taking some pains to have it just, and founded on the basis of sure experience" (1:19). Reason is here figured as a perversion from justice insofar as it relies upon principles that may be untethered to feeling. Feeling becomes a more ethical basis for action because principle may be ungrounded in anything other than reason, a tenuous form of grounding. By this logic, therefore, even sexual feelings are more reliable as a basis for action than reason. This perhaps explains why Burke has such a hard time letting go of them.

Having considered the role of sex in beauty, let us return to consider the relation of sex to the sublime. Burke's confession that sexual sensation is the highest pleasure would seem to define aesthetic pleasure as an impoverished relation to sex. Aware of this possible false hierarchy, Burke not only argues that pain and loss are more powerful than pleasure, but also that we must always turn away from the plentitude of erotic sensation to contemplating its loss. "The loss of so great an enjoyment scarce amounts to an uneasiness; and, except at particular times, I do not think it affects us at all," Burke protests (1:8).[33] The loss of sex yields no affect, yet Burke's parabasis—I do not *think* it affects us—is telling. He might not think it, but that does not stop him from saying that he doesn't feel it. One might also wonder what the "particular times" are that prove the exception.

Complicating the issue even further, Burke goes on to describe the complaints of the forsaken lover: "When men have suffered their imaginations to be long affected with any idea, it so wholly engrosses them as to shut out by degrees almost every other, and to break down every partition of the mind that would confine it" (1:8). It is the loss of sex that allows Burke to distinguish between the positive pain (empiricism/sensation) and imaginary pain (representation/the sublime). Despite the "extraordinary emotions" of love, there is no "positive pain" involved, a fact that is to the detriment of love since pain is, as Burke must insistently remind us, more powerful than pleasure. "Only in brutes is the "sensation from want . . . very troublesome" (1:9). In the end, however, Burke must admit that despite the fact that the emotions of love lack "any connexion with positive pain" (1:8), the passion of love is capable of producing very extraordinary effects" (1:8), an admission that invests sexuality with an effectivity not confined to mere sensation even as it collapses love and want.

That Burke insists that the loss of sex is not really a loss is further undercut by the fact that the normal state of man is indifference (1:3). "The mind returns to its usual state of indifference," Burke announces (1:3). If pleasure is a weak form of stimulus, and, if the loss of that pleasure isn't really a loss, what will provoke man out of his natural indifference?

Notwithstanding its essential imaginary and therefore questionable empirical status, the loss of sex to those not guided by reason enacts a virtually sublime "breakdown of partitions" caused by the violence of love, and Burke's treatment of sex as absence spills into another section. This collapse between the loss of sex and the sublime is further strengthened by the fact that both experiences rely upon a similar negation of sensation: where the sublime is a form of delight, a sensation of the idea of pain and danger "without being actually in those circumstances" (1:18), the loss of sexual pleasure is not a real pain, but is based on the idea of pain. Peter de Bolla captures some of the significance of this when he claims that "sex functions as a negative example of the kind of transport the sublime wishes to effect" (36–37). But sex is much more than a negation of sublime transport in that it grants sublime transport by way of analogy to sex the ontology and authenticity of bodily experience.

Like sexual orgasm, sublime transport overwhelms rational consciousness producing the philosophical blockage that Burke must seek to prevent. For this reason, Burke refers to the mind of the viewer of a sublime tragedy as "erect with expectation" (1:15), even as he makes the point that an actual execution will empty out the theater. By displacing erection onto the mind, Burke can imagine the effectivity of art as having a physiological effect on the body, an effect that places art, reflection, and aesthetics on the same plane as actual experience. Yet, by according the response to the theater as a form of delight, or what he calls elsewhere a negative pleasure, and by insisting that the sublime must be about delight or negative pleasure, Burke preserves the essential experience of the sublime as aesthetic, and insulates the aesthetic from the corruption of the body at the price of cutting the aesthetic off from its source. The negative pleasure that can only be imagined relies upon an idea of sensation rather than sensation itself. Nonetheless, in substituting an idea for a sensation, Burke risks pulling the empirical rug out from under his aesthetics. Such a maneuver is all the more dangerous because, as Burke admits, the "influence of reason in producing our passions is nothing near so extensive as it is commonly believed" (1:13).

But there is another perverse turn in Burke, too, and this takes place when he contemplates the relation of the sublime to usefulness. This perverse turn reminds Burke that even reproduction has its price. Burke comments, "The horse in the light of a useful beast, fit for the plough, the road, the draft; in every social, useful light, the horse has nothing sublime: but it is thus that we are affected with him, whose neck is clothed with thunder, the glory of whose nostrils is terrible" (2.5). Like the beautiful, the sublime here is antithetical to use: the figure of the horse loses whatever sublime power it might gain from its productive strength. Burke continues, "Whenever strength is only useful, and employed for our benefit or our pleasure, then it is never sublime: for nothing can act agreeably to us, that does not act in conformity to our will; but to act agreeably to our will, it must be subject to us, and therefore can never be the cause of a grand and commanding conception" (2.5). To underscore the perverse nature of the sublime, Burke announces that it "suspends" all motions of the soul (2:1) and, in so doing, yields only "astonishment" (2:1). By uniting the perverse and the sublime in the figure of an unproductive horse, Burke makes it clear that the aesthetic comes at the cost of utility; moreover, the sublime is precisely that which resists the uses we wish to put it to. Of course, since the figure of the horse has had a longstanding rhetorical function as a figure for the passions, Burke's sublime horse is also a perverted passion. It is furthermore a passion whose power always threatens "rapine and destruction" (2:5) because it refuses to be "subservient" to any master. Sublime transport is once again figured as a feminizing rape of self-mastery, one that acquires purposiveness to the extent that it is about the elevation of the mind, and one that entails liberty insofar as all forms of subservience, even generation, are rejected.

I risk flogging a dead horse when I insist there is still more perversity. Burke notes that the "nature of the language, framed for the purposes of business rather than those of philosophy, and the nature of my subject, that leads me out of the common track of discourse" (1:5). Aesthetic philosophy is thus framed as a perversion of language insofar as language is framed for business, not philosophy. Hence, if philosophical language turns away from the ordinary business of language, it must itself reject linguistic function and purpose (we call this referentiality) because those stand in the way of philosophical clarity or precision which paradoxically are achieved only through deferral. Sublime blockage in this light then is a form of aesthetic transport without rhetoric, a kind of language for its own sake. It is also very close to the obscurity required in the Burkean sublime. Where Longinus could appropriate sexuality as an aesthetic discourse insofar as Ancient Greek sex was about *Bildung*, Burke, in sacrificing the business of language, can only turn to declared heterosexuality to anchor his aesthetics in something other than perversion. Burke comes nearest to Longinus when he insists that aesthetics must exist for no other purpose than a general "elevation of mind" (1:19). Nonetheless, when Burke acknowledges women to be "an animal not of the highest order" (cited in Johnson 29), he brings heterosexuality and bestiality together, and this implies that not only that homosocial relations can be normal, but also that reproduction brings human sexuality under the orbit of crude, even bestial, purpose. In the end, then, if the separation of beauty from use allows Burke to differentiate lust (crude purpose) from love (purposiveness), animals from human beings, and sexual perversion from sexual norms, it threatens to unground Burke's aesthetics. For this reason, Burke's attempts at separation always lead to collapse.

## Richard Payne Knight and the Priapic Symbol

Where Burke considers the perversity of sexual desire as a form of purposiveness, Richard Payne Knight insists that obscenity obscures the purposiveness of explicit sexual symbolism. Roughly thirty years after Burke's *Inquiry*, the Society of Dilletanti sponsored the publication of Knight's *A Discourse on the Worship of Priapus*. The president of this society was none other than Sir Joseph Banks, who personally oversaw who got copies of this publication (Rousseau "Priapus" 122). Recipients included Walpole, Gibbon, John Wilkes, and the Prince of Wales (Funnell 58). Knight's discourse further suggests both the potentially embarrassing indebtedness of Romantic aesthetics to sex, as well as the purposiveness of a libidinal aesthetics. Knight's aesthetic interest in phallic worship culminates in a longing to return to a classical theory of the symbol, one that truly unified the representative and semantic functions of language insofar as ancient Greece and Egypt refused to see a gap between the sexual and the aesthetic. Whereas his own period imposes "prejudices of artificial decency" upon these wax and stone penises, the ancient theologies of Greece and Egypt turned to the penis as a symbol of the great Creator because it "made them partakers, not only of the felicity of the Deity, but of his great characteristic attribute, that of multiplying his own image" (28–29).[34] Sexual symbols, therefore, confer upon language and art performative powers. Knight further argues that because ancient Greek was a language based upon "imitative representations of ideas" (39) and *not* "being collected from various sources, and blended together without having any natural connection" (39), ambiguity in language could not then exist. Therefore it is no surprise that Knight's nostalgia for ancient symbols is based on the fact that symbols were then "actual emanations of the Divine Power, consubstantial with his own essence" and "treated with more respect and veneration than if they had been merely signs and characters of convention" (50). To encourage this respect, Knight reminds his Christian readers that the cross had its origins in a phallus (53).

As Knight's deliberate baiting of Christians already suggests, part of what he saw as the purposiveness of the priapic symbol was its ability to free the present from its prejudices and false notions of obscenity. Phalli, thus, are key to present *Bildung* because they frustrate contemporary purpose. Knight elaborates, "when the mind is led to the contemplation of things beyond its comprehension, all restraints [of sense and perception] vanish: reason then has nothing to oppose to the phantoms of imagination, which acquire terrors from their obscurity, and dictate uncontrolled because unknown" (26). His interpretations, he argues, by contrast, "will perhaps surprise those who have not been accustomed to divest their minds of the prejudices of education and fashion" (30). Nonetheless, "those who consider manners and customs as relative to the natural causes which produced them, rather than to the artificial opinions and prejudices of any particular age or country" (30), will see beyond the crude eroticism of these sculptures. Rightly perceived, these symbols take the viewer outside of his or her present society and force him or her to imagine long-cherished beliefs and customs as merely artificial prejudices.

If his own age could not get beyond the "prejudices of artificial decency" and understand that "there is naturally no impurity or licentiousness in the moderate and regular gratification of any natural appetite; the turpitude consisting wholly in excess or perversion" (28), the aesthetic consequences, in Knight's view, would be intolerably high. Lost to moral squeamishness was the possibility of ever again reconciling erotic sensuality with aesthetic sensation, the instinctual and passionate foundations of art and theology. At stake in such reconciliation is an end to priestly hierarchy (192), as well as a plea for religious toleration. Knight praises the Greeks for being able to worship whatever Gods were at hand; upon entering a new land, they would worship the local deity (192). Furthermore, since Christianity reformed an already austere Jewish religion by adding even more austerity, Knight's attention to the eroticism of pagan worship and its legacy within Christianity is an effort to overturn such austerity and to think about how such austerity helped to reinforce the Church's power. Thus, he highlights the fact that devices on the door to St. Peter's in Rome rival their lesbian models, that the cross developed out of phallic worship, and that the Eucharist represented the holy kiss of God (183, 184, 186). The swoon of erotic pleasure undermined the austerity and hierarchy of established religions. At the same time, by making clear that current standards of decency were artificial, Knight made it much more difficult to police the borders between nature and perversion. As I will show, when an image of bestiality can be reclaimed as an image of divinity, no sexual act speaks for itself; nothing is necessarily "unnatural" or "abnormal."

In his later remarks on the sublime in the *Analytical Inquiry into the Principles of Taste* (1806), moreover, Knight implies that, since the work of the sublime is to exalt, the true locus of the sublime is in the erotic: in the "erotic compositions of Sappho, Theocritus, and Otway" . . . the "sexual inclination is exalted into a generous and heroic passion; which when expressed with all the glowing energy and spirit of poetry, becomes truly sublime" (339). Here Knight sought to make the sublime even more physiological than did Burke, and he can do so because it fosters generosity and heroism instead of selfishness. Knight's beef with Burke was not with his tendency to materialism but, rather, that he got his physiology wrong. Where Burke claimed that terror "stretched the fibres beyond their natural tone," Knight muses, "No pathologist has . . . discovered or even surmised . . . the stretching power of terror . . . , though the laxative power of terror itself is . . . well known" (381). For Knight, Burke's notion of the sublime thus was really full of shit. Furthermore, Burke had compromised the passions of the mind by framing philosophical reflection at the expense of eroticism.[35]

If pleasure felt on the pulses might diminish the hold of the established Church, it had the added virtue of enlisting human sympathies to move the audience to some action. Rather than deny or discount the violence of the passions then as a form of the mind's energy as he felt Burke did, Knight insists that "the powers of mental feeling are as much powers of the mind, as those of thinking" (*Taste* 343). Knight warns that "those philosophers, who would exalt the one by suppressing the other, attempt to form a model of human perfection from a design of their own; which may, indeed excite our admiration, as a consummate work of art; but will never awaken our sympathies, as a vigorous effusion of nature" (*Taste* 343–44). When aesthetic pleasure is at the expense of erotic pleasure, then, the real danger is that the audience might feel mere admiration, a quality that is relatively powerless to effect change, rather than "the vigorous effusion of nature" that will awaken sympathy from its dormant state. Perhaps Knight's optimism was fueled by his conviction that even the unimproved organs of sense naturally ascend from a lower stimulus to a higher (*Taste* 105).

This is not to say that Knight believes all sexual descriptions to be exalting. In the works of Bafo, Lord Rochester, and Aretine, the sexual inclination is "de-

graded into sordid sensuality; which, how elegantly soever expressed, can never
be exalted: for mere appetite is, in its nature, selfish, through all its gratifying
and cannot, therefore, be in any case, sublime" (339). Knight's insistent caesuras
here put a stop to any false exaltation. I should add, however, that Sappho's sublimity hinges upon Knight's erasure of her sexual specificity. Glossing Longinus
on Sappho, Knight cautions that "it is not being with the particular love of Sappho, that we sympathize, . . . but with the general sentiments of rapturous and
enthusiastic affection" (338).[36] Knight turns to generalization to rescue Sappho
from "every thing selfishly low or sordid" (338). Nonetheless, Knight did allow
that "every display of perverted energy in the mind, may be, in the highest degree, interesting and sublime" (346).

Knight's relatively unapologetic devotion to sensuality has, of course, rendered him a caricature within the history of aesthetics. Coleridge dismissed
Knight's work on taste. He wrote, "Scarcely a page in his book [is] without gross
error," and "the Author of Priapus &c must needs have been ignorant in heart
of Virtue & virtuous feelings" (Shearer 71, 75). To be fair to Knight, Coleridge's
dismissal of Knight, though typical, ignores the fact that Knight sought to harness the passionate intensity of eroticism for aesthetics to the end of fostering
sympathy. Knight shows the extent to which sex did not have to result in selfishness but could lead to generosity.[37] For Knight, taste is unapologetically a
"matter of feeling" (3), and feeling what exalts sex into the aesthetic. Erotic sensuality is especially needed because "reason excites no sympathies; nor awakens
any affections; and its effect is always rather to chill than to inflame" (*Taste* 344).
"Sexual desire," by contrast, exudes "warmth" (86).

Although highly critical of Knight, Coleridge initially severs any connection
of animal appetites to the sublime, only later to reflect upon how those appetites might in fact trigger a sublime state of mind. Imagining a parched Mar-
iner who unexpectedly hears the sound of trickling water, Coleridge ponders,
"*What* will be the effect of that sound upon his mind while he is yet uncertain
whether it gives an assurance of water being within his reach, and after his
doubts pass away. The depth of interest with which he hears this sound . . . is a
sublime state of mind" (quoted in Shearer 71).[38] Upon reflection, Coleridge acknowledges that Knight does have something to offer, that appetite can lead to
aesthetics. For others, Knight's very linking of sex and taste offers ample evidence of his perverted taste. George S. Rousseau recounts the formation of a
"Committee of Taste" in 1805 in London, and it was precisely Knight's devotion to the sensual that led Joseph Farington to exclude Knight (1988 131). This
very need to exile erotic sensuousness from taste nonetheless points to the

potentially insidious power of aesthetic and sexual transport to overwhelm cognition. Knight hoped it would erase contemporary prejudices.

It did not help Knight's reputation that he not only had a perverted taste for the sexual within his aesthetics, but also that his sexual tastes were seen as perverted. Who else would have dared to imagine Edmund Burke "walk[ing] up St. James's street without his breeches" so as to ridicule Burke's connection of astonishment to the sublime (*Taste* 383)? In his later *Analytical Inquiry into the Principles of Taste* (1806), Knight went so far as to hint that the very socialization of the sexual instincts in man was a perversion: he equates "the sexual desires of brutes" with being "more strictly natural inclinations, and less changed or modified by the influence of acquired ideas, or social habits" and he declares that their desires are "less liable to be influenced or perverted by mental sympathies" (17–18). He would later insist on the need to "cultivate the pleasures of sense according to a just degree of each sensation" (Shearer 68). If, on the one hand, he made the notion of innate heterosexuality problematic because "the doctrine of innate ideas has been so completely confuted and exploded" (33), he did suggest that "there may be internal stimuli, which, though not innate, grow up constitutionally in the body; and naturally and instinctively dispose the desires of all animals to the opposite sex of their own species" (33). On the other hand, he left the door open to homosexual desire when he noted a separation between sexual aim and sexual object. He claimed that "animal desire or want may exist without any idea of its object, if there be a stimulus to excite it; so that a male, who had arrived at maturity without knowing the existence of a female of his own species, might feel it, . . . without having any determinate notion of what was proper to gratify it" (33–34). Like Burke, Knight thinks that desire is neither innately heterosexual nor homosexual but is perversely open to both. Such perversity enabled aesthetics to place at arm's length the crude purpose of reproduction, and instead, to purposefully value mutual intimacy, love, as erotic purposiveness.

This need to apprehend eroticism aesthetically and historically is invoked especially in Payne Knight's descriptions of Egyptian and Ancient Greek statues depicting bestiality. "To the Egyptians, it was . . . an incarnation of the Deity, and the communication of his creative spirit to man" (62). For benefit of his skeptical readers, Knight quotes the authority of no one less than Bishop Warburton, who proclaimed that "from the nature of any action morality cannot arise, nor from its effects" (55). As a gloss to an image of women having sex with a goat, Warburton's remarks do two things. They separate the action from questions of moral purpose, and they distance effects from morality. Knight thus demands an aesthetic apprehension of the statue, one that actively suspends moral judgments as to action and effect. He continues, "However shocking it may appear to modern manners and opinions, [it] might have been intrinsically meritorious at the time of its celebration" (55). Referring to another statue depicting bestiality in the collection of Mr. Townley, Knight comments that "Fauns and Satyrs . . . represent the emanations of the Creator, incarnate with man, acting as his angels and ministers in the work of universal generation. In copulation with the goat, they represent the reciprocal incarnation of man with the Deity, when incorporated with universal matter: for the Deity, being both male and female, was both active and passive in procreation; first animating man by an emanation from his own essence, and then employing that emanation to reproduce, in conjunction with the common productive powers of Nature, which are no other than his own prolific spirit transfused through matter" (59). Copulation, albeit bestial, symbolizes the reciprocal incarnation of the deity in man and man in deity. With that reciprocity, copulation loses the taint of selfishness.

Knight's insight that eroticism must be apprehended owes a debt to Kant's insistence that aesthetic judgment be an act of making the subjective apprehension of beauty available to universal assent. Kant was influenced by Hume, and Knight explicitly records a debt to Hume's theory that "beauty is no quality in things themselves: it exists merely in the mind, which contemplates them" (cited in Knight 16). This insight might help defuse current debates on pornography.[39] I shall allude to them here briefly because they also have something to teach us about aesthetics and erotics. In the above passage on copulation, incarnation is at the same time representation. Knight allows us to argue that nothing is inherently pornographic; pornography must be apprehended by the viewer. By shifting the locus of pornography from the object to the mind of the viewer, one is thus able to take into account the fact that, as Lynn Hunt has argued, pornography began in the eighteenth century as a means of religious and social protest and also deal with Laura Kipnis's suggestion that even pornography has an aesthetics.[40] Rather than being an object that simply speaks for itself, pornography has aesthetic effects that distance the viewer from any content that is supposedly merely literal and immediate. Kipnis argues, sometimes persuasively, that much pornography is really about the challenging of cultural assumptions of gender. In de Manian terms, pornography has convinced us of its symbolism, but not of its allegorical nature. That ancient cultures continually rework the symbols of other cultures, suggests Knight, makes these symbols necessarily allegorical.

The task of the reader thus is to bring both ways of apprehending pornography to bear upon it, along with an ironical sense that both may be wrong. The task is to read it aesthetically, in terms of purposiveness rather than crude purpose. With such an approach, for example, Sade's revolutionary manifesto that is embedded within his *Philosophy of the Bedroom* no longer seems ancillary to his graphic and sodomitic sexuality. Sade writes, "Men are incapable of obtaining true notions of a being who does not make its influence felt on one of our senses" (304), and this same hostility to abstraction underwrites both Sade's pornography and his hostility toward monarchy. Moreover, it is man's immorality—his addiction to "prostitution, incest, rape, and sodomy" (314)—that keeps him in a state of revolutionary unrest, the "necessary insurrection in which the republican must always keep the government of which he is a member" (315). Sade's folding of clause onto clause performs the insurrection he demands: subjects and objects revolve around the "of." And with such an approach, Knight can demonstrate that sex is both a creative and destructive power: Knight, for example, reads a medal of Apollo as "a union of the creative and destructive powers of both sexes in one body" (165). Especially because pornography has been legally defined as having no redeeming social value—it is, like aesthetics, useless—sexual stimulation need not necessarily be limited to selfish bodily pleasure since even that pleasure can be purposive. In fact, it can use bodily pleasure (as does Knight) to help delegitimize the church and state.

While Knight took considerable pains to remove images of bestiality from the domain of obscenity, he did not challenge cultural norms concerning sodomy. At least not overtly so. Knight makes clear that the priapic objects he so eagerly catalogues are images not of homoeroticism, but are, rather, of heterosexual intercourse. Indeed, many of them actually bear fruits in their hands, thus announcing their fertility (British Museum 1824 4–71 3, 4). For example, he notes that the "devout wearer" of the priapic symbol wore it to show herself "devoted . . . wholly and solely to procreation, the great end for which she was ordained" (*Discourse* 46). In so doing, however, Knight emphasized that women might think of their sexual objectification as the telos governing their lives, and he depicts them as "grateful to the Creator, for having taken her into his service, and made her a partaker of his most valuable blessings, and employed her as the passive instrument in the exertion of his most beneficial power" (46–47). And although Knight recognizes that many of these objects can be construed as engaging in sodomy—what he refers to as the "gratification of disordered, and unnatural appetites," as opposed to procreation (76)—because of the arrangement of the figures, he breathes an audible sigh of relief when he can invoke a

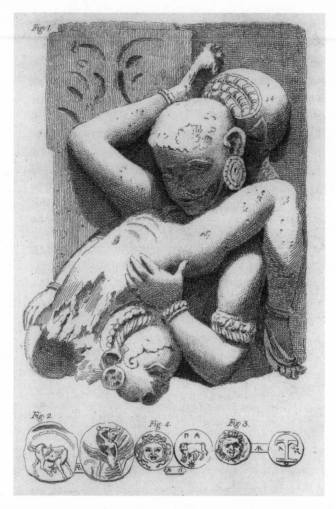

Richard Payne Knight, *Account of the Remains of the Worship of Priapus*, 1786. Plate 10, figure 1. Reproduced by permission of the Huntington Library, San Marino, California.

"learned Author" who "cleared them from this suspicion, by showing that they only took the most convenient way to get at the Female Organs of Generation" (77). Knight continues, "We may therefore conclude, that instead of representing them in the act of gratifying any disorderly appetites, the artists meant to show their modesty in not indulging their concupiscence, but in doing their duty in the best way adapted to answer the ends proposed by the Creator" (77). It is no mean feat to argue that an explicit depiction of a sexual act is in truth a

[ 195 ]

manner, without the diphthong, which was not in
ufe for many ages after the Greek Colonies fettled in
LATIUM, and introduced the Arcadian Alphabet. We
find St. PAUL likewife acknowledging, that the
JUPITER of the Poet ARATUS was the God whom
he adored ;* and CLEMENS of ALEXANDRIA explains
St. PETER's prohibition of worfhipping after the manner of the Greeks, not to mean a prohibition of worfhipping the fame God, but merely of the corrupt
mode in which he was then worfhipped.†

---

* *Ad. Apoft.* Chap. xvii. ver. 28.    † STROMAT. Lib. V.

THE   END.

Richard Payne Knight, *Account of the Remains of the Worship of Priapus*, 1786. Page 195.
Reproduced by permission of the Huntington Library, San Marino, California.

depiction of modesty. Of course, that brings heterosexual sex dangerously close
to the anus, so much so that one might be prompted to ask if Knight is indulging
in a pun on "ends." In his selection of illustrations, however, Knight may show
himself to be more liberated: he shows large-scale nonreproductive images of
cunnilingus and ends his tract with a depiction of bestiality (195), a visual ending that suggests Knight may be protesting too much that these images are reproductive rather than sodomitic.

In any case, Buffon had already argued that sex between species is by definition unreproductive. Knight attempts to get around the figure's half-beast/
half-man status by insisting that satyrs and fauns were really images of the divine uniting with the mortal (83). His original collection itself has numerous
depictions of Ganymede, the boy who was the recipient of Jupiter's love (British
Museum 1824 4–37 1–3).[41] Even sodomitic intercourse, then, could be about
love. Sodomy and aesthetics therefore unite upon a common ground of skepticism about purpose, a skepticism that leads to a kind of purposiveness with purpose. To the extent that even sodomitic images represent the mingling of the
human and divine, perversity need not be merely selfish, sordid, or pornographic. Once again sexual perversity achieves the form of purposiveness.

I am suggesting, in their mutual distrust of purpose, that perversion and aesthetics are allies rather than enemies. Because purpose is at odds with liberty
and purposelessness is at odds with the need for aesthetics to inspire *Bildung*, the
development of human potentiality, aesthetic writers such as Burke, Winckelmann, and Longinus turn to purposiveness to limit the determining force of
purpose while conferring upon aesthetics the power to educate its readers. To
see how sexuality and aesthetics meet on the ground of perversion, sex must not
be assumed to be selfish, and sex must be connected with purposeless love in the
same way that sexual sensation and aesthetic sensation are united in a common
nervous body. Perversion thus rescues heteronormativity from animality even
as it thereby acquires the aesthetic form of purposiveness. When sex and aesthetics can be about purposiveness, both can escape the tyranny of purpose
while resisting complete fecklessness through the cultivation of human potentiality. To end with a perverse twist on one of Walter Benjamin's "Theses on the
Philosophy of History": There are few documents of aesthetics that are not simultaneously documents of perversion. And such perversion is for the express
purpose of liberation from crude purpose.

# CHAPTER FIVE

# Fiery Joys Perverted to Ten Commands

William Blake, the Perverse Turn, and Sexual Liberation

Few accusations in Blake's illuminated works have the force and density of Orc's accusation that Urizen "perverted to ten commands" "the fiery joy" (*America* 8:3 E 54). Orc, Blake's symbol of revolutionary and sexual energy, here charges Urizen, Blake's caricature of reason, with perverting sexual pleasure into commands. Blake often depicts Orc with his genitals at the center of his body, a depiction that cements the connection between sex and revolution (Mitchell *BCA*). Yet, in order for readers to be able to unpack Orc's charge, they have to understand that behind Urizen's perversion of joy into hierarchy is Blake's perversion of Mosaic law. That is, Blake seeks to turn the Ten Commandments, the basis of so much Western moral virtue, on its head, and he does so by truncating commandments to "commands," linking them, in the democratic rhetoric of his day, with the illegitimate hierarchy of kings. In masking his perversion underneath Urizen's perversion, Blake shows how judgments of perversion not only assume wrong and right to be unarguable, but also assume that a stable ground exists from which to measure perversion. If the Ten Commandments are not the ground but the perversion of the ground, where is the ground? To complicate further the use of perversion, Blake inverts ordinary syntax, placing the direct object of the verb before the verb. The line begins with "the fiery joy, that Urizen perverted to ten commands," thus putting joy at least syntactically back in the driver's seat, where it belongs. The poet's perversion of ordinary syntax not only further undermines the solidity of ground, but also exploits epistemological uncertainty to the end of undermining all forms of authority, including his own.

Perversion came to occupy a central position as a concept and technique for Blake.[1] Although perversion literally means the "turning aside from truth or right," Blake demands that his readers discover the truth or right for themselves, especially when "nature" is invoked as the standard against which to measure perversion. If Foucault got it right when he claimed that the weaker perversion "is epistemologically, the better it functions" (Foucault *Abnormal* 32), then, for Blake, all perversion is strong perversion that doesn't function and this disruption of function is precisely his point because the suspension of function allows mental fight to occur. Because Blake took issue with so many of his culture's notions of "truth," "right," or what "truth" and "right" dissolve into—namely, nature—the turning of perversion allowed the poet to force readers to question the very ground upon which a charge of perversion can be made. He thus turns perversion away from ontology and toward epistemology. This turning, moreover, enacts the kind of revolution Blake wants to perpetuate and reminds us that both revolution, etymologically connected to revolve, and perversion involve turning. Much like his use of the vortex, Blake exploits the power of perversion to uproot his readers from secure ground.

At the outset of *The Four Zoas*, for instance, Enion weaves a Garment, "not/ As Garments woven subservient to her hands but having a will/Of its own perverse & wayward" (*FZ* 1:85–87 E 302). Although Enion judges this garment to be "perverse," the fact that the specter of Tharmas refuses to be subservient to Enion suggests that "perverse" is at least partly a commendable sign of individuality. Later describing the wheels of Urizen and Luvah as rolling "perverse" and "back reverse," Blake writes,

> Terrific ragd the Eternal Wheels of intellect terrific ragd
> The living creatures of the wheels in the Wars of Eternal life
> But perverse rolld the wheels of Urizen & Luvah back reversd
> Downwards & outwards consuming in the wars of Eternal Death (*FZ* 1:556–59)

This pun on "perverse" and "reverse" indicates perversion is relational rather than absolute: it depends on the vantage point of the perceiver and upon the perceiver's values. The fact that "perverse" and "reverse" bookend the line both highlights their spatiality and their dependence upon vantage point. The line literally turns on "perverse" and "reverse." Moreover, because "Terrific ragd" begins and ends the first line, Blake reminds us that revolution returns to its origin. The net effect of all this turning makes readers always question whether the ground isn't really a perversion of the ground. Is the rolling of these wheels good or bad? On the one hand, since "perverse" is antithetical to "Eternal life," and since Urizen and Luvah are aligned with the "wars of Eternal Death," perversion would seem bad. On the other hand, their reverse wheels recall Blake's own need to write backward on the copper plate[2] and thus suggest some allegiance to them. To the extent that Luvah represents desire and his wheels counter Urizen's (reason's) wheels, Luvah's reversal further moves in the right direction. Although Blake's ampersand seems to unite the wheels of Urizen and Luvah, the fact that Urizen stands for reason against desire (Luvah) hints that Luvah's wheels might be admirably "perverse." And although Urizen's and Luvah's wheels are associated with "Eternal Death" (1:574), such death precipitates Albion's "rising"—the first word of Night 2. If death is necessary for resurrection to occur, once again readerly judgment about the wheels must be suspended. Therefore, in making perversion raise so many questions, Blake disrupts its ability to function as a clear marker of morality and thus perverts the performative power of perversion—its seeming ability to deliver immediate judgment—into that which immediately provokes epistemological uncertainty. That these wheels symbolize both death and life only highlights this uncertainty.

Likewise, since the charge of perversion so often works by claiming to evade historical specificity—perversions are against nature, which is allegedly immune to history—Blake's perversion perversely insists on that history and in the process redefines that history as trauma because history has the power to show the arbitrariness of any one version of nature as well as the psychic costs of history.[3] Hence, Blake gives the Ten Commandments not the grounded authority of the Logos, the word of God, but the merely ascribed authority of Urizen ("Your Reason"). That Urizen embodies the Romantic interpretation of the Enlightenment means that he cannot be dismissed so easily as a villain.

But Orc's accusation does much more than have Urizen playing politics. To the extent that Orc is right, it suggests that liberation will be achieved when the fiery joys return, when sexual pleasure has no longer been perverted into commandments. It invites readers to consider whether they want a God devoted to joy or one insistent upon hierarchy, an illegitimate one to boot. It invites readers to consider whether commandments should be the basis of a religion as well as to consider why joy and reason became understood antithetically in the first place.

The aesthetic embodiment of perversion raised further issues for Blake: if his own words acquired the ontological solidity of the commandments, then they, too, could repress rather than liberate. Blake insists that poet/prophets are "seers not arbitrary dictators" (E 617). To make his own charges of perversion more than finger wagging, Blake made them debatable. Thus, he embodies perversion in insistently contradictory ways, often continuing to turn opposing concepts until one can see the connections between the two rather than seeing them as polar opposites. The above charge comes from Orc, not Blake, and thus Blake's distancing of himself from Orc needs to be factored into the equation, as does his ironic attitude toward Urizen and, by extension, the Enlightenment itself. Orc's charge that Urizen had perverted "fiery joys" means that Orc himself is perverted since Orc stands for fiery joy: what about perversion enables it to acquire the glue of identity? Orc's dual existence as the embodiment of joy and the perversion of it further unsettles the very ground by which one determines whether perversion exists. This duality further tempers any readerly identification with Orc and hints at the painful consequences of revolutionary instability. As Blake knew only too well, merely to substitute Orc's authority for Urizen's relocates tyranny, not does away with it.

Moreover, if reason is a perversion of joy, what role does either play in one's aesthetic? Previously I suggested that the Romantics aligned themselves with an eroticized if purposive aesthetics precisely to engage audiences otherwise abstracted and distanced by reason. Here I show what Blake's aesthetic embodiment of perversion accomplishes. And, building upon Andrew Elfenbein's insight that Romantic genius centered on the artist's ability to experiment with sex/gender roles, I ask whether perversion is the logical outcome of an aesthetics of originality and individualism. How better to set oneself apart from one's culture than to undermine the very naturalness of sex?

In short, Blake was perverse to his very core, and it is high time that we dealt with that fact along with its manifold implications.[4] My method here will be first to unpack the significance of perversion to Blake by looking closely at how the poet uses this term to open up epistemological questions rather than to close them down, then to think about the implications of perversion to Blake's understanding of body and text, and, finally, to see how he embodies perversion. I situate Blake in the medical literature of his day to show that he could not have understood the body as a fixed sign, in terms of the intransigence of materiality; nor could he have associated textuality with automatic liberation. Thus, our understanding of the body and language in Blake runs the considerable risk of saying more about our own postmodern fascination with textualism as a form of liberation and materiality as that which resists change than it does about Blake.

Textualism is here defined as the exploitation of language's "intrinsic potential for detachment from the material circumstances in which it is utilized" (Terdiman 76).[5] Blake understood the sexual body as both spirit and body and thus could make the body the ground for liberty, not its enemy. And although textualism in Blake helps to disconnect words from authority, the poet certainly recognized that the free play of language does not necessarily give anyone the traction needed to muster counter arguments (Terdiman 105). The illuminated books, thus, encode a conversionary/perversionary/transformative dimension within them yet require the readerly deconstruction of this textualism as part of their attempt to shift power from the location of the author to the reader, a maneuver which is allegorized in Blake's grounding of his mythology in the body.

At once incarnation and allegory, Blake's sexed bodies embody a flexible materiality that can ground utopia within the human body. Having defined the imagination as "spiritual sensation" (Letter 5 E 703), Blake holds onto bodies even in his concept of spirituality. These questions of the relation of materiality to text get condensed into Blake's concept of perversion. By linking the materiality of the body with epistemological questions, by giving those questions the seeming incarnation of perversion, and by reminding us that the body bears the legible signs of psychic trauma, Blake harnesses both materiality and textuality in service of the idea liberation. He thereby avoids the limitations of both: intransigence and endless vertigo, not to mention Urizenic law and impotence. Because the sexed body in Blake must always be viewed from an aesthetic stance that resists purpose, the poet is equipped to measure the forms liberation takes against any achievements.

## Perversion in Blake

Blake uses various forms of the word "perversion" nineteen times in his writings (*Concordance*), and the term offers important clues about how we are to understand Blakean sexuality and why the poet insists that "gratified desire" is key to political liberation.[6] His preference for verbal and adjectival over noun forms of the word reminds us that he understands perversion to be relational and contextual. Only three of his uses of perversion are the abstract noun forms. Although medicine and psychology were hardening perversion into deviant forms of psychological identity, Blake deploys perversion to undermine both identity and the idea of psychological diagnosis. For Blake, the problem is hardly the deviance of any individual psyche, but rather a generalized repression of imaginative vision.

I'll begin with Blake's accusation in his letter to Trusler that Trusler's eye "is perverted by Caricature Prints" (Letter 5, E 702) one of the poet's more straightforward uses of "perverted." Yet, given Blake's own indebtedness to caricature, so carefully documented throughout the Princeton facsimiles, how could the poet be sure his own eye had not been likewise perverted? Blake offers three answers. First, Trusler cannot recognize the difference between the beauty of "Michael Angelo Rafael & the Antique & best living Models" (E 702) and that of caricature. Second, Blake adds that "Fun I love but too much Fun is of all things the most loathsome" (E 702). This raises the question of how do we know when we love fun too much? Provisionally, I'll suggest here that excess fun indicates Blake's own impatience with equating a kind of aesthetic free play with liberty. Third, by linking perversion of Trusler's eye with the mass marketing of Caricature, "which ought not to abound as they do," Blake shows the dangers of commodity culture that profits by getting purchasers to pervert quantity into quality.[7]

Where Blake distances Trusler's perverted eye from his own, a distancing which paradoxically mandates an identification with Trusler in order to understand the grounds for Trusler's perversion, he deepens his idea of perversion in his annotations to Bishop Watson's *An Apology for the Bible*. Of course, if the distancing of perversion leads us back to identity, perversion is by no means simple. In the margins to Watson, Blake harrumphs, "The Perversions of Christs words & acts are attacked by Paine & also the perversions of the Bible; who dare defend [them] either the Acts of Christ or the Bible Unperverted?" (E 611). From Blake's standpoint, Watson mistakenly claimed Paine perverted the Bible when in truth Paine's argument was that the Bible was perverted to begin with, a text designed to further priestly hierarchy. So what is it about perversion that enables this kind of mistake? This is a crucial epistemological problem in Blake. How do we know perversion when we see it, and then what to do about it?

To distinguish between a perversion of something and the thing itself, one needs at very least to be able to stand outside of the thing itself. An ironic stance toward objects enables the consideration of whether one's perception of the object is distorting it; more critically, such a stance allows one to consider if the object is being manipulated in the service of specific interests. To get to the "Bible unperverted," one must acknowledge the possibility that it can be, and may have been, perverted. This means that, at least from the perspective of the fallen world, interpretations that assume meaning is fully present in the sign cannot work because they do not offer any place to stand outside the text insofar as word and meaning are welded together.[8] Instead, one needs to see the Bible as a palimpsest of texts, one whose previous interpretations mask the pure text underneath. Although my use of "pure text" would seem to reinstall the very naive logocentrism Blake denies, I want to insist upon the reader's necessarily skeptical view of all texts, even ones that claim to be pure. Here I point out that Blake uses "unperverted" rather than pure, a word choice that suggests we should initially assume all texts to be perverted.[9] As many have noted, Blake's own texts resist logocentric readings, and this is even the case when the details of the poet's printing process have been so admirably set forth, but in ways that locate Blake's meaning in materiality. I am suggesting that obsessive critical fascination with the materiality of the poet's printing process is symptomatic of, rather than counter to, the larger instabilities within Blake.[10]

Blake's resistance to logocentrism raises another and more serious problem. If the signifier only has to manage to signify the signified, how does one overcome the gap between the signifier and signified and know when a perversion has occurred? Blake offers more clues when he trumpets, "I cannot conceive of the Divinity of the books in the Bible to consist either in who they were written by or at what time or in the historical evidence which may be all false in the eyes of one man & true in the eyes of another but in the Sentiments & Examples which whether true or Parabolic are Equally useful as Examples given to us of the perverseness of some & its consequent evil & its consequent good" (E 618). Blake informs us here that divinity is grounded in neither the author nor historical evidence. He also distances perverseness from moral judgment—perverseness can have either consequent evil or good. That Blake refuses to attach perverseness to evil or good undermines the neat opposition that supposedly exists between Romantic moral perversity and Victorian perverted identities. Where Paine had dismissed the authenticity of the Bible because the actual actors had not written their own accounts, Watson argues that one must distinguish between genuineness and authenticity: although the work may not have been genuinely "written by the person whose name it bears" (Watson 11), this fact does not prevent the work form being historically true or "related matters of fact as they really happened" (Watson 11). For Watson, Paine may have shown the books of the Bible not to be genuine, but that was not the same thing as showing them to be inauthentic.[11]

Long before Foucault and Barthes would declare the author dead, Blake refutes Watson by insisting that both authorship and historical fact are insufficient grounds for truth. In other words, Blake eliminates both the bishop's genuineness and his authenticity as grounds for biblical truth, a maneuver which again insists that texts are best apprehended when they are assumed to be perverted. Such an assumption makes even sacred texts approach *jeux de vérités*, games of truth. Furthermore, what may seem historical evidence to some may not count as evidence to others; therefore, one is to understand that evidence not in terms of its referentiality, but in terms of the "sentiments and examples" that lead readers to act or embody those same sentiments. Note that Blake presumes neither the truth nor the perverseness of biblical examples: rather than presuming the exemplarity of biblical characters for good or ill, the poet again demands that we not prejudge and attempt first to gauge how the actions and sentiments of these individuals might serve as examples for others. Blake's emphasis upon "consequent" underscores that readers look to what actions and sentiments provoke. This insistence on consequence allows us to go back to Blake on Trusler's perverted eye, and to see that "too much fun" for Blake is fun without consequences. That perversion facilitates the separation of the self and other when in fact the other may define the self further calls for the deliberation that irony makes possible. Because Blake values fun but not the excess of fun, differences of kind between the poet's eye and Trusler's perverted eye begin to look like the mere difference of degree.

Perversion, then, in spite of its seeming immediacy, demands an ironic or allegorical reading of all texts. Blake enhances the ironic powers of perversion by actively distancing perversion from moral judgment and by highlighting perversion's vexed relationship to identity. Since every act or text potentially embodies its perversion, each must be actively apprehended by the reader, grounded in neither the acts nor sentiments themselves but in what those acts or sentiments lead up to. Moreover, by substituting consequences for function, Blake makes perversion into a kind of purposiveness against purpose insofar as consequences demand effects without assuming the form of them in advance. It is because Watson cannot imagine the possibility that the Bible is itself perverted that he mistakes Paine's acts for a perversion of the Bible rather than an unperverting of the biblical text. If the reader must posit the possibility of perversion, and it does not exist necessarily in the text itself, then the emphasis is not so much on the text, but in the apprehender, and in what the apprehension would achieve. Suspending judgment, Blake posits Paine to be "either a Devil or an Inspired man," and by looking at Paine through both vantages, he concludes that "Tom Paine is a better Christian than the Bishop" (E 620).[12]

Yet this final assessment of Paine is especially perverse for Blake since Paine was a professed deist, who turned to reason and science to try to explain religion. Paine read the book of nature as the only true Logos of God (*Age of Reason* 68), and Blake's beloved Book of Revelation was for Paine a mere fable (55). Blake abhorred natural religion because of its insistent materiality. Even worse, Paine denied the imagination's role in religion, and sought to debunk revealed religion because it was no more than hearsay. So why then does Blake not align himself with Watson who defends revealed religion and against Paine the deist?

The answer goes back to Blake's emphasis on consequences. While Paine was promoting equality and liberty, the bishop was merely a "State trickster" (E 612) defending the deeds of a wicked God, one who would sanction the murder of another. Blake denounces any "defence of the Wickedness of the Israelites in murdering so may thousands under pretence of a command from God" (E 614). He could also align himself with Paine because of Paine's skepticism about the Bible and its meanings, a skepticism that would allow one to choose a New Testament Christ of forgiveness over a punishing Old Testament God and see institutional religion as oppression.[13] At one point, Paine makes doubting Thomas his ideal reader (*Age of Reason* 54), and "Thomas" had the virtue of being ideal as well as real, Paine's own first name. Blake similarly takes comfort in the fact that Christ died as "an Unbeliever" in the Old Testament God (E 614). Blake also would find solace in Paine's declaration that "my own mind is my own church" (50).

In the end, because of his inability to suspend judgment and to think through the substance of Paine's arguments, Blake cannot identify with the bishop. Watson has very limited capacity for irony. He neither has a considered response to Paine's claim that the "Bible is all a State Trick" nor does he refute Paine's argument that the commentators of the Bible are all "dishonest Designing knaves" (E 616). Here the ironic distance that Blake has from Paine—Paine argues that the Bible is a state trick, not necessarily Blake—which allows the poet meaningful reflection about Paine.[14] Blake's use of "designing" above alludes to the argument from design: the very argument that Paine had used to make nature the word of God was for Blake a perverse debasement of spirituality into vegetative materialism. Hence, "designing" in this particular context is "the work of knaves." Lurking within Blake's defense of Paine is the possibility of Paine's perverseness.

Blake as reader hopes to instill in his readers this very ironic distance so that they don't mistake his words for commands. His strategy of offering disembodied quotations—Blake often does not tell us who is speaking until well after he or she has spoken—further demands readerly irony. The poet again brackets his use of perversion with irony when he states in response to Watson that "the Bible says that God formed Nature perfect but that Man perverted the order of Nature since which time the Elements are filld with the Prince of Evil who has the power of the air. Natural Religion is the voice of God & not the result of reasoning on the powers of Satan" (E 614). By emphasizing "the Bible says," and given Blake's general distaste for sacred codes, we don't know whether Blake agrees with what the Bible says. Nonetheless, the poet's attribution suspends judgment. Watson scores rhetorical points against Paine by pointing out that Paine's privileging of natural religion over revealed religion merely projects the wickedness of God onto nature. For this reason, Watson relishes the fact that by Paine's own logic, which undermined the legitimacy of the Old Testament God on the basis of his cruelty, the recent earthquake in Lisbon makes Paine's God of natural theology equally cruel. Blake retorts to Watson that one must distinguish between "an accident brought on by a mans own carelessness & a destruction from the designs of another" (E 614). Read in this light, the poet's comment that "the Bible says God formed Nature perfect but that Man perverted the order of Nature" must be ironic in that nature's perfection consists of mere accident and not design. I therefore draw attention to Blake's love of puns and the written similarity of "pervert" and "perfect" because so much hangs on two letters. Furthermore, for Blake, nature's perfection is a perversion of the divinity within mankind, the emphasis upon the vegetative at the expense of the spiritual. The key here is to remember that nature and man have different standards for perfection in Blake, and that even perfection can yield perversion. The claim of divine perfection intensifies the perversion.

Blake's willingness to think about Paine as both "devil" and "inspired man," along with the poet's positive and negative senses of devils, enables Blake to gauge if Paine's unperverting of the Bible amounts to liberation and, if so, to liberty. Moreover, by insistently deferring the adjudication of perversion onto a previous text, and by trying to understand the role of perversion in each text,

Blake makes perversion a slippery but useful critical tool against authority. Paine's unperverting of the Bible may be liberating, but that does not mean it achieves liberty. If it doesn't achieve the ultimate goal of liberty, then liberation can be a perversion. Here, lest I seem to be merely reinstalling the very terms (repression and liberation) that Foucault sought to make bankrupt, I aim to show the Romantics thinking through the limitations of liberation. By recognizing those limits, the Romantics and I can help restore credit to the concept. Often skeptics of sexual liberation miss the skepticism within the sexual liberators.[15] The Romantics recognized that liberation from something was not the same thing as liberty, yet they held onto the concept of liberation because that gave them targets to aim their revolutionary energies against, as well as a belief in a more hopeful future. Finally, Blake's emphasis on consequences offers a sobering warning to queer theorists at once intent on celebrating the disruptiveness of desire without allowing their own identities to be disrupted by that desire.

To return to Orc's charge that Urizen had perverted fiery joys into ten commands, I argue that Orc's charge of perversion enables liberation from Urizen, but to be liberated from Urizen is not to be in the condition of liberty. For one, there are Urizen's many emanations to combat. For another, the free fall of liberty, the endless turning in Blake, may liberate one from certain constraints, but it does not necessarily achieve liberty. Few would mistake vertigo or a fall into an abyss for freedom. Likewise, as Blake's Whore of Babylon and Beulah make clear, one may be liberated from the oppressive distrust of the flesh, but that is far from liberty. Whereas the whore transforms an enslavement to denial of the flesh into an enslavement to the flesh, Beulah looks like Eden only to be a vegetated Eden.

Acknowledging the liberty of the flesh to be at considerable distance from liberty itself, Blake reminds us that "the Sexual is Threefold: the Human is Fourfold" (*Milton* 4:5 E 97). If identity cannot be reduced to the sexual, nor can sexual liberation be liberty. Likewise, in *The Marriage of Heaven and Hell*, Blake distances his "Song of Liberty" from his deconstruction of sacred codes: to have profaned the Bible is not yet liberty.[16] And while Jerusalem is "named liberty," we cannot know what this means until the end of Blake's epic, and only after we measure "liberty" against how the various audiences Blake addresses construe liberty. Addressing the public, the poet, for example, explicitly distinguishes between the democratic rhetoric that amounts to the "stern demands of Right & Duty instead of Liberty" and "Love" as the bedrock of liberty (*Jerusalem* 22:11 Paley 164). The gap between liberation from something and liberty enables

Blake a standpoint outside of liberation from which to evaluate the consequences of liberation, and whether those consequences lead to love and liberty. Here since liberation takes the form of "rights and duty," the poet must ask if this form in fact achieves liberty. Furthermore, this gap enables Blake to measure the costs of sexual liberation and to think about who is really being liberated.

Now that Blake lays the responsibility for identifying perversion at the reader's doorstep, he warns that the charge of perversion can be merely a projection or transference. Blake annotates Swedenborg thusly, "Many perversely understand him as if man while in the body was only conversant with natural Substances because themselves are mercenary & worldly & have no idea of any but worldly gain" (E 606). A perverse or incorrect understanding of Swedenborg stems from the fact that one's own materialism leads one to charge others with it. A more careful reader would acknowledge that Swedenborg is never so absolute and that he insists that the mind is a composite of spiritual and natural substances, although Swedenborg does also maintain that thought derives from spiritual substances only. The very phrase "spiritual substance," however, collapses metaphysics with physics, and it is this collapse that helps make Swedenborg compelling to Blake. But perversion's ability to transfer its charge from the accuser to the accused and then to cover its tracks makes it so powerful. The accusation of perversion seems to foist perversion onto others when in fact the need to accuse others connects perversion back to the accuser's identity.

Blake will often turn to the word "perversion" when his ideal sexuality is being threatened. Perverse sexuality thus is an especially dense transfer point of power: Satan accuses Palamabron in *Milton* of perverting the Divine voice into the seven deadly sins and the "infernal scroll / Of Moral laws" (9:21, 23 E 103), when the fault is really his. Rintrah and Tirzah "perverted Swedenborg[']s Visions in Beulah & in Ulro," with Beulah and Ulro being the state of vegetative sexuality (*Milton* 22:46 E 117), while "Rahab and Tirzah pervert" the "mild influences of Enitharmon and her daughters" (*Milton* 29:53 E 128). Where the former hopes that Swedenborg takes the blame, the latter leaves Enitharmon holding the bag. In addition, sex under moral law (generation) seems to Blake a perversion of ideal sex, a destruction of the faculties of sense rather than their redemption. Blake therefore later equates the "Vegetated Mortal Eye" with "perverted & single vision" (*Jerusalem* 53:11 E 202).

But to understand more fully Blake's concept of perversion, we need to examine the complex role that generation plays in his work. Thomas Frosch is certainly right that "generation is the world of ordinary fallen experience" (187).

Indeed, the word "generation" in Blake frequently takes on distinctly negative overtones, signifying the merely material or the vegetated body so bereft of the spirit that Urizen hammers out. Blake's commentary on his "A Vision of the Last Judgment" at once links generation with the finite, temporal, vegetative, and deadly (E 555). Perhaps because "generation" evoked biblical hierarchical kin relations (Cody 21), Blake remains suspicious of it.

In *Jerusalem*, Blake condemns generation, dismissing that "false and Generating Love: a pretence of love to destroy love" (17:25–26 E 161). Moreover, "the Religion of Generation," Blake declares, ". . . was meant for the destruction / Of Jerusalem" (7:63 E150). As his symbol of liberty, then, Jerusalem must actively combat the forces of generation. Los's city of art and manufacture, Golgonooza, which literally contains the Zoas, must continually reach toward and reorient generation if such liberty is to be achieved (12:49, 61 E156). Los directs his fury against the sons of Albion, because he is afraid of the daughters, and of being "vegetated beneath / Their Looms, in a Generation of death & resurrection to forgetfulness" (17: 8–9 E 161). As Thomas Frosch ably put it, "reproduction [in Blake] carries with it the aura of meaningless, self-enclosed, and compulsive repetition that characterizes nature as a whole. The fallen world is a 'sexual machine'" (E 185); and Los says, "I hear the screech of childbirth loud pealing, & the groans Of Death" (E 175) (Frosch 161). In fact, sexual reproduction for Blake runs dangerously close to the mere reproduction of an ordinary engraver: a form of mere copying rather than imaginative recreation.

In keeping with the poet's wariness of mere sexual generation, Blake generally dismisses function and organs, which go back to the Greek word for instruments. Given his interest in perversion, Blake unsurprisingly uses the word "function" only twice in his entire work: once in his unengraved *The French Revolution* and again in his *The Four Zoas*. In *The French Revolution*, Orleans, one of Blake's ostensible heroes, rises to ask, "Can the man be bound in sorrow / Whose ev'ry function is fill'd with its fiery desire?" (182–83 E 294). By imagining desire and function as commensurate, yet opening up desire to include *every* function, Blake renders it pointedly not teleological, especially since the function of fiery desire in Blake is energy or eternal delight. Orleans's sense that every function is filled with its fiery desire makes localization conceptual nonsense. Desire is thus paradoxically detached from its instrumental function (reproduction) and turned into functions in themselves. Orleans addresses the National Assembly whose flames are "for growth, not consuming" (179 E 294), a detail which hints at the poet's democratic sympathies and his alliance with Orleans.

Blake often reminds us that the "organ" appears in organization. Los implores Vala to recognize that "Humanity is far above/sexual organization" (*Jerusalem* 79:73–74), and the poet warns us against "sexual organization," which captures both the sexing of the body into the sexes as well as the genitalizing of sexuality. Such localization moves insistently away from the integrated spiritual body that Blake hopes to achieve. Los admonishes us, for example, to "consider sexual organization & hide thee in the dust" (*Jerusalem* 34:58; Paley 184). That Luvah and Vala are relegated to servants and hierarchy implies that a reorganization of the functions will not promote liberty. Generation entails the separation of and growing friction between the two sexes, a separation that moved mankind away from fourfold vision and made sexuality necessarily a site of strife.

Perverse or functionless sexuality in Blake is potentially a form of liberation: where reproductive sex traps mankind into the material world of nature, perverse sex allows the sexual act to take on imaginative and spiritual reunification of the senses.[17] Perverse sex also resists the power of moral law. Thus, generation is on one level a perversion of joy. It is only the fall that has made generation material, painful, and sorrowful.[18] Yet, because we only know sexual nature through the fall, it is difficult to return to that original moment.

We need to keep in mind, however, that, although sex without generation is potentially liberating for Blake, it will neither restore human beings to their prelapsarian condition nor necessarily achieve or even lead to liberty. For example, in *Jerusalem*, as Los prays for the resurrection of the savior, he describes how in Beulah "the Female lets down her beautiful tabernacle;/Which the Male enters magnificent between her Cherubim:/And becomes One with her mingling condensing in Self-love/The Rocky Law of Condemnation & double Generation, & Death" (30:34–37; Paley 177). While on the one hand, intercourse represents a unification of the sexes, the fact that this takes place in vegetative Beulah, and the fact that such intercourse only leads to self-love, not self-annihilation, means that such generation, despite its double status, is deadening. Blake thought that selfhood obscured the spiritual and thus demanded nothing less than the sacrifice of the self.[19] Los fittingly concludes this prayer by asking the savior to "rend the Veil," a rending that will strip away whatever positive force double generation has.

Moreover, although the poet's negative depictions of generation imply that generation perverts fiery joy, generation cannot be subsumed under perversion because Blake paradoxically demands not only a turning away from generation but also an embrace of it. Frosch therefore tells us only half the story when he equates generation in Blake with fallen perception. Because Blake believes that one must embrace one's fallen condition in order to begin the process of self-annihilation, to imply that one must turn away from generation—that generation is a perversion—does not get us to self-annihilation. To enter into self-annihilation, one must recognize one's own sins, embrace them, and then incorporate them. When Blake foists Eve's fall onto Mary Magdalen, therefore, he makes the fall fortunate in that Mary is able to recognize her own pollution as helping to glorify Jesus's holiness. Mary says to Jesus, "If I were unpolluted I should never have/Glorified thy holiness" (*Jerusalem* 61:45–46; Paley 229). To redefine her own pollution as an amplification of Jesus's holiness is, on the one hand, positive in that Mary is recognizing her own sins. Of course, for Blake, Mary's sin is not her sexuality; it is her reduction of sexuality to moral law. On the other hand, her use of the term "pollution" still betrays the influence of moral law. The problem comes to a head when we realize that if Mary's pollution has amplified Jesus's holiness, her "pollution" is not properly pollution at all, but is instead a form of divinity. That is, she still insists that her fallen sexuality is a perversion. Blake turns to Mary to exemplify the necessity for and difficulty of self-annihilation. While Mary has taken the first step in embracing her sins by turning away from and identifying with them, she still must do more to achieve redemption. Blake thus positions generation within the realm of ordinary fallen experience, but we must both turn away from that experience and turn toward it if we are to achieve redemption.

This is why the poet praises regeneration at the expense of generation, only then to remind us that "generation" appears in both terms.[20] The fact that generation appears in both terms implies that sex under moral law can be reconceived and reimagined and that generation is a part of regeneration, not so much its opposite. Los continues, apostrophizing, "O Holy Generation! [image] of regeneration!/O point of mutual forgiveness between enemies" (7:65–66), once again connecting regeneration with holiness and forgiveness, the first step on the way to self-annihilation.

Inasmuch as self-annihilation requires the ability to reperceive selfhood as a version of generation, it demands an active negation of generation. Active negation must be more than a form of the denial of the generated self; it must also be a reperception and a sacrifice. One must have a self to annihilate it. Blake cannot ultimately choose regeneration over generation, because each makes the other possible. Hence, immediately following Lavater's statement that "the unison of various powers for one is only WILL, born under the agonies of self-denial and renounced desires," Blake writes, "Regeneration" (E 584). Regeneration is the product of human and divine will, a will that must struggle against generation, self-denial, and the suppression of desires. In this struggle generation becomes regeneration. More critically, rather than being simply enemies, self-denial and renounced desires are what give birth to the will or regeneration.

Blake's unravels this paradox more fully in his annotations to Lavater's *Aphorisms on Man*. He redefines generation as a perversion of regeneration, a conceptual redefinition that makes it difficult to divorce one from the other since a reversal in direction is not a negation. Blake asks, "But if man is considered as only evil & god only good [*sic*]. How then is regeneration effected which turns the evil to good. By casting out the evil. By the good" (E 594).[21] Regeneration turns evil into good, a reversal of Milton's Satan's perversion of God's good into evil. To the extent that perversion insists on one wrong direction, it bears the traces of previous turns in direction.[22] By acknowledging those multiple previous turns, perversion must persuade rather than insist. Refuting Lavater's praise for honesty as the absence of self-contradiction, Blake argues that this monistic way of perceiving man fails to explain how the regeneration of generated man is possible. Good can only cast out evil if man is a "two-fold being, one part capable of evil & the other capable of good" (E 594). Blake continues, "Both evil & good cannot exist in a simple being. For thus 2 contraries would. Spring from one essence which is impossible" (E 594). Blake's sense of mankind's inherent dualism means not only that the possibility of perversion is always there, but it is there twice. Because both man's capacity for good and his capacity for evil can be perverted, there is no such thing as simple perversion in Blake. Blake implies that just as the capacities for good and evil are part of man's complex essences, so must be generation and regeneration. His insistence on the potentiality within both good and evil, rather than on good and evil as essences, further ironizes the idea of either good or evil as essences.

To underscore the fact that regeneration ultimately cannot be separated from generation, Blake writes in "To Tirzah" that "Whate'er is Born of Mortal Birth,/Must be consumed with the Earth/To rise from generation free" (1–3 E 30), thus making generation, at first blush, antithetical to resurrection and liberation. Tirzah is in fact the mother of the mortal body in Blake, and thus the spiritual body who is the "I" of the poem wants nothing to do with Tirzah, having been set free by Jesus's death. Yet, rather than divorcing itself from mortality, the voice of experience must recognize that only Christ's self-annihilation of the body enables the spiritual body to rise up. Read with biblical typology in mind, as Blake's quotation of I Corinthians 15.44 demands that we do, the first Adam (generation) must pave the way for the second, Jesus (regeneration) (Lincoln 201).[23] Blake, of course, conflated the two in time and space, at times giving Adam the halo of Christ (Genesis Manuscript, First Title Page). Blake's illustration for "To Tirzah" foregrounds a pitcher of water being held over the pieta of Christ's body, and this reminds readers that only self-sacrifice of the generated body can lead to baptismal rebirth. Thus, Blake suggests that the speaker's need to separate generation from regeneration is really a perversion of regeneration. Blake takes the mortal body down off the cross and highlights that body to undercut the speaker's need to divorce himself from it.

In a stroke of brilliance, Blake culminates *Jerusalem* with an image of "the all tremendous unfathomable Non-Ens/of Death . . . seen in regenerations terrific" (98:33–34) precisely to insist upon the connection of generation or death (sex under moral law) with regeneration. Line number 33 makes death occur precisely at the age of Christ's self-annihilation, and turns the unfathomable Non-Ens of death into a meaningful sacrifice of selfhood, a combination that forcefully reminds us that self-negation of the generated self is necessary for resurrection to occur. Blake hated the idea that Christ had been a passive victim of his crucifixion, and so he stresses the activeness of self-sacrifice. Thus, to transform generation, one must initially turn away from it and then value it. That Jesus "must create Luvah" (lust) so that "banished [desire] can return before the resurrection (62:20; 22 Paley 230), brings self-annihilation perversely close to orgasm. The turn of line 33 into 34 also occurs when the Non-Ens/of Death is no longer seen as nothingness but is miraculously transubstantiated into regeneration. With regeneration, death becomes cognizable instead of unfathomable. As the very last word of line 33, Non-Ens, juts out to the very edge of the plate and signifies the nothingness that can be changed into regeneration. Blake tellingly surrounds "Non-Ens" with leafy decorations. The significance of this visual representation is threefold: first, the absence of Non-Ens is countered by the emphatic presence of the word which pushes itself into the margin, thus calling attention to itself. Death is only absence from a fallen perspective. For Blake it is an active negation. Second, "Non-Ens" is surrounded by the vegetative death represented by the leaves and thus begs for regeneration. And, third, the proximity of the Non-Ens to the edge of the plate reaches out to the reader who must activate it into regeneration. Death can be positive as long as resurrection is in sight. Yet, if resurrection is in sight, the Non-Ens of death is the fecklessness of death: death has been reduced to nothingness as opposed to

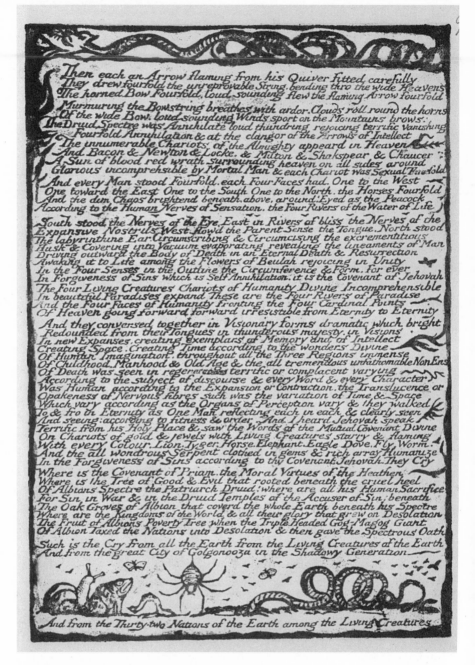

William Blake, *Jerusalem*, plate 98 (Rosenwald 1811). Courtesy of the Lessing Rosenwald Collection, the Library of Congress, Washington, D.C.

being the condition of nothingness. Blake's perverse turn here suspends the reader between these two meanings of death with the end goal of bringing him or her to the state of self-annihilation. He counters that suspension with his incarnation of Christ, an incarnation that closes much of the gap between generation and regeneration.

This transformation also incarnates the awakening of Jerusalem into his (Jesus's/Jehovah's) "Bosom in the life of Immortality" (99:4–5). Of course, Blake emphasizes the simultaneity of the Non-Ens of generation with regeneration in his insistence that the one "is seen in" the other. What appears to the fallen senses as necessarily unfolding through time, Blake reminds us is actually revealed instantaneously. That we are finally told that Jerusalem's emanations are named Jerusalem enables us to close this temporal gap even as it unifies the emanations of liberty. Elsewhere, Blake's insistent pun between consume and consummation, linking the physical act of eating with the spiritual act of attaining divinity, also transforms physical orgasm—consummation—into simultaneous religious experience. Indeed, the illustration to plate 99 depicts Jehovah sensuously embracing another: their approaching lips look as if they might kiss, one groin is pulled near Jehovah's groin, and Jehovah's hands caress the male—Is that the idealized face of Blake on the nude figure?—or female figure's left buttock. All of this physicality reminds us of the divinity even within generation.

In Blake's hands, perversion is an exceptionally flexible instrument, one that announces a turning away but that also demands that readers themselves reevaluate the standards by which perversion is measured. To the extent that perversion can turn and yet suspend moral judgment, the turn of perversion must be initially unpredictable. Because Blake's ground shifts, the turning of perversion has the possibility of developing into a full-blown vortex. Whereas perversion often works by grounding itself in nature, in Blake, nature is not a stable construct. Los and Urizen constantly hammer nature into form. Not only is nature always shifting because it is continually generated, but also Blake replaces the already shaky ground of nature with the imagination. By making the creative imagination a type of Christ (Tannenbaum 74), and by making the imagination the bridge between Christ and man, Blake argues that nature perverts spirituality. Moving the ground of perversion from nature to the imagination, of course, enables Blake to pervert perversion.

Moreover, the minute that the reader understands generation to be negative, Blake insists that regeneration is positive, leaving the reader grasping at what might possibly distinguish the two. This leads to a necessary reevaluation of generation and the body. Note the multiple movements here. Generation initially looks perverse in Blake because it is material, divisive, and merely reproductive. Although most would understand sexuality with reproduction as normal, Blake's sense of generation as being a mechanical and vegetative process turns the normal provisionally into its perversion or sex under moral law. If regeneration forces the reappraisal of generation, since generation is contained within regeneration, generation can no longer be intrinsically perverse. Rather, generation only becomes perverse when it is the ultimate end of sex and does not lead to self-annihilation. As long as generation leads to regeneration, generation is not perverse. This means that although one must initially turn away from generation by recognizing it as a perversion of fiery joy, to turn away from generation blocks regeneration in that one must embrace generation in order to be resurrected. Thus, an initial turning away must lead to an embrace of one's errors, sins, sex as moral law because that is the only way to regenerate. In sum, by defining moral law as a perversion of joy, Blake has us turn away from moral law and toward joy. But this turning away does not enable regeneration, because regeneration can only be achieved through embracing one's sins. As he puts it in *Jerusalem*, "Forgiveness of Sins . . . is Self Annihilation" (98:23 E 257). Thus, Blake has us turn back to the moral law we had rejected so as to incorporate our generated selves back into ourselves so that we can annihilate the self.

If generation is not necessarily a perversion of the imagination, the narrative arc of liberation in Blake is nothing so simple as a liberation from generation to regeneration. Instead, self-annihilation demands that liberation go through the body, not above it. This journey through the body must entail both a rejection of generation as well as an embrace of it. In this way, one can be truly liberated from generation and that liberation can lead to self-annihilating liberty.

We can now perhaps understand why Blake so insistently stages and restages the battle between sexual pleasure and sex under moral law: there are many levels to his argument, self-annihilation occurs in stages, no one character can capture the numerous ways in which generation is maintained and regeneration is facilitated, and self-annihilation demands that we both reject and accept generation, along with the self that is part of generation. Consider the range of characters who represent sexual energy of one kind or another. A preliminary list would include Orc, Luvah, Leutha, Jesus, Antamon, Ahania, Enitharmon, Oothoon, Ololon, Tharmas, Rahab, Reuben, Vala, Tirzah, and the Whore of Babylon. In Blake, furthermore, sexuality and the division of power extend to the particularity of individuality. This divisive individuality cloaks power under identity. Therefore, Blake's concept of self-annihilation dissolves both sexual division and identity. If self-annihilation is literalized in orgasm, desire disrupts the power that comes with sexual individuation, the power that is cloaked under identity so that it does not seem like power. In *Milton*, self-annihilation takes the form of fellatio, an act that Blake undercuts with the words a "fallacy (phallusy) of Satan's churches" (plate 44 E 141) in the plate immediately before. This reminds us of how easily orgasm can enhance selfhood rather than undermine it.

Thus, sexual liberation in Blake offers a number of key cautions to queer theory. For one, as Jonathan Dollimore argues, queer theorists regularly celebrate the inherent disruptiveness of desire only then to recontain that disruptiveness within identity (homosexuality, queerness, bottoms, or tops) (Dollimore *Sex* 26–29). Blake, by contrast, uses sexual desire to dissolve identity because he recognizes that identity is a powerful cloak for power. As Elfenbein argues, following traditional male gender roles often reduces male characters to "ineffective heaps of egomania" (*Romantic Genius* 153). The overwhelming thrust of *Jerusalem* is the dissolution of individuality. Blake's insistence that we must consider the consequences of any act of liberating or perverting resists an identity politics that equates one's own outing from the closet as intrinsically liberating. He knows too well that declaring one's identity in terms of one's desires tends to tame the disruptiveness of desire. Finally, if liberation is held up to higher standards of liberty, self-annihilation, and love, the mere approval of perverse sexuality cannot in itself be necessarily liberating because approval does not dismantle the logic of perversion; it merely reverses the direction of perversion.

For Blake, perverse sex by itself had no necessary connection to liberty. Even though perverse forms of sexuality fly in the face of moral law, the rejection of moral law in itself does not lead to the poet's ultimate goal of the rejection of selfhood. For self-annihilation to occur, one must reject and embrace moral law. Blake therefore can both celebrate homosexuality in *Milton* and conceive of Satan's homosexuality as Leutha's "stupefying [of his] masculine perceptions, and keep[ing] only the feminine awake" (12:5–6).[24] As a symbol of Blake's weak patron Hayley, Satan allows himself to be made effeminate by no less than Leutha, representing sexual guilt and sin. Blake renders homosexuality as a form of stupefying of Satan's masculine perceptions so that the feminine perceptions can take over, a representation that offers a universalizing narrative of homosexuality insofar as we all have masculine and feminine perceptions.

True, this characterization is Leutha's, and because Leutha represents sin, critics have dismissed the possibility that Blake is thinking about homosexuality in terms of effeminacy. But any clear distance between Leutha and Blake is undercut by the fact that Blake considered the male allowing the female to be on top as a form of foppery and that he wrote of Hayley, "Of H s birth this was the happy lot/His Mother on his Father him begot" (E 506). Blake does at times think like Leutha. Elfenbein demonstrates how effeminacy/foppery got "pushed closer" to sodomy in the Romantic period (21), and such rapprochement meant that same-sex acts were in part forms of gender deviance.[25] Blake writes, "Unappropriate Execution is the Most nauseous of all affectation & foppery" (E 178). While foppery here stands for civic decay, the sodomite was the very embodiment of the ultimate civic decay, and thus Blake draws upon a chain of signifiers that show ambivalence to some forms of "perverse" sexuality. Yet this ambivalence is not hypocritical because Blake never argues that perverse sex is intrinsically liberating: the suspension of function/reproduction must have consequences in order to be liberating. Once again Blake's emphasis on consequences rather than function transforms perversion into a kind of purposiveness. The couplet seeks to understand something about Hayley's nature in light of Hayley's mother's sexual assertiveness. In taking the top position, she did something to Hayley. Blake demands that we think of the consequences of perverse sex rather than embrace it as a good in and of itself. That Leutha annihilates herself for her father's (Satan's) sins in *Milton* further indicates that Blake embraces rather than rejects Leutha, an embrace that symbolizes his own self-annihilation as well as his own embrace of his own sin. To the extent that Leutha models self-annihilation—sin embraces sin so that she may redefine it—Blake recognizes the costs of his gender attitudes. Self-annihilation, moreover, has the potential to counter the poet's phallocentrism even as the poet unsexes strength and "punctures constricting gender roles" when characters keep up with "exhausted conventions" (Elfenbein *RG* 153).[26]

Because he mistakes approval of perverse sexuality in Blake for liberation, Christopher Hobson is thus forced to argue that Blake eventually approves of masturbation. To equate perverse sex with liberation in Blake is to ignore the poet's insistence on consequences. Where function welds sex to reproduction, consequences allow for results that are not always known in advance and redefine function as being too narrowly construed. Hobson writes, validation of masturbation in turn leads to "validation of other types of perverse sexuality, and then to an incomplete revision of his idealization of the male" (36). Although Blake would have had little truck with the demonizing of masturbation, the problem is that it tends to lead to self-love, which is antithetical to self-annihilation. To wit, Blake's descriptions of masturbation in the *Visions of the Daughters of Albion* emphasize not the liberation of desire but rather the religious constraints that pervert "the moment of desire" into the "creation of an amorous image / In the shadows of his curtains and in the folds of his silent pillow" (7:3–7 E 50). These are precisely the "places of religion," Blake wryly comments (7:8). Blake thus sees masturbation as the inherently paradoxical "self-enjoyings of self-denial" (7:9), a formulation that enables religion to perpetuate its power as pleasure.[27] Hence, he objects to masturbation because it can use orgasm to consolidate the self: it may look like self-annihilation but often achieves its opposite.

Blake further harnesses the disruptive turning of perversion by emphasizing that moral categories are really false names for things rather than essential descriptions of truth or right. In *The Marriage of Heaven and Hell,* Blake insists that conventional morality is merely language, words that have lost any connection to the thing itself. John Mee reminds us of the antinomian resonances of *The Marriage,* where Blake so celebrates the spirit over the letter of the law that he "represents grace as the reward of transgression" (58). Hence Blake insists that from reason and energy, attraction and repulsion, "spring what the religious call Good & Evil. Good is the passive that obeys Reason. Evil is the active springing from Energy. Good is Heaven. Evil is Hell" (3). By making good and evil mere words used by the religious, Blake demands that readers reassess why they value one at the expense of the other. In the process, "religious" has become a mere word, too. Blake then perverts Evil into a Good by making evil active rebellion as opposed to passive obedience. But he does not stop turning there. Blake then equates good with Heaven and evil with Hell, an equation that merely substitutes one empty signified for another. Now that Heaven is twice removed from good, insofar as it now stands for passive obedience and that passive obedience is what the religious label good, Blake can further destabilize perversion by making it merely a word used for good or ill. As my use of the *Marriage* suggests, Blake valued perversion when it prompted mental revolution.

## Body, Medicine, and Text

Beyond Blake's concept of perversion, his very idea of the term demands our rethinking of how body and text work. For Blake, perversion is about epistemological uncertainty, and thus he transforms the function of perversion—the delivery of immediate and unarguable moral judgments that are often grounded in the body—from performative immediacy to performative vortex. The twists and turns in Blake's treatment of generation and its relation to regeneration imply that the body is an especially flexible form of materiality, as does his sense of orgasm as bodily sensation that can lead to self-annihilation. Performative vortex then leads to incarnation into the holy lust of Christ. Blake's paradoxically uniting self-annihilation with incarnation indicates his skepticism about perfect embodiment. Again, rather than being pure, Blake regards texts as being "unperverted." And, because Christ is for Blake the very embodiment of perversion—Blake takes especial pride in the fact that Christ broke every one of the Ten Commandments and that "no virtue can exist without breaking these ten commandments" (*MHH* 21 E 43)—incarnation into Christ is simultaneously incarnation into perversion. Perverse incarnation, thus, enables Blake to move beyond Urizen's naive incarnation; where Urizen not only believes his brass books to be perfect incarnations (fully embodied meanings that would deny the transformative powers of perception), but also that his children incarnate his will (thereby denying them free will), Blake yokes together incarnation and self-annihilation, generation and regeneration, along with Christ's sins and mercy to preserve a gap between incarnation and meaning. Such a gap demands an aesthetic apprehension of embodiment, one that gauges the extent to which the form of liberation yields liberation. His concept of perverse incarnation thus harnesses the disruptive powers of deferral and the incarnational powers of reference because the self under moral law must be embraced so that it can be annihilated.

I have already hinted that our postmodern faith in textualism—"that language has an intrinsic capacity to detach itself from material circumstances" (Terdiman 76)—has led us to overestimate the intransigence of materiality and to underestimate its capacity for change.[28] Textualism has also led us to misunderstand how body and text function in Blake, a misunderstanding that has, in turn, led to the belief that sexual liberation in Blake can only be achieved by transcending the body (see Porter and Hall 32), or to the idea that Blake thought that the deferral of language was inherently liberating. Rather than seeing liberation as working from the body into speech, from materiality into malleable text, Blake recognized that the body was a crucial agent and object of change, and that speech was not the same thing as liberty. And rather than emploting liberation along a predictable narrative arc from body into text—one that testifies to our postmodern faith in textualism—Blake, by contrast, sought to harness the liberating possibilities within both bodies and texts, along with both the incarnational and deferring capacities of language itself, a dual capacity writ large in the idea of Christ as the incarnation of perversion. Blake reminds us of Christ's perversions when he praises him for refusing to convict Mary of adultery, and when he delights in Christ's "lay[ing] his hand on Moses Law [*sic*]" ("Everlasting Gospel" f E 521). Christ's defiance of Moses results in "The Ancient Heavens in Silent Awe/Writ with Curses from Pole to Pole/All away began to roll" (ibid.). In the process, the Ten Commandments can now be seen for what they are: curses. Finally, if orgasm leads to self-annihilation, the body can be a site of both incarnation and deferral, the recognition of the difference (generation) within the self even as the self is reincarnated into the perverse body of Christ.

Textualism has also blinded us to the differing possible outcomes of linguistic embodiment. While the Romantics generally sought a kind of natural sign that would contain the arbitrariness of Lockean signs, they could also turn to language as Logos to counter our fallen condition even as they dismantled it to get rid of tyranny. If the arbitrariness of the letter helped to disconnect language from authority, then incarnation could bring the ideal within human reach. While our faith in textualism has engendered blindness to the fact that both language as deferral and language as embodiment can be put to liberating or tyrannical ends, our amazement that Blake united conception and execution in his printing process, making his direct composition onto copper plates into autographic sketches, has blinded us to Blake's perverse incarnations, bodies that resist perfect embodiment even as they attempt to transform word into flesh. Joseph Viscomi's magisterial *Blake and the Idea of the Book* is in part driven by a polemic against *différance*, the theory that language defers meaning. On the one hand, Viscomi emphasizes Blake's autographic hand uniting conception and execution; on the other, he tames the gaps between word and thing by reminding us that Blake's works were produced in editions, and this meant that the illuminated books could not have had the individual intentional instabilities that critics have celebrated. By contrast, Morris Eaves's caution that Blake actively orients his aesthetic "toward conception and away from execution" (179) is much more forgiving of *différance*. Blake's antinomian background, moreover, meant that he recognized that the letter could obfuscate the spirit, especially when the letter became law, and explains why he attempts to quicken the spirit at the expense of the letter (Mee 58). That "fiery joy" can so easily be translated into the fires of Blake's acid baths further blinds us to how Blakean incarnation resists logocentrism. After all, acid annihilates and thus allows meaning to occur. Linguistic deferral, fueled by antinomianism, can help undermine authority from within, just as the differing editions of the illuminated books reinscribe that deferral onto Blake's rhetoric of unifying composition and execution.

Our distrust of materiality, furthermore, has meant that we underestimate the capacity of Blake's bodies to deliver change, even as we substitute the body of Blake's printed texts for the physical body.[29] Thus, in a suggestive study of the body in Blake, Tristanne Connolly underestimates what the fallen body in Blake can do (71), and embodiment, whether Urizenically fixed or Reuben-like in its flexibility, only leads to fallen generation.[30] In his Genesis manuscript, Blake titles chapter 3 "Of the Sexual Nature and Its Fall into Generation and Death,"[31] a title that insists "sexual nature" predates the fall of man, and thus there is nothing intrinsically wrong with sexual nature, and by extension the human body. The fact that Blake thinks regeneration stems from generation means that bodies have as much potential for liberating pleasures, which may or may not lead to liberty, as they do Urizenic oppression. *Jerusalem*, after all, ends with a celebration of the "Human Form" and imagines the awakening of those forms into Christ's bosom. If Blake's "Life of Immortality" goes through Christ's bosom, and the illustration reminds us that Christ has a real bosom, the body is the ground for utopia, not its enemy.[32] To the extent that the generated body grounds Blake's utopia, he is neither a strictly utopian thinker (Williams) nor an ideological escapist turning toward idealism when the French Revolution gets too bloody. If transcendence in Blake goes through as opposed to above the body, we will also have to learn to see Blake's idealism as nothing less than a thorough social engagement with the body. And, although Blake is acutely aware of what can go wrong with the body in that the senses can constrict him into a caverned man, situating him within the medicine of his time can remind us that he knew what could go right.

This distrust of materiality has also led Blake critics to underestimate the force of language as incarnation, the word as Christ's flesh, while trust in incarnation has led to overestimation of what embodiment can do. That textualism and incarnation both want language to foster liberation—one sees liberation from authority within linguistic difference, the other sees liberation from our fallen condition in incarnation or in words as Christ's perverted body—suggests that neither texts nor bodies have any monopoly on liberation. Leslie Tannenbaum has argued that Blake's sense of incarnation was "broadly conceived" in that he equated Christ with the poetic imagination, thus allowing the prophet to both communicate the word and be the word (74–76). Incarnation, however, raises a problem, one that Tannenbaum sleights, in that how do we reconcile language as incarnation with language as deferral with the fact that Blake distrusted the notion of language as Logos because it inevitably led to tyranny?

I suggest that whenever language threatens to become law, Blake seeks to remind us of the spirit that perverts the law. Urizen's tablets of brass indicate Urizen's naively incarnational view of language because he does not acknowledge the possibility that the tablets themselves might be perversions of God. By contrast, Blake relies on a paradoxical view of Christian incarnation, one that recognizes the capacity of deferral to ironize what is being incarnated. Because Christ perverts each of the Ten Commandments, incarnation into Christ mandates the supplementing of the Ten Commandments into art of writing. As the very incarnation of perversion, Christ embodies both sin and the forgiveness of sin, generation, and regeneration. Nonetheless, whenever language seeks to reunite and expand the senses into Christ's body, language results in a liberating incarnation as long as Christ perverts Urizen. By allowing forgiveness to triumph over law, as when Blake rereads the mark of Cain not in terms of God's curse but rather in terms of God's forgiveness, Blake enables Urizen's naive incarnationalism to become incarnation into Christ. Blake demands that we too filter our Old Testament God through a God of love and forgiveness, so that we can see the true significance behind the Old Testament. Hence, the pencil sketch shows that Blake's mark of Cain is really God's kiss (Genesis Manuscript 11). By emphasizing New Testament spirit over Old Testament letter, Blake enables naive incarnationalism to become incarnation; now the son can regenerate the father. Thus, even generation (sex under moral law) can become regeneration by an imaginative act, one that reminds us of the spirit that has always been within the letter but, since the fall, obscured by the letter.

Blake's insistence upon consequences, furthermore, helps us further to distinguish between naive incarnation and perverse incarnation. Because one must stand outside the immediacy of even sexual experience in order to evaluate the consequences for that experience, Blake demands an ironic stance to even incarnation. To the extent that words lead to law and punishment, and therefore deny the need for interpretation, that is naive incarnation. To the extent that words lead to forgiveness and self-annihilation, that is perverse incarnation, an embrace of one's sins so that they can be forgiven and a simultaneous disembodiment of the generated body and regeneration. Readers are obligated, moreover, to recognize naive incarnation as a perversion of incarnation, to then convert that naiveté into Christ-like incarnation, by turning away from it and then embracing it. We can do so by suffusing ourselves with the spirit and not the law and by rereading the Old Testament as a type of Christian forgiveness.

Consequences, moreover, provide the poet with an aesthetic stance from which to gauge perversion and to see if perversion amounts to sexual liberation or even liberty. Just because Blake valued a flexible body does not mean that he could not see the limitations of the body: sexual pleasure leads to re-enslavement in Beulah, and selfish sexual pleasure moves away from self-annihilation and love, not toward them. By reminding us that the ground may be the perversion of the ground, Blake warns us that what looks like liberation and the free expression of desire may not be terribly liberating. Earth answers the Father of Ancient Men that his "free love [is] with bondage bound" (E 19), and Blake here insists that the forms that free love must take must be scrutinized. For whom is free love free? Moreover, if perverse sex (sex without reproduction) does defy moral law, the defiance of moral law is not in and of itself liberty. Getting rid of moral law only produces liberty if there are no other forms of repression. To wit, Blake describes masturbation as the "self-enjoyings of self-denial," a definition that insists not only that pleasure has failed to escape moral law but also that moral law intensifies pleasure. Getting rid of moral law, of course, will not achieve self-annihilation.

Now that I have laid out many of the unfortunate consequences of our inability to come to terms with Blakean materiality or textuality, let me unsettle once more Blake's concept of perversion, by putting Blake's bodies in a contemporary medical context.[33] Medicine grounds Blakean optimism that the fallen body can be regenerated and that the body under moral law can become the incarnation of Christ, liberty, and divine imagination. More crucially, contemporary medical and botanical understandings of the body would allow Blake to collapse body/utopia, body/text, body/allegory, real/ideal, materiality/transcendence, and feminine/masculine, thereby making the ideal attainable within the body and regeneration possible.

Blake's optimism that the generated body could be regenerated in the same way as naive could become perverse incarnation was intensified by the fact that regeneration was a hot topic in the burgeoning biological sciences. Building on Bonnet's work on regenerating polyps and Reamur's work on earthworms' ability to regenerate lost parts, Abbe Spallanzani demonstrated in 1769 that lower forms of life like salamanders, slugs, tadpoles, and earthworms could literally and repeatedly "regenerate" lost or missing limbs or tails.[34] Spallanzani marveled at how the salamander could regenerate its tail, legs, and jaws: "this regeneration is so much more surprising than that which takes place in the craw-fish and small lizard, as the structure of these parts in the salamander is infinitely more complicated and refined" (58). Spallanzani ends this treatise by asking if "the flattering expectation of obtaining this advantage for ourselves be considered entirely as chimerical?" (86).

Spallanzani was not the only scientist of the period interested in the body's ability to regenerate itself. Monsieur Le Cat published an article in the Royal Society's 1766 *Philosophical Transactions* on the regeneration of human bones in a three-year-old French child and in a forty-one-year-old soldier. Blake was apprenticed to James Basire, the official engraver to the Royal Society from 1772 to 1779, and perhaps had access to the *Philosophical Transactions.* Le Cat urged surgeons not to amputate limbs "when there is a possibility of bringing about this sort of regeneration" (277). Here, regeneration is both divine and human, brought about by the surgeon's knowledge and nature's help. In 1785, Charles White published a pamphlet "On the Regeneration of Animal Substances," based on a paper he read at the Royal Society on December 1782. Citing the work of Le Cat, Monro, and William and John Hunter, White concluded that "in the human species, not only flesh, skin, bones, may be regenerated, but membranes, ligaments, cartilages, glands, blood vessels, and even nerves" (16). Moreover, he posited that this might be explained by the ability of "coagulable lymph, which is poured out, and becomes vascular, and forms organized parts" (17). He concluded, "In some animals, we see this regenerating, and living principle, carried still to a much greater length, where not only whole limbs, but even the more noble organs are reproduced" (17). Blake uses "lymph" only once in his entire works, and like White understands it to be a basic building unit of the body. In *The Book of Urizen*, "the void shrunk the lymph into Nerves" (13: 56). For Blake, it would seem that "lymph" is not only ontologically prior to the void, but it is also a unit of the body that has not yet been localized or specialized into organs. "Shrunk" depicts this biological specialization in terms of loss.

Seen in light of Spallanzani's, Le Cat's, and White's scientific studies of regeneration, Blakean regeneration becomes less ideal and more immediate: less theory, and more actuality. Although the poet certainly associates generation with the material world of pain and death and regeneration with the spiritual, he often reminds us that generation is literally within regeneration. That is, the physical and spiritual bodies are one. Hence, in *Milton*, Blake envisions the moment when "Generation is swallowed up in Regeneration" (41:28 E 143). Of course, the word "generation" is already literally swallowed up by "regeneration." Indeed, "swallowing up" reminds us of the body even as it depicts resurrection. Notwithstanding the fact that Blake insists that the "Religion of Generation . . . was meant for the destruction/Of Jerusalem," he later suggests that "O holy Generation! [Image] of regeneration" (*Jerusalem* 7: 63–64 *E* 150). The parallelism of the phrases recalls the sublime of the Bible and suggests that the one is contained within the other. Very close to the end of *Jerusalem*, Blake describes "the all tremendous unfathomable Non-Ens/of death was seen in regenerations terrific" (98:33–34 E 258). Because the nonentity of death can now be seen within regeneration, Blake reminds us that body and spirit are not at odds as long as perception does not obfuscate one within the other. Shot through with regenerative powers, then, the mortal body is holy.

Furthermore, since biological sex was a much more mobile set of categories than it is now, the poet could justifiably hope for the end of sex under moral law. Sexual division could be overcome if sexual difference was still in the state of flux. That the Romantic period worked through competing models of sex—from one sex to two—meant that sexual difference had not yet hardened into stone. Indeed, Blake can image the vanishing of the sexes (E 252) because they were a construction very much in formation.

Orc, we recall, gets to work at the age of fourteen, and since puberty was in the Romantic period a state of dynamic change from two feminized sexes into masculine strength and female weakness, not to mention a window of up to twenty years, the body was literally in transition. Orc is revolution in puberty, perhaps recalling the French medical descriptions of puberty as revolution, making him an embodiment of revolution not yet fully sexed. Just as puberty shows the body to be capable of enormous change, so does revolution foster bodily change. As the flexible if material embodiment of revolution, puberty helps explain why Blake celebrates the androgynous, why he is obsessed with hermaphrodites and equates them with being a two-fold form (*Milton* 19:32),[35] why a part of *Jerusalem* takes place in Middlesex, and why the fall of man begins in puberty in *The Four Zoas*. The medical discourse about hermaphrodites sought to make sex not a problem of ontology, but rather a problem of epistemology: how do we know that we have a real hermaphrodite, especially since the culture thought of the penis and clitoris as relatively interchangeable organs? Understanding the human body to be in transition between sexes not only enhances epistemological uncertainty about sex itself, but it also enables Blake to see sexing of the body as part of a fallen condition rather than a given, just as it offers hope that the sexes can be reunited into one. It is not as far from

Middlesex in England (plate 90) to the Jerusalem of the everlasting imagination: indeed, we have only to turn ten plates to get from one to the other. Without being able to see the generated bodies within Blake's regenerated bodies, we misread idealism as escapism, when in fact nothing could be further from the truth. The poet's critique of sexual organization and genital sexuality could well have been informed by Albrecht von Haller's relocation of the sensations of the erections of the penis and breast nipple from the organs of generation to the soul/mind/brain. In his *Memoirs of Albrecht von Haller*, for which Blake engraved a frontispiece portrait, Thomas Henry rehearsed Haller's distinction between mechanical muscular irritation, not under control of the will, and the sensible activity of the brain/nerves, the organs of pleasure (72–75). Therefore, when Blake has Urizen command Luvah and Vala to be "servants" and "return O Love in peace/Into your place the place of seed not in the brain or heart" in Night Nine of *The Four Zoas* (9:363–65 E 395), Urizen turns back to a physiology before Haller, one that sought to limit sexuality only to the genitals, and only to mechanical processes. By equating such a return with servitude, and by connecting such servitude with being "thrown down from their high station/ In the eternal heavens of Human Imagination" (*FZ* 9:367–68 E 395), Blake suggests that the furnaces Urizen repeatedly uses to lock up Luvah allegorizes the return of the seed to the genitals even as it allows Blake's acid baths to restore lust to its rightful place: throughout the body and particularly to the brain, the place where the soul resides. Indeed, whereas Urizen thinks furnaces are forms of containment, the poet connects their fires with "Mental flames" (E 39), thus ironizing Urizen's repressive desires. Haller thus allows Blake to connect sexuality with the immaterial mind/soul, enhancing its potential divinity, and to refuse the sexual organization that comes with reorganizing Luvah into the organs of generation and the body as machine. Henry referred to Haller's *Dissertation on the Sensitive and Irritable Parts of Animals* as having achieved a "revolution in anatomy" (75), one that Urizen seeks to overturn. Should Urizen get his way, the body will revert back to a mechanistic materialism and away from one that understood the body as suffused with a vital principle both within and above matter.[36]

From the standpoint of Romantic medical terminology, Blake's negative treatment of generation actively seeks to pervert what were known as the "organs of generation"—the genitals—into fiery joy. Organs of generation that do not generate are ontological oxymorons. To the extent that scientists in the Romantic period actively showed how sexual pleasure had no necessary connection to reproduction, Blake's hostility to limiting the genitals to generation was part of a larger cultural hostility of limiting pleasure to function. Indeed, Blake never uses the term "organs of generation," preferring instead to invoke the genitals or the loins.[37] The closest he comes is to refer to "some organs for craving and lust" in *The Book of Ahania*, but that is to empty out the genitals of generation. Blake makes these organs part of Urizen's "army of horrors" (4:6): having cast out Ahania or pleasure, Urizen now seeks to repress mankind through the body. Thomas Frosh has argued that genital sexuality in Blake is a form of tyrannical centralization, and this suggests another reason why Blake eschews the term "organs of generation" (162–63).

The fact that Blake describes Orc at his birth as a worm (Urizen 19) and then as a serpent connects Orc physiologically to the sperm. Spallanzani had proven that generation could not take place without physical contact between the female organs of generation and the semen, and Erasmus Darwin had referred to the sperm as "spermatic worms." Orc thus acquires a powerful, if phallocentric, but continuously shifting form of embodiment, one that could provide a material ground for Blakean idealistic revolution. Because worms are etymologically related to snakes,[38] Orc's transformation from worm to serpent allegorizes the body's embryological development, albeit in a masculine one, and gives Orc's revolutionary fires transformative embodiment.

Blake's emphasis on the consequences of unperverting the Bible in his annotations to Watson might have come from his reading in physiognomy and phrenology, and the general wariness many scientific writers had have toward materiality lest they be accused of ascribing to French atheism. Thus, Lavater insists that facial features only indicate potentiality, while Spurzheim and Gall relentlessly generate organs of the mind but then have to insist that the mere existence of those organs will not determine one's actions, and the organs are really more ideas than organs. Rather, the presence of organs only amounts to a predisposition toward the particular behavior, not the material embodiment of the behavior. Might not Blake's awareness of the capacity of evil and the consequences of actions done in the name of liberty owe something to the physiognomical and phrenological idea of a predisposition or propensity? Likewise, Blake's ability to see generation as having the capacity for regeneration suggests that generation can have a predisposition to regeneration, especially if one recognizes that Christ dwells within the human body. By so insisting upon gaps between the material body and human behavior, Gall and Spurzheim attempted to deflect charges of materialism. Gall and Spurzheim's ideas were widely diffused in the Romantic period, appearing, for example, in Henry Crabb Robinson's article for *Rees's Cyclopedia* (Richardson 2001 36), and Blake prepared multiple illustrations for this work. Robinson sought out Blake in the spring of 1810 for his German article on Blake (Bentley 296). We know that Blake read Spurzheim's 1817 *Observations on Insanity*, and Spurzheim insisted that both "external impression[s] and internal predispositions of the mind" combine to reduce the mind to insanity (154).

Blake filled the margins of Lavater's 1788 *Aphorisms on Man* with much praise, and engraved four plates for Lavater's 1788 *Essays on Physiognomy*. In his "Public Address," we can hear Blake's bravado when he claims, "It only remains to be Certified whether Physiognomic Strength & Power is to give place to Imbecillity" (E 571). Lavater writes in his *Essays* that "certain situations of mind frequently repeated, produce propensities, propensities become habits, and passions are their offspring" (1:135). On the one hand, propensities insist on a gap between the material shape of the head and the immaterial mind. Materiality is thus distinguished from immateriality in much the same way that Blake initially separates generation from regeneration. On the other hand, propensities are the link between materiality and immateriality and thus Lavater explains how the material interacts with the immaterial, how generation can lead to regeneration. That the body was so malleable as to "assume the habits, gestures, and looks of persons with whom we live in close harmony" (3:195), made it at least partly capable of realizing Blake's ideal of the unification of the sexes. While Blake would certainly have objected violently to Lavater's attempts to make perversity (sexual immorality, criminality) visible on a person's face, Lavater does say that "I have seen men the most perverse . . . all their malignity, all their blasphemies, all their efforts to oppress innocence, could not extinguish on the faces the beams of divine light" (2:41). Blake would have found especially provocative the fact that perversity could not extinguish divinity; by analogy, no amount of generation could extinguish the capacity for regeneration.

The poet's connections to the radical Joseph Johnson circle meant that he potentially had access to much of the key medical literature of his day. Johnson was one of the three major medical publishers in London. While I do not have the space to survey this vast literature, I want to suggest at least one cross current. The poet's imagery of childbirth resonates differently in light of the 1790s dispute between men-midwives Thomas Denham and William Osborn, both published by Johnson. What made their dispute so vitriolic was the fact that they had once practiced midwifery together. Where Osborn insisted that women's generation was necessarily painful, and so mandated by God, Denham, by contrast, insisted that parturition was a "natural" process, "not . . . generally requiring assistance" (*Introduction* 2:1). At issue are two competing understandings of nature: Osborne's, which distrusted nature, and especially female nature, arguing for example that the intricate passage of the pelvis made it impossible for childbirth not to be difficult and painful (14), and Denham's, which urged that men-midwives restrain themselves from intervention because nature "should be suffered to have its own course" (2:1). Osborn therefore emphasized the need for active male control over female childbirth. Read in light of this controversy, Blake's depictions of childbirth remind us of the falleness of generation and childbirth in that they are generally accompanied by pain. But they also remind us of the reasons why he could think of generation as not being too far from regeneration. Denham's view would have helped him to see that generation did not have to imply either the curse of God, or male dominance over the female body, or the necessary falleness of nature.[39]

The degenerating and rheumatic body, moreover, could be regenerated by electricity, once again grounding utopia within the living body. Blake was in fact a witness to just such a transformation. Blake's own and his wife's physician, John Birch, was a leading practitioner of medical electricity. Blake refers to Birch's "Electrical Magic" in his letter to Hayley of December 1804 and to the fact that his wife had discontinued these treatments in these three months, indicating that Catherine had been under his care earlier in that year. In October 1804, Blake had indeed rejoiced in his wife's recovery: "Electricity is the wonderful cause; the swelling of her legs and knees is entirely reduced" (E 756). This was, of course, also the year in which Blake inscribed on the title page of *Milton*, and in that work, Blake describes, "Albions sleeping Humanity began to turn upon his Couch;/Feeling the electric flame of Milton's awful precipitate descent" (20:25–26). Viscomi informs us that "*Milton* was not in draft or in production before 1804" (315). Electrical shock is precisely what the sleeping Albion needs to regenerate his body; one might even imagine Blake watching Catherine on the couch while undergoing Birch's therapy. That Blake compares Milton's descent to an electrical flame links the onset of self-annihilation to electricity. In 1802, Joseph Johnson reprinted Birch's 1792 *Essay on the Medical Application of Electricity*, and in it Birch marveled at the fact that "so mighty a power, capable of extinguishing life at a stroke, may with discretion, be passed through the tender fabric of the brain!" (iv). Birch himself described his application of electricity: "When I wish to apply the fluid, I connect by a smooth wire the glass-mounted director to the conductor with a point at it's [*sic*] extremity, and the radii are projected from it to the part affected. When desirous of propelling the sparks, I change the point for the ball. When the shock is intended, the circuit of the Leyden jar must be made" (Adams 522). Electricity was helpful because it acted as a "sedative, stimulant, and deobstruent" (Adams 521).

Blake's symbolic use of medical electricity thus occurs just at the moment when the narrator reminds us that "thou art cloth'd with human beauty O thou mortal man./Seek not thy heavenly father then beyond the skies" (20:31–32). Blake urges us to look within our own bodies for God, and electricity reinforces the divinity within man. Birch thus framed electricity between annihilation and miracle cure. Because electricity was thought to be either a subtle ether that could permeate porous matter or an electrical fluid that revealed the Promethean spark to be real (Fulford 16–17), electricity thus helped to restore belief in regeneration of man's otherwise dead flesh. As the prototype for Albion, Catherine Blake hints that women are not beyond divinity and redemption.

John Hunter's 1794 *Treatise on the Blood, Inflammation and Gun-Shot Wounds*, published by Joseph Johnson in the very same year that Blake produced the *First Book of Urizen*, informs Blake's depiction of the "red globules of life blood" of Urizen. Hunter challenged Hewson, who claimed the globules of blood were not really globules at all (40). Blake may have known Hunter and he satirizes him in *An Island in the Moon*. Not only did Hunter think the blood held the principle of life (it was the vital fluid), but also Hunter made it clear that globules of blood were a particularly flexible form of matter. Blake alludes to a "red globule of blood" twice in *Milton;* indeed, Blake's point that the microscope and telescope "alter/the ratio of the Spectators Organs but leave Objects untouched" (*Milton* 29:16–18 E 127) specifically recalls Hunter's warning about how magnifying glass in particular distorts the perception of objects. Comparing how the eye sees to how objects are seen through a magnifying glass, Hunter notes: "In such a situation, respecting our eye, all the relative objects by which the eye, from habit, judges with more nicety of the object itself, are cut off; the eye has likewise a power of varying its forms, adapting it to the different distances of the parts of an object within its compass, making the object always a whole; but a magnifying glass must be made to vary its position, and bring in succession the different parts of the hemisphere into so many focal points" (*Treatise* 42).

Hunter claimed that "to conceive that blood is endowed with life, while circulating, is perhaps carrying the imagination as far as it well can go; but the difficulty arises merely from its being fluid, the mind not accustomed to the idea of a living fluid" (77). Hunter explicitly invokes the "imagination" here, and calls upon it to help make a connection between life and fluid; matter does not preclude imagination. Blake also equates blood and life, insisting upon the "trembling" "globe of life blood" twice in *Urizen* (15:13 E 78 and 18:1 E 78). The immortals behold this trembling, and the fact that this trembling enjambs over three plates, and that such trembling culminates in the branching out of the blood into roots and fleshly fibers, further indicates Blake's physiological debts to Hunter. Indeed, Hunter suggested that although "the coagulation of the blood, would seem to be unconnected with life, yet life could not go on without it; for as all the solid parts of the body are formed from the blood, this could not take place, if there did not exist in it the powers of coagulating" (17). For Hunter, blood provides the basic building materials for the body. "Trembling" further signifies a complete and living body because for Hunter, bodies must contain "body, blood, and motion (circulation)" (86). "The three make up a complete body," he concludes (86). Urizen's failure to recognize the life within blood thus is an imaginative failure, and it is one that even medicine tried to forestall in its insistence upon the gaps between dead anatomy and living physiology, body parts and body. It is no surprise that the bodies Urizen creates are by Hunter's standards incomplete, more dead than alive.

Hence, in *Urizen*, blood mediates between the abstract and brooding Urizen and the creation of material bodies. The outset of Urizen emphasizes abstraction and shadows and void, but when the heavens awaken, "vast clouds of blood roll'd/Round the dim rocks of Urizen" (4:40 E 71). The presence of blood as an especially flexible form of materiality even within the void means that there is nothing about materiality itself that makes it fallen. To the extent that one can imagine a materiality that is not bereft of spirit or life, even bodily materiality need not equate to fallenness. More to the point, blood offers a kind of corporeal materiality that can counter abstraction yet not ossify into fixity and, as such, clues us in to how the body can provide a via media between shadows and substance. Urizen's creation of a dead womblike structure "vast, petrific around" (*Urizen* 5: 28–29 E 73) shows his failure to grasp the difference between living bodies and the dead. His womb therefore entombs and petrifies rather than generates life.

When Urizen takes the "globe of fire" to light his journey—an image that recalls globules of blood and anticipates Los's globe of light—he is annoyed by the "forms of life on his forsaken mountains" and by the "fawning portions of life;

similitudes of a foot, or a hand, or a head/Or a heart, or an eye" (21:1–5). These are further described as swimming "mischievous Dread terrors! Delighting in blood" (21:6–7). Here again blood symbolizes a living material potentiality, a potentiality that is fundamentally disturbing to Urizen because it cannot be pinned down and measured. Unsurprisingly, Urizen immediately sickens "to see/His eternal creations appear" (21:8–9). In connecting the red blood globule to the globe, Blake reminds readers once again of what Urizen cannot see: the universe within the grain of sand, and the metonymic connections between globe and globule, globule being the diminutive form of globe. The ability to perceive this connection—one theorized by medicine—is what enables a blood globule to become a globe of enlightenment. Quite literally so: the globule as a symbol for life embodies that life and points to its possible physical manifestation in the world even as it does not mistake the physical manifestation with life. The gap between the fallen and unfallen body thus can be traversed in Blake by material bodies, but only ones that see that the structure of a body is not the same as life.

Blake's debt to Hunter, however, is more subtle and specific. Hunter argued that "matter continually passes between solid and fluid" and that "no species of matter can assume solid form, without first been in a fluid state; nor can any change take place in a solid till it be first formed into, or suspended in a fluid" (12). In Hunter's view, bodily matter fluctuates between liquid and solid and back again, and his interest in the coagulating powers of blood as a means of healing the body's wounds meant that both solidity and fluidity were necessary for corporeal health. Read in this context, Blake's having Urizen and Los hammer bodies into form shows that they do not grasp the need for the body's fluidity. At the same time, if "coagulation is an operation of life" (Hunter 26), flesh is not so much the enemy to imagination but rather its enabling vehicle. Precisely for this reason, Blake takes an epigraph from the Bible, "For we wrestle not against flesh and blood, but against principalities, against powers, against the rules of the darkness of this world, against spiritual wickedness in high places," and makes this a gateway into *The Four Zoas*. The fact that Christ's blood was yoked to his incarnation further reminded Blake that even flesh could be divine. Although the development of the body in *Urizen* seems equated with fallenness, the problem is that all Urizen and Los seem to care about is the hardening, delimiting, measuring, imprisoning, and chaining of the body, and thus it is no surprise that the senses harden into dumbness. Blake reminds us that they "forgot their eternal life" (23:42). With this forgetting, the chords and meshes of the human brain devolve into "the Net of Religion" (23:20–23). Hunter insisted that the principle of life was not indebted to organization, that "life can never rise out of, or depend on organization" (78), and his separation of the living principle from materiality and organization helped to reinforce Blake's sense of a possible gap between corporeal organization and life. Hunter likewise reminds us that without the living principle of blood, all we have been examining "is like dissecting a dead body without having any reference to the living, or even knowing it had ever been alive" (76).

The globular form of the red part of the blood had "something like the nature of a solid body, yet the particles seem not to have the properties of a solid," Hunter declared (40). He concludes that these globules are fluid. How then to account for the shape of the blood globule? Hunter surmises that the shape was due to "a fixed principle in the globule itself" (40). Hunter's theory of the blood supports Blake's sense of the dynamic materiality of the body by making the body and life essentially fluid, by connecting idealized principles like the life force to the body of the red blood cell, and by bridging the fixity of shape with the fluidity of the globule. Orc's red fires are the fires within our blood, only waiting to be reactivated. Also, as the agent of growth and repair in the blood as well as the agent of coagulation, Hunter's red globules imply that generation has within it regeneration. Los, by contrast, does not appreciate the flexible materiality of these globules: he wants to hasten their progress to fibers (*Urizen* 18:1–3 E 78). Moreover, Los's fixing "englobing" is antithetical to the flexible globes that are within the human body. Hunter also argues that these red blood cells are the source of strength, and this perhaps explains why Urizen arose at the beginning and end of night six of *The Four Zoas*, "gorgd with blood" (6:322 E 352). Orc's fires recall the strength that is within our very blood.

Recently, we have discovered that Blake owned a copy of John Quincy's *Pharmacopoeia Officinalis & Extemporanea; Or, a Complete English Dispensatory* (1733).[40] I have been unable to consult the ninth edition of this work, but I have read the tenth edition, which has the same number of pages. From this, Blake would have understood the body as an amalgam of processes, and Quincy lists "fermentation, calcinations, digestion, incorporation, filtration" as processes common to both pharmacy and the body (n.p.). Quincy theorizes that "there is an attractive force in all bodies whatsoever; or, that all the parts of matter are mutually drawn towards one another" (1), thus emphasizing the mobility of matter.

Quincy not only helped reinforce Blake's faith in the regeneration of matter, but also detailed how to make and dilute *aqua fortis*, the substance Blake used as the acid in his relief etching process. Robert Essick argues that Blake was innovative in using a much weaker acid than normal (*Printmaker* 99), and thus Blake would have found Quincy's directions for manipulating the strength of this acid especially helpful.[41] Quincy, moreover, stresses that *aqua fortis* had its place "as a Menstruum for other pharmacological preparations" (288), thus making its corrosive powers curative. Insofar as his acid baths could both corrode and heal, Blake could harness this dualism in service of the regeneration of matter.

Through Erasmus Darwin, Blake learned of the perverse sexuality of plants,[42] how so few plants were monogamous. For Darwin, plant sexuality allegorized human sexuality, one that did not have to confine itself to monogamy or marriage. While Darwin helped to expand the range of natural forms of human sexuality, he also depicted a world rife with fecundity and desire. These medical and botanical contexts also help explain the relentlessly allegorical nature of Blake's bodies. Body fits with allegory in that both can be flexible. Bodies in Blake can be fallen and unfallen, and this means that his depictions of sexuality are necessarily allegorical. Because natural history, comparative anatomy, and botany of the period so relentlessly allegorized animal and plant bodies in terms of human ones, bodies were profoundly like texts. This simultaneous incarnation and allegorization of bodies meant that Blake could at once harness the immediacy of incarnation (performative vortex), and the reflexiveness of allegory, giving him the space from which he could evaluate who is being liberated and from what and to what.

Blake's textualized bodies, therefore, demand careful scrunity. For example, before we can assent to Brenda Webster's claim that Blake is misogynistic, we must be sure to have factored in the poet's insistent perversities. Webster's comment that Blake comes to "see women as responsible for the Fall" (209) ignores the multiple significances of the fall to Blake, along with the possibility that Blake's fallen women are only seen from the vantage of the fall. Although the flexibility of his bodies further undercuts any stable vantage point from which to level a critique, I am also mindful of Tristanne Connolly's point that "the fallen/eternal distinction in Blake can be a convenient trapdoor to save him from many sins: anything unpalatable can be explained away as fallen" (ix). I therefore side with Helen Bruder's more nuanced claim that Blake recognized the costs of his gender attitudes, because that position, at very least, recognizes the value of Blake's perverse turns.

## Blake's Perverse Aesthetics of Incarnation

I have thus far laid out the many ways in which Blake uses perversion to intensify epistemological uncertainty to the end of undermining all forms of authority including his own. I have also considered how medicine made it possible for Blake to see regeneration even within the mortal body. I now examine ways in which he embodies perversion in his aesthetics.[43] Here my focus is less on how perversion leads to skepticism, but more on how he goes about delivering his perverse ideas. Blake embodies perversion in such a way as to undermine its ability to deliver immediate moral judgments, thus perverting the function of perversion from condemnation to questioning while harnessing the immediacy of perverse judgments in the service of epistemological uncertainty. Embodiment of this uncertainty in the reader makes the reader's self-annihilation possible. To the extent that the moment of self-annihilation is, for Blake, the moment of perverse incarnation—the moment when readers recall that they are already the embodiment of Christ who in turn embodies perversion—then Blakean incarnation recognizes the pitfalls of naive incarnation, and it does so by remaining skeptical about incarnation as perfect embodiment. That is, Blake recognized that without deferral, language must take part in an authoritarian metaphysics of presence, Urizen's tablets of brass and sex under moral law. Through perverse incarnation either via Christ, because Christ negates the Commandments and died as an "unbeliever" in the Old Testament God ("Annotations to Watson" E 614), or through bodily orgasm as a kind of unknowing or forgetting or *jouissance*, Blake maintains skepticism about perfect embodiment. Indeed, because perfect embodiment would obviate the need for interpretation, not to mention cleansing the doors of perception and epistemological uncertainty, the poet must hold on to that skepticism.[44] If I have until this moment described what perversion in Blake does, I now consider how he gets the job done.

Perversion is also essential to understanding Blake's aesthetics. The turning of perversion is manifested in texts that resist stabilization: a resistance that is simultaneously articulated and performed. Performance helps to give perverse turning the ontology of direct experience.[45] Turning the page in Blake literally becomes a potential act of perversion. For example, copies of the *Book of Thel* that end with Thel's motto, which might refer to the motto for *The Book of Thel* or that of Thel, redefine the opening of the poem as its conclusion. Copies A–M and P–R (P and Q have been untraced) open with the motto, while the "final" copies N and O end with it. Given that the journey of Thel is one of sexual awakening, one especially called for by Thel's virginity, the placement of the motto is either previous to that awakening or after it. If previous to that awakening, then Thel cannot be aware of the sexual innuendos in the golden bowl or phallic rod. And if she cannot see sexual innuendo, it stands to reason that she must be equally incapable of skepticism about such forms of sexual embodiment or restriction. Moreover, the motto's placement at the end suggests that Thel's awakening into sexuality is much more than an awakening into Thanatos and that, rather than being soundly denounced by her critics, Thel should be praised for her ability to see beyond mere generation and death. By plate 8, Thel only sees sexuality in terms of vegetative and mortal generation, and thus she flees back into the Vales of Har, or self-love. The ending motto gives Thel the final words and suggests she is more than a failed heroine who has fallen into silence or self-pity.[46]

Finally, where the motto at the outset frames the text with the language and message of the preacher in Ecclesiastes—that all is vanity and that human desire must give way to duty and to the commandments (12:13)—the one at the end undermines the voice of the preacher with his very own words, suggesting that love cannot be put into a golden bowl in much the same way as the preacher wants to confine desire to the commandments and duty. Again we can only credit a critical skepticism to Thel's motto if she has been awakened to sexuality and if she can maintain an aesthetic stance vis à vis the forms that sexuality and love take. Should love take the forms of duty or should love transcend those forms? I am suggesting then that Blake's decision to end with the motto perverts not only his previous reading, but also the underlying message of Ecclesiastes itself.[47] Marjorie Levinson's reminder that Thel is etymologically rooted in desire, coupled with her sense that "for desire to know itself as desire, hence to be felt, it must, in some tenuous, incomplete, or unconscious way, have assimilated its object" (292), means that this desire suspends reproductive purpose, and is akin to purposiveness.

In placing so much emphasis on the placement of the motto, I am guided by Blake's critique of sexuality as mere generation and his sense that sexuality needs to awaken spirituality or it will be perverted from its true essence. Thus, Thel's sexual awakening is only partial; while she "saw the secrets of the land unknown" (8:2 Eaves, Essick, and Viscomi 100), she sees only the generative aspects of sexuality since the underworld can only show death. Hence, Blake initially concludes that she "fled back unhindered till she came into the vales of

Har" (8:22), leaving her still hindered. In the final copies N–O, however, we turn the page to find Thel's motto, giving Thel the last word. Here, the motto occurs after Thel's admittedly partial awakening, but it now holds the promise of a fuller awakening, a recognition that sexuality must lead to something more than mere generation, regeneration. Her motto reads,

> Does the Eagle know what is in the pit?
> Or wilt thou go ask the Mole:
> Can Wisdom be put in a silver rod?
> Or love in a golden bowl?

When the motto follows Thel's journey into the underworld, it offers the possibility of the higher knowledge gleaned from the descent. All epics demand that we descend before we can ascend, and the motto offers a possible ascent from the depths of death. Although Thel does insistently question, her questions throughout *Thel* are prompted by a lack of knowledge rather than a skeptical questioning of the answers that she is being given as truth.[48] The cloud, for example, reminds her that she "know'st thou not. [*sic*] our steeds drink of the golden springs" (5:7). The experiences chronicled in her book enable her to move from innocent to informed questioning as she does in the motto's final questions.[49]

By thinking about the vantage point of the eagle in her motto, Thel recognizes the possibility that sexuality means more than reproduction and generation. Instead of simply taking in the information without considering her source, Thel now wonders what wisdom would look like if it came from the eagle's perspective. Would the eagle even be able to hear the voice of sorrow that is in the pit of plate 8? Only after the lily and the cloud introduce her to sexual pleasure can Thel read the innuendos within the phallic rod and the vaginal bowl and see that these containers are limited. Sexuality cannot be reduced to genitality; desire refuses to remain localized anatomically. Thel's rhyme between "bowl" and "mole" introduces what Blake would later call the "bondage of rhyme": rhyme highlights her awareness of these limits.[50]

Blake's tail-piece depiction of a naked Thel riding a phallic Orc-like serpent further supports a general movement from descent in plate 8 to ascent in the motto. Blake often symbolizes a rejection of materiality and fallen sexuality by a stripping off of garments: both *Milton* and *Jerusalem* show us his correlation of spiritual and sexual enlightenment with nakedness. Blake's rendering of bodies with transparent skin suggests that nakedness is the start of a journey within.

Whereas many have taken the snake as an emblem of "infantile regression," the fact that Blake elsewhere links Orc to the serpent connects Thel with the liberating energies of Orc. And although Thel does seem to be holding a rein over the snake, the rein connects Thel to Orc's tongue, limiting the potential restraint. That the rein is slack and does not bind the serpent's neck further implies that it is a relatively ineffective form of restraint if indeed it represents restraint. If the serpent represents Orc-like rebellion, the final words of the plate, "the end," indicate not a termination, but the purposiveness of an enlightened and liberating sexuality.[51] My sense of the significance of the motto's [re]placement at the end of *Thel* further supports this dual meaning of end as goal, but one that remains to be achieved.

To the extent that the motto stands for the knowledge of epic ascent, Thel's criticism of Ecclesiastes now becomes clear. Her motto replaces that of the preacher. Although the preacher's sense that all is vanity helps undermine worldly materiality, his desire to break the golden bowl and loosen the silver cord amounts to a denial of the flesh rather than the recognition that one must attain regeneration through the flesh. He concludes his book of the Bible with a clear motto: "Let us hear the conclusion of the whole matter: 'Fear God, and keep his commandments: for this is the whole duty of man. For God shall bring every work into judgment'" (12:13–14). Not only do Thel's first two questions in her motto demand that readers consider their source, but they also strongly indicate her recognition that material embodiments for love, desire, and wisdom are themselves inadequate. Her questions further show that she knows sexuality must partake of both love and wisdom. Here Thel recognizes she has only been given the generative understanding of human sexuality, one that is subsumed by death. To ask whether wisdom can be put in a silver rod is to ask whether metaphor is an adequate container. It is also to see the absurdity of fixating on the "little curtain of flesh on the bed of our desire" (E 6) as if the hymen is really the embodiment of the moral virtue of chastity. The preacher of Ecclesiastes, by contrast, is only too happy to contain desire in duty and the commandments and ends his book in the certainty of God's judgment. Thel, by contrast, resists judgmental closure, offering questions in the place of conclusion, summation, and judgment.

Thus, when we turn to Thel's motto as the final plate of the book of Thel, we overturn readings of *The Book of Thel* that emphasize the weakness of Thel and see her as an anti-heroine, that see sexuality as Thanatos and spiritual death, and that remain blind to how this illuminated text so thoroughly undermines

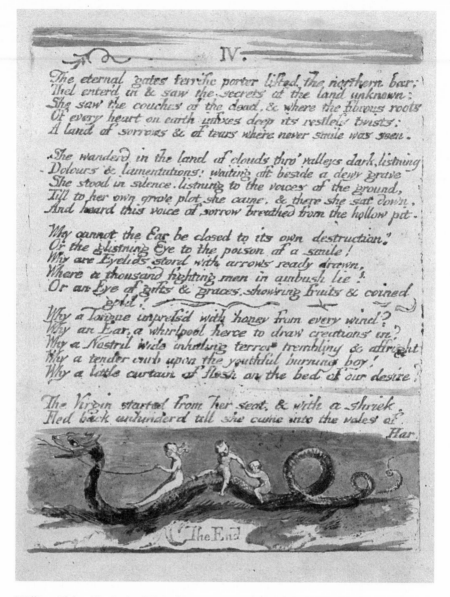

William Blake, *The Book of Thel*, plate 8 (Rosenwald 1798a). Courtesy of the Lessing Rosenwald Collection, the Library of Congress, Washington, D.C.

the Book of Ecclesiastes. Without the motto at the end, we miss Blake literally perverting Ecclesiastes by ending the final plate with an image of a serpent instead of a judgmental God. At very least, Blake found ironic the fact that the preacher of Ecclesiastes stipulates all to be vanity yet concludes the book by demanding that we "Fear God, and keep his commandments: for this is the whole duty of man" (12:13). We also miss a glimmer of Thel's sexual and spiritual awakening to a sexuality beyond Thanatos, to the regenerative possibilities of sex construed without purpose. And we miss the perverse heroism of Thel herself, her transformation from a passive and silent listener into an active and skeptical questioner. If plate 8 ends where Thel began in the vales of Har, a place no different than Thel's own grave, the motto, by contrast, signals an awareness of the limited perspective provided by the Clod, Cloud, Lilly, Worm, and the Voice of Sorrow. In turning the page to the initial beginning of the book, a beginning that is now properly its end, less in the sense of a terminus but more in the sense of a goal, Blake has transformed the act of turning the page into an act of perversion. We turn the page to the end that was once the beginning, an ending which ironizes the very idea of endings. Sexual awakening is a process rather than a product. That the motto is written in the relative freedom of Blake's calligraphic hand as opposed to the alienating block letters of the title page further marks transition from alienation to awakening and supports the significance of the motto's placement at the end of the book.

Before leaving behind the *Book of Thel*, I want to highlight the role that orgasm plays in Blake's aesthetics because minute descriptions of sexual acts are often taken to be aesthetically perverse. Saree Makdisi has lamented the lack of attention to joy in Blake (xiii–xv), and I would simply add that much of the poet's joy is sexual. But orgasm has an even more important resonance in Blake in that it is the closest thing our bodies experience to self-annihilation. Blakean orgasm has the potential to destroy selfhood. That this destruction of selfhood is a form of forgiveness, whereby one both forgives errors of the self and no longer blames others, adds a key ethical dimension to perversion. Hence, the cloud in the *Book of Thel*, Blake's *Vade Mecum* of pleasure, anatomizes orgasm as the loss of self:

> O virgin thou know'st not. Our steeds drink of the golden springs
> Where Luvah doth renew his horses: look'st thou on my youth,
> And fearest thou because I vanish and am seen no more.
> Nothing remains; O maid I tell thee, when I pass away,
> It is to tenfold life, to love, to peace, and raptures holy: (3:7–11)

The cloud's steeds drink in the golden springs. Gold often in Blake has sexual resonance. Not only does Luvah symbolize lust, but also the horses are a long-standing image of the passions. Upon drinking from the stream, the cloud is "seen no more," "nothing remains," and the cloud "passes away" into the petit mort that is orgasm or "holy raptures." Even as Blake here equates orgasm and self-annihilation, he calls attention to the benefits of that annihilation: "tenfold life . . . love, . . . peace . . . and raptures holy" (5:11). Orgasm is precisely the knowledge that the virgin know'st not; Blake's twist on sexual knowledge is that it leads to unknowing, the process of self-annihilation. For Thel, such knowledge comes at too dear a price, at least until her motto. Her immediate response to the cloud is to declare that she is "not like thee" (5:17). She reimagines herself at her death as the "food of worms," solely in the terms of generation rather than in the terms of the absence that the cloud uses, and this implies that she has not yet grasped how self-annihilation demands a regeneration of generation.

In giving self-annihilation the physiological experience of orgasm, Blake again grounds the real in the ideal, the erection within resurrection[52] and the resurrection in bodily experience. But this is an especially powerful if paradoxical bodily experience. If orgasm is a form of self-annihilation, it is experienced as a dissociation of the body. Thus, when the nameless shadowy female experiences orgasm in *America*, Blake describes that sensation as the womb's sensation: "it joy'd" (2:4 E 52). The "it" insists on the gap between the womb and the self and ruptures any metonymy, any connection between the part and the whole. As Blake defines it, orgasm is the sensation that leads to the breakdown of the self. So if the poet turns to physiology to ground his concept of self-annihilation in the body, self-annihilation in turn grounds the regeneration of the self. Where Robert Essick argues that linguistic performance in Blake is not about the deconstruction of the transcendental, but about the "celebrat[ion of] the engendering powers of language" (*Adam* 239), I want to consider the power of orgasm in Blake to perform both engendering and division. The traffic in Blake's performative language goes two ways: it is a highway to transcendence and to the generated body. Such duality allows Blake to harness the liberating capacity of incarnation (recall that Lavater helped Blake to see that generation gives birth to the will or regeneration) as well as the liberating capacity of deferral.

Perversion further operates at the level of the poetic line in Blake. Milton taught Blake to think of the line as a means to liberation. On occasion, Blake will use the word "pervert" as either the final foot in the line as when "Rahab and Tirzah pervert" the "mild influences" of Enitharmon and her daughters (*Milton*

29:53 E 128), or in the first two feet, as in "to pervert the Divine voice in its entrance to the earth" (*Milton* 9:23 E 103). The turn of the verse ("verse" comes from *versare*, to turn the plow) is also the turn of perversion. In this second example, the infinitive form reminds us that although Satan tries to fob his perversion onto Palamabron, the perversion is his. Blake will at other times put perversion smack in the middle of other turns. In *The Four Zoas*, for example, Urizen invents "harsh instruments of sound/To grate the soul into destruction or to inflame with fury/The spirits of life to pervert all the faculties of sense/Into their own destruction" (8:18–21 E 374–75). Note how Blake puts "spirits of life" into an ambiguous position just after the turn of the end of the line, hovering between the objects that are being inflamed and the active perverters of sense. This epistemological uncertainty—enhanced by the parallelism of "to grate" and "to pervert," which not only suggests that grating and perverting are synonymous, but also figuratively moves pervert to just after the line break in the position of grate—demands that readers actively apprehend who is doing what to whom. Insofar as the "spirits of life" have been perverted into death, the truth is that they are both the victims and agents of their own perversion. Where the charge of perversion is usually an attempt to absolve the self from blame, Blake makes clear that perversion simultaneously moves toward and away from the self. That Blake uses the physical layout of the page to break lines into subunits amounts to what Susan Wolfson has called a perverse "performative antiformalism" in Blake (2003 64–65).

John Hollander has noted "the conscious formal perversity to [his early] Spenserian imitation, . . . in which every stanza is 'defective' if taken from one point of view, or 'adapted' if from another" (205). From the standpoint of Blake's early neoclassicism, which understood originality in terms of the conscious choosing of which models to imitate rather than the Romantic transcendence of imitation, Blake has been perverse in the sense that he demands that the reader recalibrate the very standard by which one measures metrical perversity.[53] If judged from a Romantic perspective that values innovation, Blake's departures look innovative and demand to be seen as positive adaptations. But such departures imply the limitations of the source and beg the question of why imitate Spenser anyway. If judged from a kind of neoclassical originality, Blake has chosen a potentially good model but then needs to explain what licenses his departures, else his departures look like perversions. Blake, thus, raises multiple standards for assessing the differences between his and Spenser's lines precisely to undermine the single and stable uniform standard that perversion demands.

In terms of the metrical fourteeners of Blake's longer works, the poet turns to structural parallelism to pervert the balance and smug witty antithesis of Augustan verse (Hollander 208). Few of his lines are end stopped, and thus the termination of the line rarely equates with a semantic unit of meaning. Where other poets exploit the tension between the line's ending and the unit of meaning, Blake typically layers line upon line so that the lines themselves threaten to become the poetic equivalent of a vortex. This layering is all the more overwhelming in light of the fact that meaning in Blake so depends upon a "network of interactions within [and between] texts" (Makdisi 7). Where John Hollander stresses Blake's metrical contract of the fourteener, albeit one tempered by his free accentualism, I want to emphasize the impotence of this contract to assist us in unraveling Blake's meanings. This impotence is especially acute when dealing with Blake's long catalogs of "nouns, phrases, or whole clauses [that] tend to form a succession of brief, more or less equally weighted elements distributed isochronously along an indefinitely extended line," which reduce particulars to "virtually atomic units of significance" (De Luca 68).[54]

Even in his depictions of the figures, Blake exploits the turning of perversion. He often depicts figures in *contrapposto*, in the act of turning from one stance to another. Moreover, sequential plates can sometimes rotate a particular figure, a rotation that allegorizes how readers are to engage with the figure or to reflect upon the limitations of perspective. For example, in *The Marriage of Heaven and Hell*, Blake depicts a resurrection through fire (plate 3) only to give us the obverse of that image eleven plates later (plate 14 Eaves, Essick, and Viscomi 167). Why would he invite the reader to recall the former image eleven plates later, and why does he turn that image 180 degrees? While the earlier plate 3 announces that the "new heaven is begun," an assertion that implies the apocalypse has already taken place, plate 14 insists that the apocalypse is still in the offing, as the world, we are told, "will be consumed in fire at the end of six thousand years" (14). Moreover, the cherub with his flaming sword "will come to pass by an improvement of sensual enjoyment" (14). Important clues appear at the bottom of the earlier plate. Although the poet here emphasizes the now of the apocalypse, he shows at the bottom of the plate a woman giving birth to a child (bottom left) along with a couple in sexual embrace (bottom right). Combined, these images suggest that the real improvement of sensual enjoyment has not yet taken place in the earlier plate, given that sexuality is still subsumed under generation, the reduction of sexuality to reproduction.

In the later image (plate 14), by contrast, Blake shows us that behind the image of resurrection of the flesh is precisely the generated dead body, a death that was obscured in the earlier plate by the flames. What the earlier image neglected to mention was the price of apocalypse, the death of the generated self. The improvement of sensual enjoyment thus cannot truly come to pass until one recognizes the price of regeneration, self-annihilation, as well as how reproduction confines sensual pleasure unnecessarily to the physical body. What looked like the apocalypse in plate 3, then, was merely the first stage of it, the recognition of the pleasures of the flesh. But Blake warns us not to mistake generation for regeneration. Hence, in the earlier plate he ironically alludes to the resurrection of Swedenborg, when his audience would have known immediately that, when Swedenborg's tomb was opened, the only thing discovered was his dead flesh. When we reperceive the earlier plate in light of the later one, we must come to terms with the fact that the dead body was there all along. Taken together, these plates insist that regeneration must entail generation and that regeneration is not without its costs.

Furthermore, the poet's valorizing of nudity over clothing equates nudity with holiness and thus attempts to reverse Christian distrust of the flesh. As Blake put it in his accompanying aphorisms to "The Laocoön," "Art can never exist without Naked Beauty displayed" (E 275). His rendering of characters such as Los, Thel, and Milton in various states of undress as they go through experience reminds us that maturation is at the same time a process of self-annihilation in Blake, a willing surrender of selfhood. In *Milton*, that surrender is achieved via fellatio when it had previously been accomplished by intercourse, suggesting that self-annihilation takes multiple forms and that these forms declare a gap between form and meaning.[55] Once Blake connects maturity with the surrender of selfhood, the adolescent search for identity becomes a perversion. Furthermore, the difficulty of being able to see nudity as holiness—the difficulty of stripping off one's garments, especially to an eighteenth-century audience—is nothing compared to the difficulty of taking off of one's selfhood.

Armed with these ways of thinking about perversion in Blake, let us now return one final time to *America* and to Orc's claim that Urizen has perverted man's fiery joys into ten commands. Again, rather than merely taking Orc's word for it, because authorship or speaking are not in and of themselves guarantees of truth, we need to think about why we should believe Orc. We should note the ways in which Blake makes it hard for us to take anyone's word as the unequivocal truth. That he so often identifies the speaker only after he or she

has spoken, and even then not always, means that statements have to be interpreted at least initially without speakers behind them. Moreover, his speakers
so insistently change states from the elect, redeemed, or reprobate, or specters
or emanations, or even identities as when Luvah becomes Christ; Blake insistently disembodies words. Finally, the poet's illustrations fail to embody the
words on the page insofar as they often have little correlation to what the words
say. Even when we can finally identify a visual rendition of a character and thus
begin to attribute speech to a depicted speaker, that identification often comes
after or sometimes well before the speech itself. The nude male perched atop
Blake's words on plate 6 of *America* is only identified as "his" in the plate, and
we can only later begin to identify this male as Orc.

Certainly from the perspective of Albion's angel, whom Orc addresses at this
moment, the claim that "fiery joys" have been "perverted into ten commands"
seems absurd and furthermore supports the angel's feeling that Orc must be
stopped at all costs. "Angel," of course, seems to load the deck against Orc; the
angel's accusations that Orc is "serpent-formed" and is "standing at the gates of
Enitharmon, ready to devour her children" doesn't predispose readers to accept
Orc. Nor does the angel's charge that Orc is the Antichrist. But readers can become more sympathetic to Orc once they see that Albion's angel is no angel: he
is motivated by wrath, and the fact that he is "wrathful burnt" (7.1 E 53) suggests that he is unbeknownst to himself already tainted with the Orcan fire of
rebellion. Blake's illustration of children lying peacefully down with a sheep undercuts the angel's view of things, allowing Orc to then score some rhetorical
points by converting the angel's wrath into a wreath: Orc describes himself as
being "wreath'd round the accursed tree" (8:1 E 54). Portraying himself as a victim, Orc has been both wreathed and accursed, and we have only to conclude
that the angel's wrath has led him to do these things to Orc while maintaining
the illusion of angelic innocence. If Orc is now serpent-formed as the angel declares, the angel has made him so, for the angel has converted pleasure into a
kind of satanic evil.

Blake's play on wrath and wreath hearkens back to Milton who in Book 6 of
*Paradise Lost* wrote,

> So spake the Sovran voice, and Clouds began
> To darken all the Hill, and smoke to roll
> In dusky wreaths, reluctant flames, the sign
> Of Wrath awak't: (6:56–59)

In *Paradise Lost*, as God mobilizes his troops to defeat Satan, the wreaths materialize God's voice into the smoke of fire and awaken the Old Testament God's wrath. In Blake's *America*, the wreath emphasizes Orc's status as victim—he is, after all entwined around a tree—even as it suggests that Urizen's torture will awaken the wrath of Orc. We should note, however, that Blake values the mercy, forgiveness, and love of God, not the punishing angry Old Testament Urizen. So while Orc's "wreath'd" status brings him closer to God, it brings him to the Urizenic God of the Old Testament, not the divine mercy of Christ. The Miltonic allusion further complicates our identifications with Orc: we turn toward him when he seems God-like, only to turn against him when he looks like Urizen. Hence, when Orc speaks, cursing Urizen, Blake gives us an illustration of Urizen (Blake's plate 10). In linking our identification with Orc with our potential perversion, and in linking Orc with his nemesis/father Urizen through pèr(e)/version, Blake demands that we wean ourselves from his revolutionary energy and manifest our own.

The charge of the angel's hypocrisy accrues more weight when Orc denounces "that pale religious letchery, seeking Virginity,/May find it in a harlot, and in coarse-clad honesty/The undefil'd tho'ravishd in her cradle night and morn" (8:9–11). Where Christian asceticism tries to pawn virginity as one of its highest virtues, Blake has Orc call attention to the seeking of that virtue as a form of lechery. The denial of the flesh does not remove the influence of the flesh; rather, it forces the cloaking of desire in the name of virtue. Such cloaking only intensifies eroticism rather than does away with it. Hence, religious lechery can find virginity in a harlot who remains undefiled although she is repeatedly ravished in her cradle. That the angel's words fall on deaf ears doesn't invite readerly sympathy either; even though the angel thrice demands the sounding of trumpets of war, he is greeted only by silence: "No trumpets answer; no reply of clarions or fifes,/Silent the Colonies remain and refuse the loud alarm" (10:3–4). As Blake's annotations to Watson insist, we must be attentive to consequences as part of evaluating who is perverting what. Where Orc achieves nothing less than revolution, the angel's words and trumpets are mere sound and fury, signifying nothing.

We are now in a position to believe Orc when he says, "The fiery joy, that Urizen perverted to ten commands" (8:3). Having earned this right, readers now can admire the crispness of this accusation, how it in a single stroke threatens to undermine the very foundation of Western morality. Although the commandments seem to be a set of rules that provide a social contract between God

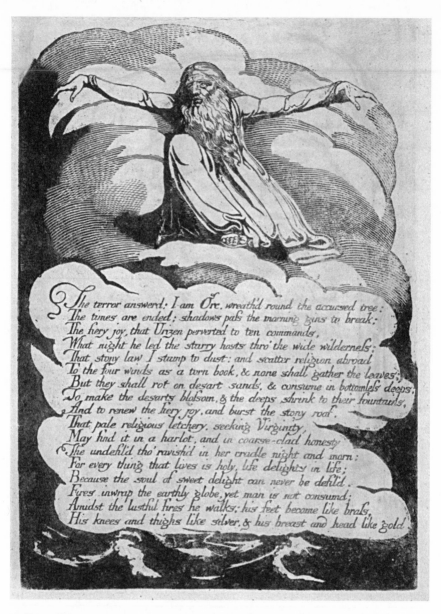

William Blake, *America*, plate 10 (Rosenwald 1804). Courtesy of the Lessing Rosenwald Collection, the Library of Congress, Washington, D.C.

and his worshippers, Blake underscores the tyrannical authority of it; he also comments on how the denial of the pleasure of others actually consolidates power. Shortening commandments to commands allows him to insinuate illegitimate kingly authority: didn't American democracy show precisely the futility of such commands? Later, of course, Blake will inform us that the writing of the Ten Commandments was really the means by which God gave humans the art of writing; such an interpretation makes the actual referentiality of the commandments beside the point (*Jerusalem* 3:4).

Nonetheless Orc's charge of perversion only holds up if the Ten Commandments can be seen as an authoritarian document of illegitimate authority. The obstacles to such a reading are enormous, but this is precisely where Blake performs perversion in addition to writing about it. Blake critics frequently remark how the poet must get rid of his audience's mental furniture in order to raise its levels of perception. How then does Blake propose to make it possible to think of Mosaic law as a perversion of pleasure? Here John Mee, Vincent De Luca, and Steven Goldsmith can help, insofar as each shows how Blake took advantage of prophetic, democratic, and sublime language to help deliver his point.[56] But Blake's syntactical ruptures further model the kind of epistemological rupture he wants to achieve. Tannenbaum stresses that Blake turned to Isaiah and the apocryphal Second Book of Esdras to depict Orc as demonical Christ coming down with his sword (124–33), a yoking together of opposites that hints at the syntactical perversions to come. The object of the sentence, "fiery joy," appears at the outset of the line, whereas the subject, Urizen, has through a distortion of syntax almost become the unwitting object of the joy. The syntax in other words prompts a reversal of Urizenic perversion by putting joy back in the driver's seat where it belongs.

Let's now examine the complicated phrasings that surround Orc's accusation of Urizen's perversion:

> The terror answered: I am Orc, wreath'd round the accursed tree:
> The times are ended: shadows pass the morning gins to break:
> The fiery joy, that Urizen perverted to ten commands,
> What night he led the starry hosts thro' the wide wilderness.
> The stony law I stamp to dust: (10:1–5 Paley edition)

Note Blake's insistent colons here, and how those colons shape the reading of these lines. Because of those colons, this passage is difficult to understand insofar as the relationship of one phrase to its previous phrase is unclear, and colon piles on top of colon before the reader can process the syntactical relationship of each phrase. This piling fosters the reader's self-annihilation insofar as it takes the reader outside him or herself in order to process this. Yet if the colon signifies the elaboration of "I am Orc," a declaration of identity that appears in the very center of the first line indicating its importance, the statement "the fiery joy, that Urizen perverted to ten commands" must likewise amount to a declaration of identity. While "perverted" is shunted into a restrictive clause, Urizen's perversion runs the danger of subsuming Orc's identity, and to the extent that both are simultaneously possible, Orc and Urizen begin to fold into one another. Indeed, Orc's actions are merely a père/version, a version of—and structured by—his father's.

Orc is not without limitations, as his raping of the shadowy daughter of Urthona further shows. Orc perhaps reasons that rape is the best way to show Urthona (earth owner) that he does not own America. Likewise, Orc's regenerating powers are not outside of Urizen, but they burn within, a fact that explains why *America* opens with "Albion's fiery Prince," Urizen's agent, "burning in his nightly tent," who is its mistaken "Guardian" (3:1, 5) and "Angel."[57] The question is how can Urizen be forgiven and redeemed if he lacks the capacity for regeneration from within? That Orc's claim of identity leads to a breakdown of identity furthers the reader's process of self-annihilation, a process intensified by the fact that although perversion foists commands onto Urizen, Orc is not free of commands either. Blake thus renders the Orc cycle itself as a perversion simply because the son's activities are merely reactions rather than essential displays of fiery joys unconditioned by Urizen.

At the risk of breaking the camel's back, I might add that Urizen/Orc embodies a perversion of reason on at least two levels. Urizen perverts reason into taxonomy, systematicity, and a body based on organs. And as the embodiment of the Romantic understanding of the Enlightenment, Urizen cannot accurately capture the Enlightenment, because he must offer an interpretation of the period that enables Romanticism (fiery joy) to differentiate itself from its predecessor (reason). Such an interpretation of Romanticism was under considerable pressure, given the fact that "revolution" then straddled an Enlightenment sense of turning back to an origin and the sense we now have of revolution as a turning away (M. Brown 46). Blakean perversion thus acquires an additional epistemological certainty at the moment when one must define the kind of turning that revolution demands, a definition whose stakes are raised when the Romantic must differentiate himself or herself from an Enlightenment past.

Where Orc stamps "the stony law . . . to dust," are we likewise to smash the past into bits, or are we to gather up the past toward revolution? By showing ultimately that fiery joy (Orc) was within (Urizen), however, Blake acknowledges that the Enlightenment sets into motion the revolution that is Romanticism and suggests that Romanticism is a regenerated form of Enlightenment. Reason thus has the capacity for liberation, just as fiery joy has the capacity for repression.

Blake's decision to print the bulk of *America* in recto/verso format literally makes Orc the obverse of Urizen and further underscores their connectedness. Through perversion, manifest in Orc's charge of Urizen and in turning the page, Blake reminds us of these dual capacities. In Blake's plate 9, Albion's angel accuses Orc of being the Antichrist, while the on the obverse (plate 10), Orc accuses Urizen of perverting fiery joys.[58] Critics have been at a virtually complete loss to explain Blake's illustrations. Not only do Orc's and Urizen's mutual accusations make one not unlike the other, but if the cuddly image of the children lying down with the sheep (plate 9) is Blake's ways of refuting the angel's accusation, this Edenic image stands for Orc even by way of negation. Blake demands that we pay attention to who delivers each perspective. Meanwhile, Blake illustrates Orc's charge with a Urizen-like figure, whose outstretched arms prefigure his arisen status, his Christ-like crucifixion and resurrection (his body is in the shape of a cross). Urizen too will be arisen; such a prophetic hint implies that plate 9 foretells the regeneration of Orc from destroyer to forgiver. Within plate 10, Orc's speech appears below an image of Urizen, juxtaposing these contrary figures. As we turn plate 9 into plate 10, the pastoral image (refuting the angel's description of Orc) gives way to Urizen (the master of the angel appears while Orc speaks). When we factor in that Orc's accusation of Urizen leads to Orc's recognition that the perversion of fiery joys has perverted him into the Ten Commandments, we have a sense of what Blake may be up to. Urizen is the generated self that must be regenerated into Orc. Given that Urizen also represents Blake's Old Testament God, the son, Orc, who is surrounded by Christ imagery (Tannenbaum 141–42), will rise from the dead to replace Urizen's sexuality under moral law/reason with Christ's holy lust.

At the same time, since Urizen has Orc within himself, generation can partake of regeneration as God generates the son. Urizen's Christ-like arms hint at the regeneration to come even as the generated body must be actively crucified/annihilated in order for regeneration to take place. To the extent that plate 9 represents the regeneration of Orc, his demonic anger has been transformed

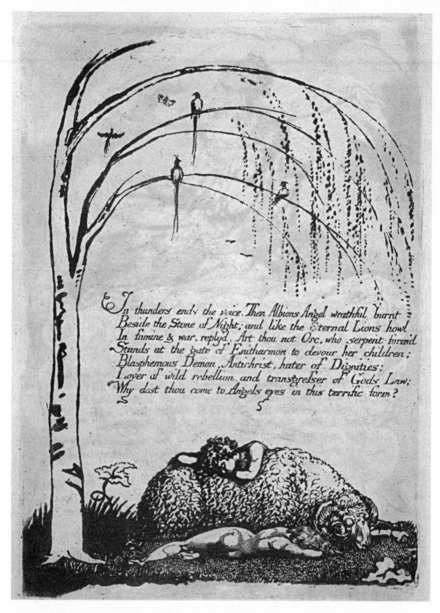

William Blake, *America*, plate 9 (Rosenwald 1804). Courtesy of the Lessing Rosenwald Collection, the Library of Congress, Washington, D.C.

into peace and love once he has gotten rid of sex under moral law. Furthermore, the poet's acknowledgement that, while the charge of perversion promises to foist perversion onto the other, the accusation itself must on some level bespeak identity, and we come to the conclusion that Urizen and Orc are but names for the dual capacities within each of us—what Blake elsewhere calls "the self-enjoyings of self-denial" (E 50)—that we must break through to get to true liberty. Blake equates Christ with liberty in *Jerusalem*. Urizen represents the law over the spirit and thus generates through the Immaculate Conception, while Orc represents the spirit over the law. Hence, Blake makes one the obverse of the other, and the act of turning the page is potentially our regeneration of generation, our choice of spirit rather than law. But he reminds us simultaneously that each has the capacity for law and holy spirit.

What, we should ask, is the consequence of all of this perversion? On one level, words have bodily consequences in Blake insofar as Blake can get us to rethink the role and value of sexual pleasure. If sexual pleasure and orgasm lead to both division and regeneration, they cannot be intrinsically liberating. On another level, Blake's sensuous embodiment of perversion enacts a turning within the reader, a violent shifting vortex of concepts and their relation to value that is both articulated and performed. Nelson Hilton has argued that Blake's vortex "signals either a passage into transcendence or, in its vaginal form, a return to generation" (165–66). I would adjust Hilton to say that the vortex signals both a regeneration that looks like a transcendence of the body and a return to generation that does not preclude a later return to regeneration. If Orc is within Urizen, their external struggle allegorizes a battle within the human psyche and that they are part of the dual capacities of mankind for generation and regeneration. Similarly, the capacity for liberty and the capacity for repression are simultaneously within. Blake's insistence upon consequences mandates that perverse sexuality be neither intrinsically liberating nor necessarily meaningfully pleasurable.

Blake was not merely being idealistic when he imagined the transformation of the generated body to the regenerated one. He was taking part in a cultural understanding of the body that saw the body, even the sexed body, as open to change. Eve Kosofsky Sedgwick asks social constructionists what makes them think culture can be more easily changed than biology (1990 41). Biology in the Romantic period insisted upon the interrelations of nature and culture, and this meant that since Blake did not need textualism and free speech to liberate bodies from materiality, the body could ground change. Of course, because sexual liberation too was not yet liberty, the body could not guarantee liberty either, but a medical understanding of the body along with a recognition of the poet's perversity could certainly rewrite the narrative of Blakean liberation: instead of bodies becoming speech or speech incarnating into bodies, the false naive incarnation of the judgmental Old Testament (Urizen), where language is law, could become the true yet perverse incarnation into a merciful yet sinning Christ (Orc), where language is forgiveness. Whether through Erasmus Darwin's botany, physiognomical propensities, healing acid, fluid blood, or medical electricity, Blake's bodies could continually regenerate themselves until they attained liberty. Blake did not need Judith Butler to remind him that bodies matter. But Blake can remind us that bodies are flexible, and that bodies, not performance, are the grounds for change. To the extent that perversion in Blake would allow him to harness the liberating capacities of text and of bodies, not to mention the text's multiple bodies, the many twists and turns of perversion could help the reader reclaim and incarnate the divine imagination within the body.

# CHAPTER SIX

# Byron, Epic Puberty, and Polymorphous Perversity

Puberty is hardly a poetic subject, much less an epic one. Nor does it seem particularly Romantic. Christopher Ricks has shown us why: it embarrasses.[1] Against the maturity required of the epic, puberty seems hopelessly jejune. Yet I shall argue that puberty is not only Lord Byron's epic subject in *Don Juan*, but also its truest one. As a volatile moment of bodily transition, puberty threatened categories of sexual and gendered identity. This threat was exacerbated by the fact that puberty was at once a natural and a perverse shift. On the one hand, puberty was a universal "natural" rite of passage. On the other hand, puberty hinted at the perversity of the body, its resistance to neat sexual and gendered categories. By foregrounding puberty, Byron hopes to liberate human beings from the normalizing force of these categories. Puberty allows Byron to question the value of maturity and conventional masculinity; more important, by stretching puberty over seventeen cantos and by making it epic, he insists that, although male/male love has its origins in puberty, it cannot be reduced to adolescent behavior.[2]

Simply put, biological difference was an insecure ground and thus could neither form the reliable basis of gender nor sex. As a moment of biological potentiality in all bodies, puberty allows the youthful body to be read as full of perverse potentiality. The body thus becomes a paradoxical ground of latency. Moreover, because puberty frustrated the sexual categories then available—heterosexual, homosexual, molly, effeminate, male, or sodomite—none of these could accurately capture one's sexual desires and identities. Even worse, insofar as the norm is itself mobile, neither normality nor perversity could confer stability. Puberty enables Byron not only to make the epic epicene—partake of the characteristics of both sexes (*OED*)—but also he connects sexual perversity with aesthetic purposiveness. That is, he embodies the contingency of bodily sex in an epic form whose contingent rhymes eschew purpose in favor of purposiveness in much the same way that the narrator of *Don Juan* eschews reproduction in favor of the mobility of desire. Put another way, rhyme enables the poet to redefine liberation in terms of choosing and shaping the causes one allows oneself to be determined by. Puberty then allows Byron to intervene in compulsory heterosexuality even as it undermines sexual complementarity from within.

Because male puberty presented two very different norms of masculinity—an effeminate norm appropriate for a boy and indeed ontologically prior to a second manly norm—it was the moment in which normality was indelibly tainted by the perverse. The famous eye surgeon William Lawrence captures this belated sense of difference when he remarks that, "in the first years of life, the individuals of two sexes do not differ from each other at the first view; they have nearly the same general air, the same delicacy of organization" ("Generation"). In sum, they are both "innocence joined by weakness." In puberty, however, "his limbs lose the softness and the gentle from which he partook with the female" (ibid.). Because they were published in Rees's *Cyclopedia*, Lawrence's remarks achieved wide diffusion. To the extent that effeminacy is the norm prior to manliness, masculine strength can appear to be abnormal. Consequently, any law of gender could seem arbitrary.

Because puberty was thought to be the moment when one feminized sex became two, the manly man cannot escape from his effeminate shadow in this period. The fact that Lawrence is less interested in changes in the female body during puberty (Buffon insisted that women matured much more quickly than men and put great emphasis upon menstruation) indicates the legacy of the one-sex model in England, which tempered differences between the sexes under an essential similitude. Peel back the layers of complementarity and find homology, if not one sex. John Hunter's conviction that the sexual character was annulled in old age further supported this essential similitude. And if male-male love was the open secret of sensibility, the sensitive man was doubly cursed. Thus, for example, throughout *Don Juan* Byron understands gender in terms of a "she-condition," denominating the whole circumstances under which femininity exists (*OED*), rather than in terms of any clear universal essence.

In part a nostalgic look backward to his own adolescence, a time of sexual play unencumbered by the demands of marriage, *Don Juan* allows Byron to turn back the clock, away from the burdens of his own mature strength—including a sexual narrative that must culminate in marriage—and away from a moment in history in which sex was being embodied in two newly incommensurate sexes.[3] Verging on the carnivalesque and the masquerade, *Don Juan* amounts to much more than return to libertinism because Byron is after the recently acquired power of biology to ground sexual difference. For Byron, biology could not ground difference if it itself was vitally dynamic. Moreover, even though Byron could be hopelessly conventional in his gender attitudes, his Brunonian understanding of the body enabled him to challenge biological complementarity, the idea that male strength prepared men for public life while women's delicate nerves better suited them for the domestic sphere. Based on John Brown's theory that excitability was the key to bodily health or disease, Brunonianism had the potential to equalize the genders because excitability had no dependence upon structures of the body (neither penis nor clitoris) and because both muscles and nerves had vital power equally distributed (C. Lawrence 9–11). Tellingly, Brown treats delayed, suppressed, or impaired menstruation in women not specifically in terms of the female body but rather of a generalized debility (*Elements* 2:184–85).[4] Like men who suffer from "indirect debility" when they have too many evacuations, women suffer the same debility when their evacuations are irregular in quantity or in duration.[5] That Brown suggested the consequences of vice were physical and medical and not theological further made his ideas attractive to Byron.

Byron was schooled in the principles of Brunonian medicine by his physician, George Pearson, and by Sir John Sinclair's *The Code of Health and Longevity*, of which Byron owned no fewer than two copies.[6] The fact that Brown insisted that life was dependent upon external causes, a main concern in *Don Juan*, undermined any biological essentialism. As the material equivalent of improvisation and digression (digression also means deviation), moreover, puberty is the moment when bodily semiotics strive to catch up with cultural gender. This gap between the two semiotic systems enables Byron to question the role and value of gender and of sex, along with its political investments. Insofar as Brunonian medicine understood the body in terms of an economy of excitability where excessive stimulation could lead to debility, it further suggested that any strength gained by men during puberty could be easily lost. Because masculinity was always under threat, Byron can be both more sympathetic to the plight of women, and alive to the costs of reducing male/male love to immature sex.

In calling attention to the role of puberty in *Don Juan*, I aim to complicate our understanding of the poet's gender attitudes[7] and to revise our understanding of Byron's perversity. Puberty means that the body does not become fully sexed until age thirteen or fourteen or even later, and puberty thus throws a monkey wrench into any one-to-one correspondence between sex and gender. Genitals cannot fully signify sex if masculinity is understood, as it was in the Romantic period, in terms of strength. Whereas Jerome Christensen links Byron's perversion most closely to his oriental tales—arguing, for instance, that Byron did not engage in homosexual acts before visiting Turkey when the geography permitted it and declared it to be normal—the fact that effeminacy is a normal stage of development that all boys undergo means that it will not so easily be written off as perversion. And whereas Christensen argues that Byronic homosexuality cannot be liberation because any such liberation must be regional, and therefore only valid for a particular kind of sexuality, and because such liberation does not represent a "final break with a prior repression" (55), I argue that puberty makes such liberation a process open to all men and that even women are not necessarily excluded if femininity or softness can be redefined and revalued. What's more, because "liberate" means to free from something, the fact that liberation is never complete—it cannot represent a final break with repression—means that Christensen, following Foucault, is setting an impossible standard for liberation. In the process, he underestimates the good that can come from taking care of obstacles to liberation one by one.[8] Those obstacles include regulatory categories like sodomite, effeminate, heterosexual marriage, and male, and Byron's point is that personal bodily experience so often resists or exceeds political co-optation and regulation. Furthermore, as Moyra Haslett reminds us, "the poet's attempt to excuse its libertine hero was therefore in itself a political act because it contradicted the increasing hegemony of moral and political conservatism" (166) as well as the sanctity of property (185). Finally, the fact that Byron at times identified with "softness" instead of with strength underscores the limits of seeing masculinity in terms of "consequential action" (Christensen xviii) and suggests a fundamental ambivalence to class privilege.[9] By indicating that Juan's softness is the reason why he is an erotic object for men and women alike, Byron calls attention to the differing forms masculinity and desire may take.

Thomas Laqueur, Ludmilla Jordanova, and Londa Schiebinger have argued that around 1800 a one-sex Galenic model whereby the female was an inferior and inverted version of the male sex gives way to a two-sex model whereby the sexes are incommensurate. In the one-sex model, a penis is not what Robert Stoller has called the "absolute signature of maleness" because women have penises too—just on the inside—and genitals cannot ground gender. For Laqueur, the notion of a passionless woman becomes evidence for this newly incommensurate way of thinking about the sexes since the notion of a passionless male was presumably an oxymoron.

For Jordanova, the evidence lies within nascent connections between musculature and masculinity and nervousness and femininity. And for Schiebinger, the male body—in particular, the male skull—remained the paradigm of human anatomy throughout the eighteenth century, thus illustrating the profound legacy of the one-sex model. This model would only be ruptured by the French Revolution and its emphasis upon egalitarianism (*Nature's Body* 156–59). As democracy and equality put pressure on difference, sexual differences are reconfigured so that they underwrite hierarchy that does not look like hierarchy. In the name of separate spheres, difference is allegedly equalized and each sex is given its separate but equal and proper domain. Within medical treatments of puberty in the Romantic period, one can discern the collision of these models, and Byron's focus on puberty—the moment when one sex becomes two—enables him to put pressure on cultural understandings of masculine strength. He can thereby also take issue with notions of female passionlessness as well as the alleged equalizing gesture of the separation of spheres. Puberty enables sexual difference itself to come into crisis. Is there one sex or two? Is the foundation of difference gender or sex? Is sexual desire based on a desire for difference or similarity? What happens when a feminized male desires another feminized male?

If complementarity was an improvement over the one-sex model by which femininity simply meant inferiority to a male, it was undercut by the value that Romantic culture placed on feeling, and even the man of feeling. Claudia Johnson has shown how men declared feeling and sentiment to be their legitimate province in the Romantic period, and this meant that women's feelings had to be shown to be inferior to men's and pathological. One way to accomplish this goal was to make women's bodies hostage to their nerves and reproductive organs in ways that men's weren't. Likewise, Lisa Cody has argued that fathers in the eighteenth century were expected to be more compassionate (303) and that men-midwives helped to straddle the demands of science and of sympathy. The fact remains, however, that feeling was ambiguously gendered. Biological complementarity was under further threat by the medical understanding of genius. Because sensibility was both a delicate sensitivity and brilliance, effeminate men were considered to be creative geniuses who treaded gingerly the line between masculinity and femininity. As John Sinclair put it, the "man of brilliant talent" was cursed with a "delicate frame" (1:79). Andrew Elfenbein has argued that genius was homosexualized in the period, and the price of such brilliance was pathology. Finally, since the one-sex model relied upon the homology of the penis and vagina or penis and clitoris, locating sex in the structures of the genitals, theories of vitality that downplayed the role and influence of localization and anatomical structures undermined the idea that sex could be localized in different—male and female—genitals. In short, vitality threatened to undermine the metonymies by which body part subsumes erotic identity.[10]

At first blush, puberty offers a rather meager nail on which to hang one's hat in *Don Juan.* Indeed, Byron uses "puberty" only once, contrasting it with philosophy: "If you think 'twas philosophy that this did,/I can't help thinking puberty assisted" (1:93). "This" refers to Juan's thinking of Donna Julia's eyes. Yet such a witty couplet sets up a pervasive concern: the role and the needs of the body over that of the mind, social categories, or even language. Byron put it this way in his "Detached Thoughts," "Man is born passionate of body—but with an innate though secret tendency to the love of Good in his Main-spring of Mind—But God help us all!—It is at present a sad jar of atoms" (*Byron's Letters and Journals* [*BLJ*] 9:46). Whereas the stanzas preceding the one that plays with puberty and philosophy deliberately inflate our expectations to metaphysical heights—Coleridge's "condition," we are told, is that he has become a "metaphysician" (1:91)—Byron turns to puberty to suggest the biological bases of any metaphysical speculation. The gulf between reader (what you think) and the poet (I) can only be closed by admitting not only that puberty and philosophy have a common ground beyond consonance, but also that the energies of a sensate and desiring body are perhaps more real and more philosophically consistent than metaphysical speculation. Puberty's role, moreover, does not have to wait for the poet to realize that he must think about it.

In his distrust of metaphysics, Byron would have agreed with Humphrey Davy's argument that "man, in what is called a state of nature, is a creature of almost pure sensation" (15). As Byron shows in his famous shipwreck episode, beneath his or her civilized veneer, humankind is very much a creature of sensation. Davy continues, "Called into activity only by positive wants, his life is passed either in satisfying the cravings of the common appetites, or in apathy, or in slumber. Living only in moments, he calculates but little on futurity. He has no vivid feelings of hope, or thoughts of permanent and powerful action. And, unable to discover causes, he is either harassed by superstitious dreams, or quietly and passively submitted to the mercy of nature and the elements" (15–16). In his "Detached Thoughts," the poet recalled having hung around Davy, and Byron met up with "the man of chemistry" in Ravenna (7:78). If unbridled sensation might liberate mankind from the dictates of civilization, it might substitute one form of tyranny—civilization—for another, nature.

The role of puberty in *Don Juan* looks even more substantial once we consider that Byron insists throughout much of his epic upon crossing genders and upon Juan's boyishness or even girlishness. He is described as having been a "pretty child" (1:69). Although he is sixteen at the start of Byron's epic, and despite the fact the narrator supposes him to be "then grown up to man's estate" (1:85), Juan is manhood manqué. "Every body but his mother deem'd/Him almost a man" (1:54). Antonia, Donna Julia's maid, wonders if Juan's "half-girlish face" could possibly be worth all the trouble (1:171). Insofar as Juan straddles boyishness and girlishness, he is in the midst of puberty, when manly strength fully transforms one effeminate sex into two.

After the shipwreck, Juan "buoy'd his boyish limbs" (2:106). The pun between buoy and boy reminds us that boyhood is a state of suspension between two sexes. Like women, boys are economically dependent upon men (T. King 67). Puberty therefore also reminds us of how Byron's serial narrative suspends telos. The narrator insists both Juan and Haidee "were children still" (4:15). One canto later, we are reminded again that "Juan was juvenile" (5:8). One might add like Juvenal: though he condemns effeminate men who engage in same sex acts, in Satire 2, Juvenal praises Peribomius, because he is subject to the "workings of fate" and whose "obsession secures indulgence."[11] The chain of signifiers—Juan, juvenile, Juvenal—yokes together Juan, youthfulness, and perversity, and implies that youth is a natural breeding ground for perversity. Especially so, in light of the role of the classics in upper-class British education. The sultan refers to Juan as "this boyish, new, Seraglio guest" (6:115). Juan is at once "blushing and beardless" (9:47); while both adjectives make him effeminate, in "beardless," the sign of masculinity is at least present by its absence. Juan is described as being "in the bloom . . . but not yet in the blush" (10:5), adjectives that again remind us of puberty. Even as late as canto XVI, Byron catalogs the things which "kindle manhood" (16: 108); moreover, in the very last canto, Byron alerts us to Juan's "virgin face" (17: 13).

In his own life, Byron found puberty particularly traumatic. He writes, "It was one of the deadliest and heaviest feelings of my life to feel that I was no longer a boy,—From that moment I began to grow old in my own esteem—and in my esteem age is not estimable" (*BLJ* 9:37). Byron once again explicitly refers to puberty in his epic when he states,

> Juan, I said, was a most beauteous Boy,
> And had retained his boyish look beyond
> The usual hirsuite seasons which destroy,
> With beards and whiskers and the like, the fond
> Parisian aspect which upset old Troy
> And founded Doctor's Commons:—(9:53).

On the one hand, Juan is a boy. On the other hand, the poet informs us that he has passed the "usual hirsuite seasons which destroy" boyhood; yet, he retained his "boyish look." Byron's enjambment here extends Juan's boyishness into the next line, even as he suggests Homeric epic to have likewise been engendered by Paris's puberty. The question is, is he ontologically a boy, or does he just look like a boy still? To make matters worse, since boyishness at times is equivalent to effeminacy, is Juan more like a girl? When Juan cross-dresses as Juanna, no one doubts her sex: "no one doubted on the whole, that she / Was what her dress bespoke" (6:36).[12] My point is that as a dynamic and variable biological process, puberty raises problems for gender insofar as it takes longer in some than others, it does not have the exact same signs in everyone, and the process can at times remain incomplete. Byron's narrator no sooner reminds us that Juan and Haidee are "children still" (4:15), than he insists upon their "mix'd all feelings, friend, child, lover, brother" (4:26). Despite our need to demarcate clearly defined categories of identity, Byron reminds us that feelings and bodies defy such categories. By calling attention to the anomalies within puberty and Juan as an anomaly, he insists upon a gap between sex and gender. His allusion to "Doctor's Commons"—the legal court devoted to separation and divorce—further implies that even the marital norm has its problems. As Jonathan Gross puts it, "the whole poem is written against 'straight' life: against stifling marriages like Julia's; polygamous one's like Gulbeyaz's; and sexless, and more importantly, soulless, one's like Adeline's" (144).

Susan Wolfson has shown the surprising ways in which gender is transgressed in *Don Juan*, and she suggests that Juan's intersexual character allows the poet space for "homoerotic material in disguise" (1987 592), not to mention active questioning of the "she condition" (597). Wolfson insists that Byronic gender transgression is associated with "anomalies of nature" and "monstrosities" (595). Rather, I think, in highlighting a moment of biological transition, Byron is much more radical in his gender attitudes than he has been given credit for, because he exploits the dynamism of puberty to undermine any stable or unitary notion of monstrosity or anomaly. Given contemporary debates about how monsters do not refute God-like design even in their imperfection—they, quite to the contrary, often show the designed developments of the species (see chapter 2)—monsters themselves in the end could prove normality rather than undermine it. Whereas Wolfson insists that "Byron senses the fatal consequences when the law of gender is violated: the annihilation of self in both its social identity and psychological integrity" (601), I argue Wolfson puts too bleak a spin on the loss of identity. Because the breaking of the law of gender is the source of so much of the poem's comedy, and since Byron knew too well that a sodomitical identity could be imprisoning if not deadly, I emphasize the ludic possibilities in the loss of identity and the gains of what Byron terms "mobility."[13] In satirizing cultural notions of gender, then, and in showing how the body resists the stability of gender, Byron insists that any law of gender will ultimately be incommensurate with the body, be it monstrous or normal. Puberty is such fertile ground for Byron because it pushes the line between monstrosity and normalcy, not to mention between male and female, in the direction of undecidability. The normalizing categories that society uses to arrest sex and gender always have the potential to be frustrated.

The Compte du Buffon understood that in order for the organs of generation to mature, the process of growth had to be over, and he conceded that many men continued to grow until 23 years of age. "The growth of the body must be nearly complete before a superfluous quantity of organic juices can be accumulated in the parts still undergoing puberty destined for generation" (2:411), Buffon wrote. Byron owned Smellie's 18-volume translation of Buffon (Munby 1:211), and Buffon's remarks on puberty were rehearsed in Sinclair (1:48). Buffon also argued that growth lasted in a man until 22–23 years of age (2:436), and that men did not acquire their "most perfect symmetry until age 30" (2:436), and this meant that puberty in man lasted as long as twenty years. Juan therefore is potentially undergoing puberty from start to finish of *Don Juan*. John

Brown likewise insisted that puberty was "a time of great change over the whole system. Now the desire for coition, a stimulus, never experienced before, produces a commotion over the whole body; and in preference to other parts, in the genitals of both sexes" (2:186). The poet credits the Persians with having the right attitude toward this commotion because they teach boys only "to draw the bow, to ride, and speak the truth" (16:1) as they grow from age five to age twenty.

Buffon also argued that the "marks of puberty" are "not always uniform," highlighting variability in an already dynamic process. The beard, for example, does not always appear precisely at the age of puberty: there are "whole nations who have hardly any beard" (2:411). Juan's beardlessness thus is normal in some contexts and abnormal in others. To make matters even worse, "beards" were sometimes used in the erotica of this period to refer to female pubic hair (Harvey 97), and thus were hardly unambiguous signs of masculinity. Although perversion assumes a single standard of normalcy, Byron points out that perversion is contextually dependent and therefore far from a universal standard. In his *Observations on Madness and Melancholy*, which Byron owned (Munby 1:240), John Haslam warned that during the "interval between puberty and manhood, I have painfully witnessed this hopeless and degrading change, when in a short time has transformed the most promising and vigorous intellect into a slavering and bloated idiot" (66–67). Clearly puberty was a time of volatile biological change, changes which threatened the very idea of a norm.

This variability of puberty helps explain why the poet links genitals with both presence and absence insofar as a penis requires the testicles to begin their work in order to transform boys into men. Buffon makes it clear that the onset of women's menstruation too is highly variable and contingent upon the quality of diet (2:411). Indeed, women who do not get enough iron in their diet have delayed puberty. To wit, not only does Byron align Lord Henry's erect "perpendicular" with a lack—"something wanting on the whole" (14:71), but also such a mathematical term inevitably recalls his mathematical genius of a wife, his "princess of parallelograms." A penis, cannot guarantee manhood because in a one-sex model, women have them too. Moreover, men are always in danger of losing them either through castration or through the loss of manly strength consequent to excessive emission. Byron reminds us of this potential loss when he feminizes even this paragon of male handsomeness, and notes that his perpendicular remains "preserved" despite "each circumstance of love and war" (14:71). Presence is presented as being only momentarily present: absence is always in the offing. The culture's obsession with male impotence, not to mention venereal disease, underscores further the potential loss of virility.[14] Byron's play on even the male genitalia as being both presence and absence is heightened by the fact that only recently did women and men acquire genitals of their own: instead of having genitals within their bodies as opposed to without as Galen thought, women's vaginas were no longer considered to be internal penises, women's uteruses no longer thought to be scrotums, and women's ovaries were no longer considered testicles or stones (Laqueur 1990 78–93). Furthermore, external signs of sexual difference—namely beards—have no necessary connection to genitals since genitals do not necessarily presage absolute difference. Recall once more Juan's pointed beardlessness. "Perpendicular" reminds us as well that the penis can only symbolize virility when it is erect. In much the same way that a perpendicular line needs other lines in order to prove its perpendicularity, Byron suggests that the penis cannot be a self-sufficient sign of masculinity. The gap between the penis and the development of manly strength furthermore undercut the significance of the genitals as the marker of sex. Finally, if geometry leads us back to Byron's "Princess of Parallelograms," what is the difference between a parallelogram and a perpendicular? Both terms share consonance, the same number of syllables, and a similar geometrical origin.

Nor can the vagina function as the sign of absolute difference. Byron acknowledges this most clearly when he euphemistically refers to the vagina as an "affair of women" in canto 6, stanza 2 (Haslett 153). While one must concede that the poet does align women's affairs with "strange whirls and eddies," making the vagina a place of mystery that surpasses the reveries of Jacob Behmen, and while he does suggest a dichotomy between what men do with their heads and what women do with their hearts, any absolute difference is undercut by the fact that Byron uses "affair" in the first stanza of this canto to refer to male orgasm. "There is a tide in the affairs of men" too. "Few have guess'd/The moment, till too late to come again" (6:1), Byron chortles. While Byron's enjambment defers the moment, his medial caesura, coming in the middle of the second foot, enacts the onset of orgasm whose timing cannot be known in advance. Although aligning the vagina with mystery runs the danger of fueling misogyny, Byron emphasizes as well the unknowability of men's affairs.[15] Byron may be alluding to the fact that the vagina and women's reproductive system were very much terra incognita since the human female ovarium was not discovered until 1827. Not only do few guess the moment of no return, but also Byron concludes the stanza devoted to men with "Of which the surest sign is in the end:/When things are at the worst they sometimes mend" (6:1). Although "surest sign" suggests some certainty, that certainty is undermined by "sometimes" as well as by the circumlocution "of which" which has no clear referent. My point here is that Byron uses the same term "affair" to refer to men's and women's genitalia, and this hearkens back to a one-sex model in which the vagina is an internal penis. "Tide" also insists upon fluidity of both organs. As a metonymy for the public sphere, "affair" for both sexes is reduced to sexual affairs, and both sexes are thereby stuck in the private and domestic realm. The dichotomy between women's hearts and men's heads is further undermined by the fact that Byron ends the stanza with "heaven knows what!" (6:2). Furthermore, the line, "But women with their hearts or heaven knows what!," lacks a verb, leaving any dichotomy hanging in mid air. The "or" enhances this dangling, as does the fact that "know," while ostensibly a verb, here functions as an adjectival modifier to heaven.

Of course, "affair" refers back to Shakespeare's *Julius Caesar*, when Brutus proclaims "there is a tide in the affairs of men/Which taken at the flood leads on to fortune" (4:3). Though Brutus thinks that now is the time to act, he is on the cusp of his downfall. The point of the allusion is to further undermine any epistemological certainty when human sexuality is at issue. In this light, Byron's comment that the "able seamen" who navigate the affairs of women have charts which "lay down its currents to a hair" (6:2), pokes fun at the very idea of anatomical localization since all the precision of the charts leads to no knowledge whatsoever. No matter how carefully anatomists map out the contours of the female body, their enthusiasm for cartography outweighs any knowledge gained. How does one chart tides anyway? "Men's reflection" (6:2), therefore, is essentially impotent. Byron suggests that even the trope of metaphor itself is powerless; not even the "strange whirls" of Behmen "can compare" (6:2). His invocation of the imprecise pronoun "it" in both stanzas—"most of us have found it" in the former, and "lay down its currents to a hair" in the latter—takes away from anatomy's power to locate sex in the body.

To add to all this uncertainty, Byron's preface about the suicide of Castlereagh suggests yet another referent for "affair." Like Brutus, Castlereagh kills himself. Unlike Brutus, Castlereagh kills himself because he fears he will be exposed as a sodomite. Byron's wry comment—"he was an amiable man in *private* life, may or may not be true" (Steffan and Pratt edition [S&P] 3:2),—hints at Castlereagh's sodomy.[16] The line, "of which the surest sign is in the end:" (6:1), thus takes on the specificity of sodomy, and to the extent that this is true, the typographic colon after "end" represents an anatomical colon. One's anatomical part predicts neither the sex of one's object of desire, nor the means by which one satisfies those desires. "In the" reminds us that this end is to be penetrated. As Byron puts it in Canto 1:

Man's a strange animal, and makes strange use
Of his own nature, and the various arts,
And likes particularly to produce
Some new experiment to show his parts; (1:128)

Byron heightens the strangeness of mankind, thereby normalizing perversion, and suspends the uses to which parts/genitals are put through his medial cae-suras. Indeed, *coitus* has been so interrupted that reproduction is no longer a clear use. He suggests that sexual experimentation is a particularly human predilection. That Byron links Castlereagh to the Bishop of Clogher, another sodomite, further clues us in to Byron's innuendo (Crompton 1985 310). In his rejected stanza 76, canto 11, Byron had rhymed the line, "Some, for having turned converted Cullies," with "while Clogher's Bishop sullies/The Law." Be-cause "Cullies" contains the French word for arse, cull, Byron links the passive recipient of sodomy with the sullying power of shit.

Jonathan Gross has shown how Byron equates beginnings and endings with sexual acts. Thus when Byron instructs his readers to "Commence not with the end—or, sinning/In this sort, end at least with the beginning" (5:13), the poet suggests his anatomical book is male but not to be penetrated (Gross 138). However, the fact that Byron's prohibition deals with beginnings—anal inter-course cannot be a beginning—suggests that sodomy might properly be the cul-mination of sex. Byron's placement of "turned" and "converted" near the turn of the verse not only implies that such a perverse turn is as easily achieved as the turn of the verse, but it also hints that such conversions might be easy. Just as the reader is now confused about beginnings and endings—which end are we looking at?—sexual positioning too can be ambiguous since it is dependent upon one's vantage point. Finally, insofar as seriality in *Don Juan* frustrates be-ginnings and endings, not to mention conventional epic purpose, sodomy as anal intercourse is the logical sexual correlative to aesthetic purposiveness. By making this end teleological, Byron thus frustrates the end of reproduction.

The poet's explicit and repeated pun on "adulteration," moreover, highlights puberty as the natural process of coming into adulthood even as it makes this natural process one of degeneration rather than growth or maturity. John Brown likewise considered life a process of degeneration since we are born with a certain amount of excitability and eventually lose it. Byron initially confines puberty to the ages between thirteen and sixteen (1:69), and he frames this change neutrally in terms of an "alteration" (1:69). Later, however, Byron pokes fun at Lady Adeline by comparing her to a bottle of decanted wine: "both upon occasion,/ Till old, may undergo adulteration" (15:6). If Buffon declared marriage to be the next step after puberty, Byron suggests that puberty and marriage are not mutually exclusive. In the same way that the adulteration of wine is an unpredictable process, so too is puberty. Byron too hints that the scythe of time has gone rusty, and now may go slower and to shave us more smoothly (14:53). "Shave" suggests that Juan's beardlessness may be less natural than it is willful. Linking adultery, sexual experience, and the coming into adulthood—can one be an adult without adultery?—Byron undermines as well societal emphasis upon a woman's honor as being solely localized in her private parts. Here, the poet may be recalling Buffon's remark that it was jealousy alone which "bestowed a physical existence upon female virginity" (2:414). The metaphor of adulteration implies that like a bottle of wine that will inevitably and eventually go bad, even honorable women are destined for adulteration. Describing the flirtation of a "cold coquette" in terms of "not quite adultery, but adulteration" (12:63), Byron once again naturalizes adultery as a process of social and sexual maturation. Perhaps one reason that adulthood is like the corruption of adulteration is that desiring bodies then further rigidify into cultural identities. In terms of the male sex, "adulteration" suggests masculine strength to be a spurious admixture to a pure but effeminate male body. Not only does this strength make Lord Henry less attractive rather than more, but also it defines that strength—usually considered as a presence into an absence of effeminacy. "Something was wanting" (14:71). The consequences of this point are that masculinity as strength can be understood as a perversion of an original male effeminate norm, and that the effeminate can become a legitimate object of sexual desire. Indeed, the narrator makes Don Juan the subject of his erotic gaze (Gross 137).[17]

Just as adulteration intertwines the normal with the abnormal, and just as puberty reminds us that normal biological growth is bound up with deviation, Byron suggests that sexual perversion is an error that has as much moral weight as a typesetting error. Perversion thus is to be expected. Describing Queen Semiramis, Byron muses,

> That injured Queen, by Chroniclers so coarse,
> Has been accused (I doubt not by conspiracy)

Of an improper friendship for her horse
(Love, like religion, sometimes runs to heresy);
This monstrous tale had probably its source
(For such exaggerations here and there I see)
In printing "Courser" by mistake for "Courier":
I wish the case could come before a jury here. (5:61)

By comparing love to religious heresy, Byron makes sexual perversion the logical outcome of any freethinking individual. No sooner is the category created—proper friendship, let's say—than the category will be exceeded. Formally, Byron hints at his support for the improper by making lines two and four exceed their syllable count, by interweaving enjambment and end-stopped lines, by having the parenthetical aside threaten to overtake this stanza, and by stretching the final rhyme between "Courier" and "here." While it seems as if the parentheses and the colon will arrest any heresy, Byron suggests that this could not be further from the truth when he equates the sins of improper friendship with a graphical error or even a printing error. The early draft of this stanza had "printing" in the place of writing and noted "an erratum of her *horse* for Courier" (S&P 5:61). The poet's equation of a sexual sin with a printer's mistake, inevitable so long as books were typeset by hand and by printer's devils no less, gives perversions of print and sex the equivalent moral weight. In his review of *Ireland's Neglected Genius*, Byron mused that "the malicious fun of the printer's devil in permitting it [the error] to stand, for he certainly knew better" (Nicholson 19). Somewhere between inadvertent error and conscious choice, the Queen's rumored bestiality is as commonplace as an erratum, just as monstrosity originates in a typesetting mistake. Since genitals can predict neither sexual aim nor object, heteronormativity lacks both logic and inevitability.

Moyra Haslett has argued that Byron's coarseness and sexual innuendos are part of a larger strategy by which the poet makes fun of the gendering of contemporary reading. Byron found absurd the notion that women were to be chivalrously protected from carnal knowledge, and despite knowing the fact that he had attracted a wide female readership, the poet refused to bend to notions of delicacy (221–25). Because the Queen Caroline Affair made the sexual lives of the royals common knowledge, Byron sees little point in decorousness. Moreover, if women are as sexually passionate as Byron claims, then his work would teach them what they already knew. Indeed, the stanza above on printing mistakes alludes to Queen Caroline's trial for adultery. Byron thus wonders why the Queen is to be punished for her alleged sexual intrigues while the Prince Regent literally gets off scott free.

Byron undermines the ability of biology to ground sexual difference in a number of ways. He highlights the dynamism of biological change to show that biology is a precarious ground of difference. Because puberty cuts across gender lines, lines demarcating biological sex, and lines dividing natural and unnatural forms of sex, it is rife for comedy and political subversion. Thus, for example, Byron ponders which pronoun accurately captures Juanna, the cross-dressed Juan, and remarks,

> And next she gave her (I say her, because
> The Gender still was Epicene, at least
> In outward show, which is a saving clause)
> An outline of the Customs of the East,
> With all their chaste integrity of laws,
> By which the more a Harem is encreased,
> The stricter doubtless grow the vestal duties
> Of any supernumerary beauties. (6:58)

At a superficial level, Byron exploits the comedic potential of drag. More deeply, his choice of "epicene" derives from the Greek *epikoinos*, which means "upon the common," and thus seeks to understand gender not upon the ground of difference, but upon similitude.[18] The epicene nature of gender itself is enhanced by Byron's addition of "supernumerary" letters to Juan, the "na," as if gender itself is so easily changed. Juan is made equivalent to Juanna by Byron's use of "or" (6:57). Although he claims that gender here is only epicene in its outward show, by calling attention to this clause as a "saving clause," Byron takes away any readerly satisfaction in the outward show when he hints that an outward show (dress) may disguise an inward one (the body); show and disguise are thus hopelessly entangled with one another. The fact that Don Juan's boyish body lacks the hirsute outward form of manhood, coupled with the fittingness of his feminine disguise, shows that Juanna, and even Juan, exceed the binary demands of gender along with the heterosexual imperative. Juan's ambiguous gender extends to his body and not just to his clothing, frustrating the need for even cross-dressing to reinforce heterosexuality: cross-dressing was legitimate during this period so long as it furthered heterosexuality (Harvey 99). Insofar as Byron here describes a seraglio—a place where women do indeed occupy the position of Lacan's "phallus" since they "circulate in patriarchal societies as visible and acquirable symbols of masculine power" (Yiu 86)—epicene enacts itself by taking on unexpected forms of figural embodiment. Brunonian medicine would suggest as well that growth could be advanced or hindered by the balance or imbalance between the body's internal excitability and its external stimulation. By rendering the body as much of a garment as the dress, the poet suggests that gender may resist bodily superimposition.

In his original draft, Byron wrote that "The Gender[s] still [were] Epicene" (S&P 3:35), and this suggests that although "epicene" can be used to indicate effeminacy (*OED* 2nd ed.), Byron is after a collapsing of gender difference itself, one whose ontological equivalent is the body in puberty. The fact that "epicene gender" applies to Latin and Greek grammar, indicating nouns which, "without changing grammatical gender, may denote either sex" (*OED*), enables linguistic perversion (the phrase is nonsense in English) to take on sexual perversion. Such a collapse is furthered by the poet's playing with the chastity of a harem and the lewdness of the East: as comical as the notion of a harem devoted to vestal duties is, so too is the idea that Eastern harems are about profligate sexuality untainted by the leering gaze of the West. Byron's play on "supernumerary," a word that highlights Juanna's surplus status along with his supernumerary member, deflates a sign of virility into an excess supplement. That his final couplet has supernumerary syllables further renders gender into textual play: the feminine rhymes (duties/beauties) not only enhance Juan's cross-dressing, but also literally effeminize him.

Byron further undermines confidence in gender binaries by calling our attention to the addition of a third sex, the eunuch. He wonders if all the money the Pope makes in a year will allow him to find "three perfect pipes of the third sex" (4:86). That the perfection of the pipes must come at the expense of the mutilation of the male body allows Byron to ask if the gains are worth it. Nor does Byron miss an opportunity to foist perversion onto the Roman Catholic Church. Now one might ask on what grounds can a castrated male be another sex, especially if sex is taken to be an ontological given. Yet to call an eunuch a "third sex" is to situate sex somewhere between nature and culture.[19] In order to be able to map gender onto the body, a third gender that suggests effeminacy must be available, else the third sex will have no gender that corresponds with it. This is the reason why Randolph Trumbach labels the effeminate sodomite as the third gender in the eighteenth century. As heterosexuality became the mark of the true gentleman, the bisexuality that was accepted among men of rank since the Elizabethan period became redefined as effeminacy (Cash 35;

Trumbach chaps. 2 and 3). The problem is that although an effeminate male might be analogous to a eunuch, gender can only map itself onto sex if, in the case of men, castration acquires both literal and figurative ontology. In other words, for a third sex to correspond to a third gender, it must be possible for a man to castrate himself figuratively, and if this is so, figuration will always demand at least a slight gap between gender and sex, else the figure is no longer a figure. Perhaps this explains why the poet refers to the "confusion of sorts and sexes" (11:3). "Third sex" is also open to women to the extent that they have masculine traits. The Duchess of Fitz-Fulke's dressing up as a male monk implies that women too can exceed the binaries of gender.[20] Byron's use of "third sex" thus moves sexuality beyond complementarity and symmetry and toward contextualization (Garber 1995 12), and his emphasis upon context can be seen especially in his yoking of gender and condition as in "she-condition" (14:24). To the extent that there is a third sex, one that exceeds male and female, sex must take on other disciplinary forms beyond binaries.

When Byron lists the kinds of love, he reminds us that behind the "third sort" of love, "Marriage in Disguise," lies a third sex. Ostensibly "marriage in disguise" refers to a now outlawed clandestine marriage, usually a marriage between a man and woman of a different social class that would not have parental approval. In as much as "disguise" also metonymically names Juan's effeminacy, Byron exchanges one form of prohibition for another, homosexual love. "Disguise" is thus a metonymic closet for all forms of clandestine desire.[21] This allusion gains credence when we consider that the poet begins the stanza with the line, "the noblest kind of Love is Love Platonical" (9:76), and Byron recalls Plato's sense that sexual relations between males is the highest form of love since only men can represent intellectual beauty. Byron's careful qualification of the kinds of love to be "noted in our Chronicle" further implies that there are kinds of love he dare not catalogue, although his mention of "burning Sappho" hints at another form that he cannot enumerate. In his early draft of this lyric, Byron wrote the "Lesbian Sappho" (Isles of Greece 1) further making explicit the object of Sappho's passion, along with the possibility of the dispensability of men in matters sexual.[22] Men might be irrelevant when it comes to sexuality. Although the epic catalogue relies upon enumeration as knowledge, Byron suggests that this trope falsely assumes that cataloguing is a form of knowledge, since there are kinds of love which resist naming.

Because Byron sees a culture's gender attitudes as a crucial index of the legitimacy of governmental authority over the individual (Franklin 116), he is especially wary of how women are socialized into being women. He actively wonders if any woman would truly choose the "fetter" of domesticity over public life when he states, "but ask any woman if she'd choose/(Take her at thirty, that is) to have been/Female or male? A school boy or a Queen" (15:25).

Byron's sustained focus on effeminacy in *Don Juan* affords him space from which to undermine sex as a given fact about the human body. Unlike the Romans who associated effeminacy with political, social, and moral weakness (C. Edwards 65), Byron can be more ambivalent about it because effeminacy makes clear that neither masculinity nor femininity have exclusive purchase upon gender.[23] In suggesting that gender is not a binary opposition, Byron challenges the conventional understanding of gender. In much the same way that there are three sexes—men, women, and eunuchs—there are at least three genders—masculine, feminine, and some combination of the two, sometimes referred to as "she-men." Byron also confesses that Juan is "warm in heart as feminine in feature" (8:52). To be sure, Byron can be virulently homophobic, and his favorite strategy of delegitimation is to demasculinize his political targets. Bob Southey is a "dry bob" (Ded. 3), meaning that he partakes of coition without emission, and Lord Castlereagh is an "intellectual eunuch" (Ded. 11) because of his excessive despotism. "Eunuch" obliquely refers as well to the fact that Castlereagh thought he was about to be exposed as a sodomite, and thus committed suicide.[24] As Southey's employer, Castlereagh shares his subordinate's fate.

Gary Dyer has shown that although the references to sodomy "are read most easily as being unsympathetic," Byron's homophobia is directed toward the passive recipient of the act, not the act itself, and the poet allows readers to take the subject position of the active sodomite (573). Because the potential price of homophilia was death at the hands of an angry mob, one's declared homophobia could protect oneself, leading readers away from thinking about Byron's obsession with Juan's pretty boyishness. Indeed, Don Juan is continually presented as an object of erotic interest. Although wary of effeminacy, Byron is most open to it when effeminacy becomes a matter of individual choice rather than a prescribed identity, because effeminacy gives men a vantage point from which to choose or reject strength, a sense of the limitations of strength, and an aesthetic that redefines agency in terms of choosing and shaping the circumstances that one is to be determined by.

Effeminacy is furthermore the male's first natural state, and Byron makes this clear by foregrounding Juan's original pre-pubescent and feminine body. To the extent that effeminacy is a normal point of origin for a man, then strength threatens to become a potential deformation. At the outset we are told that everyone, except his mother, deemed Juan "almost a man" (1:54), and deep into the next canto we find him in "very spacious breeches" (2:160). Because his spacious breeches will eventually fall down, Byron here may be coding Juan's sodomy (Dyer 572). The implication here is that if clothes make the man, Juan does not quite measure up. As a long-standing sign of the proper beginnings of boyhood (Fletcher 297), breeches further mark culture's false imposition of gender on the male body. The poet's awareness of the gaps between breeches and Juan's body, therefore, exposes breeches as a sign of aristocratic wish fulfillment. Marjorie Garber further reminds us that "boy" in and after the Renaissance referred to the players who took the parts of women on the Renaissance stage, and that "boy" became a code word for males homoerotically attractive to male spectators (*Vested Interests* 10). That is, "boy" could also be code for effeminacy.[25] Garber implies that boys and women are somewhat interchangeable objects of desire, an interchangeability that further mucks up the binary of gender. The Sultan thinks Juan is a "pretty" girl (5:155). Trumbach argues that since in the eighteenth century, middle-class men had to see prostitutes in order to prove themselves not sodomites, heterosexuality was potentially a closet for sexual perversity. He further suggests that the eighteenth-century marks the beginnings of compulsory heterosexuality. By emphasizing Juan's pubescent gender ambiguity, Byron at least momentarily considers that male strength is a belated addition to an otherwise effeminate norm. When Lord Henry's strength (14:71) makes him less attractive, not more, Byron links that strength with adulteration, not purity. And when we factor in Byron's antipathy to war, Don Juan's relative passiveness within it potentially serves as a critique of epic values, heroism, and martial forms of manliness. In any case, the ontological priority of effeminacy to strength undermines the normality of that strength.

When Byron terms Juan quite "a broth of a boy" (8:24), he turns to an Irish colloquialism, but he does so in such a way as to empty out its certainty. Steffan and Pratt gloss this line as meaning "what a real boy should be" (S&P 3:171). But what exactly should a real boy be, especially given that Juan has shown himself to be more passive than active (even in the heat of battle), looking the part in his feminine disguise, and more infantile than boylike. The fact that Byron himself was taken for a beautiful boy at 21 underscored the fact that "boy" was more of a relative than absolute term. Ali Pasha's ability to consider Lord Byron a child even in spite of his strength implies that the narrative of Greek homonormativity left plenty of room for interpretation. Byron recounted this meet-

ing to his mother, "he told me to consider him as a father whilst I was in Turkey, & said he looked on me as his son.—Indeed he treated me like a child, send-
ing me almonds & sugared sherbet, fruit & sweetmeats 20 times a day" (*BLJ*
1:227–28). Pasha, moreover, was "pleased" with Byron's "appearance and garb"
(*BLJ* 1:227). Although Byron may have identified himself as a man—he is especially happy that Pasha recognizes his aristocracy—that self-identification did
not prevent others from foisting its opposite upon him. Byron obliquely re-
members in *Don Juan* the fact that Ali Pasha admired "the delicacy of [his]
hand" (4:45). When he met Pasha's son, Veli, Veli called him a "beautiful boy"
in Greek and threw his arm around Byron's waist (cited in Crompton 1985 149).

As late as canto 15, Juan is still being described as "soft" (15:14), and Byron
himself confesses that he might have made a better spouse if he weren't in a "soft
condition" (15:24). Despite the fact that Byron acknowledges that in England
Juan's mind "assumed a manlier vigour" (15:11), he immediately compares him
to Alcibiades, who was know for gaining men's affections, not to mention his
lust for Socrates. Of course, "*ass*umed" reminds us that manliness is a garment
even as it exposes the male ass.[26] Although in the first example "soft" literally
modifies Juan's "whole address," Byron places the adjective before the noun it
modifies to suggest that his address is not the only evidence of softness. The
connotations of "soft" run the gamut from pleasant to "weak, effeminate, and
unmanly" (*OED*). As Byron's own journal notes reveal, he recognized softness
of voice itself was sign of effeminacy. The poet records hearing a "beau" asking
"in a very soft tone of voice" for a "glass of Madeira Negus with a Jelly" (*BLJ*
9:29). This prompts a "Lieutenant of the Navy immediately [to] roar out
"Waiter—bring me a glass of d——d stiff Grog—and rub my a——e with a
brick-bat" (*BLJ* 9:29). How quickly signs of softness can fade into effeminacy,
which itself so easily becomes sodomy. Why else would the lieutenant have
asked for his arse to be rubbed with something no less phallic than a brickbat,
a fragment of brick? I note here how easily the body you don't fuck with is
imagined as the body to be fucked.[27] Nonetheless, since brickbats were sometimes hurled by mobs (*OED*), the soldier might allude to a veiled threat: punishment by the pillory, where an accused attempted sodomite would be subject
to whatever the mob decided to throw at him.

But whereas the Lieutenant's response seems little more than virulent homophobia, Byron cops to the fact that his "soft condition" has been "proved," and
he admits that his softness is precisely what made him an indecent spouse (15:
24). For a poet who so prided himself upon his aristocratic strength, what could

possibly make him identify with softness? Byron writes, "I think I should have
made a decent spouse,/If I had never proved the soft condition" (15:24). Given
the poet's hostility to marriage generally, it is not clear if Byron is apologizing
for or proudly declaring his softness—or the proof of it—as a badge of honor.
In any case, softness is framed as the antithesis to decent marriage, and, by logical extension, becomes indecency. Of course, since it is the reader who must extend this logic, Byron can once again claim that any indecency is the reader's not
his. Given Juan's and his own declared softness, when Byron bemoans the fact
that "few of the soft sex are very stable/In their resolves" (15:6), it is not clear
to which sex he is referring. Although this stanza alludes to Lady Adeline, Byron
refers to Juan's natural softness a mere eight stanzas later. Toward the end of
stanza 24, Byron links softness with poetic ability, the wearing of "the motley
*man*tle of a poet" (15:24, emphasis mine). When coupled with the poet's own
declared soft condition, "*man*tle" again deftly transforms the essence of manhood into a garment that can be taken on or off. I might add that "condition"
fudges the ontology of softness; he may have been in the condition of softness,
but that does not mean softness is an inescapable essence. The poet's linking of
softness with both sexes, his use of garment imagery, and his emphasis on "condition" implies that effeminacy is a choice, and to the degree that Byron sees liberation in terms of "personal relationships that will extend the boundaries of
the self" (Franklin 132), even effeminacy plays a key role in that extension. In
defining the "motley" garb most appropriate to the poet, and in making gender
clothing, Byron hints that part of the poet's role is to confuse gender and sexual
laws, to mix them up.[28] Susan Wolfson argues that Byron's softness is at times
equivalent to the humane (*Borderlines* 148), and I would simply add that softness
enables the poet to see masculinity as a lack.

In addition to the fact that effeminacy is a boy's normal state, James Sinclair's
*Code of Health and Longevity* may help explain why Byron could value softness
even in men.[29] Sinclair argued that vivacity was associated with the softness of
bodily fibers and vessels, and the fact that women had softer fibers showed why
they generally lived longer than men. Sinclair writes, "in the human species, in
particular, the male is commonly not only larger than the female, but his muscular fibres are firmer, and more compact, and his whole frame indicates a superior bodily strength, and robustness of texture. But as in women, the bones, cartilages, the muscles, and every other part of the boy, are softer, and less solid
than those of men, they must require time in hardening to that degree which
occasions death" (1:63–64). Sinclair continues, suggesting that "men who have

a weakly appearance, and who, approach the nearest to women, often live longer than those males who are more robust" (1:64). When we consider that Sinclair credited women as the origin for a child's "talents and . . . structure of mind," arguing that "the abilities of many families may be traced to one distinguished female, who introduced talents into it, or, according to a common expression, mother-wit" (1:42), we recognize that softness and effeminacy could have their strengths: vivacity, intelligence, and longevity. Moreover, since death was a process of hardening of the fibers, women would eventually lose their softness, making even feminine softness inherently unstable.

If Sinclair gave women too much credit for wit by gendering it as feminine, the fashionable doctor J. M. Adair insisted that "every faculty of mind is equally dispensed to both sexes" (11). In September 1812, Byron wrote to John Murray, asking him to send him "Adair on Diet & regimen just republished by Ridgway" (*BLJ* 2:191). Perhaps with an eye toward flattering his wealthy female patients, Adair insisted that "the apparent superiority of our sex, in other mental accomplishments, proceeds entirely from difference of education" (11). Hence, the poet not only emphasizes Haidee's intelligence, but also makes it clear that Haidee and her father are "alike, their features and/Their stature differing but in sex and years;/Even to the delicacy of their hand" (4:45). I note that sexual difference is confined to features and stature; that sexual difference alone doesn't explain these differences, age plays a role too.[30] Byron minimizes sexual difference in an age that sought to maximize them. He relegates differences to a parenthetical clause. Difference is, moreover, surrounded by and even perhaps dwarfed by likeness. Contributing to this minimizing of sexual difference is the fact that "delicacy of hand" recalls the Ali Pasha's admiration of Byron's own hand. The hand bridges any gap between male and female. Despite Byron's disparagement of bluestockings and of "ladies intellectual," he was much more sympathetic to Aurora and Adeline and took care to situate their intellectual equality within the context of their upbringing (Franklin 162).

The norm of male strength was under further threat by the popular notion that luxury and civilization had conspired to make men generally more effeminate. Luxury is, for example, much to blame for Sardanapalus's effeminacy: Salemenes points his finger at both "the weakness and wickedness of luxury" and "the evils of sensual sloth" (1:ii). In *Don Juan*, Byron puts it this way: whereas in previous eras men made manners, now "manners make men" (15:26). Luxury and excess combine to demasculinize men; yet that demasculinization can appear to the poet as more erotic. On the negative side, this means that effeminacy and its growing links to sodomy[31] are a majoritizing threat to all men. As Caroline Franklin argues, against a narrative of the French Revolution that sought to essentialize the ancièn régime as effeminate, Byron insists Europe's post-Revolutionary leaders are no less effeminate (116–17). Byron's majoritizing of effeminacy seeks in part to normalize it. Moreover, since he refutes the relegation of effeminacy to the aristocratic past, he does not allow the end of it to underwrite a narrative of liberal progress.

Unlike the effeminacy of Castlereagh or Southey, and despite Juan's own disavowals of the effeminate, Juan's effeminacy thus can be potentially positive as long as it is about agency. Effeminacy not only allows Byron to critique the martial emphasis of the standard epic, but also enables him to consider whether feeling is necessarily a feminine characteristic. Like Horace, whom Byron emulated, Byron turns away from warfare his and other masculine exploits, preferring instead to write about such feminine subjects as love. Aligning feeling with femininity or even feeling with masculinity does not allow one to consider the possibility that the display of feelings can be a highly manipulative process. Thus, Byron wryly notes that men who display their sympathy for the plight of women may be doing so for the sole purpose of seduction. "Man's very sympathy with their [women's] estate/Has much of selfishness and more suspicion" (14:24). Feeling is thus best divorced from gender so that one might consider what is being gained by the public display of any one feeling. At the same time, just as the *OED* reminds us that effeminacy "did not have to imply reproach," suggesting compassion and sympathy, Byron suggests that men need to have compassion especially when they consider how a woman risks everything in falling in love. Donna Julia pleads that men have the world of resources while women have "but one,/To love again, and be again undone" (1:194). Here, Byron undermines the naturalness of the separate spheres by noting the inequalities they actively perpetuate. Because he occupies both the position of effeminacy and masculinity, Byron undercuts the logic behind separate spheres.

It is only fitting that, if gender and sex are shown to be malleable essences, so too is effeminacy. Already in *Sardanapalus*, Byron shows the effeminate tyrant to nonetheless be capable of martial heroism. The fact that he is effeminate does not preclude his acting like a hero in battle. Byron makes this clear from the very outset of the play when Salemenes declares that in "his effeminate heart/ There is a careless courage which corruption/Has not all quench'd" (1.1). While effeminacy is thus framed as a luxurious corruption of masculinity, Sardanapalus's enemies make the mistake of seeing his effeminancy as a depletion of masculinity when in fact he is capable of "re-manning" himself so long as he is determined to do so.[32] Arbaces sneers that "the she-king,/that less than woman, is even now upon/The waters with his female mates" (2.i). I want to suggest that modern critics make an analogous mistake when they too easily solidify the links between effeminacy and a passive sexual role. Sinclair, after all, suggests that softness could paradoxically imply mental strength and even corporeal longevity. As he grieves, Sardanapalus fears that he "grows womanish again" and vows to "learn sternness now" (4.1). Indeed, Sardanapalus claims that "all passions in excess are female" (3.i). By making his declared gender a willed choice—sternness, we cannot forget, must be learned—*Sardanapalus* reminds us that effeminacy to Byron is overwhelmingly about the choices one makes rather than an ontological state. To support this, Myrrha, Sardanapalus's lover and female slave, imagines the mind as being essentially unembodied, "all unincorporated" (4.i). In death, corporeality will at most be "a shadow of this cumbrous clay," flitting and stalking, yet no longer beholden to the fear of death. That effeminacy is about choices is furthermore in keeping with a post-Revolutionary view of health that defined it as an ideal to be striven for instead of an ontological condition (Outram 47). Health became an assertion of control over one's own environment, over the "non-naturals" like "air, food and drink, motion, rest, sleep and waking, evacuation and retention" (ibid.). Despite Byron's emphasis upon the mind's ability to assert gender, his emphasis upon the symmetry between Sardanaplus's effeminacy and his self-immolation, like Indian widows undergoing sati, implies that, at very least, the male mind has considerable work cut out for it if it is to escape the pejorative associations of effeminacy.

Not only did all males begin with effeminate bodies, but also a prevailing medical belief in a spermatic economy meant that vigorous masculine bodies could revert to a literal state of effeminacy at any time with too much expenditure of semen. Not enough expenditure was also unhealthy: for this reason, Byron stipulates that "health and idleness to passion's flame" are "oil and gunpowder" (2:169). By equating health with oil and idleness to passion with gunpowder, Byron seeks to make sexual activity a sine qua non of health even as he implies that restraint will only add to the explosiveness of passion, not diminish it. Hunter's anatomy collection, with his filigree of sperm ducts filled with quicksilver, and the famous surgeon Astley Cooper documented the elaborate and intricate pathways for the semen to travel, and they proved semen to be an especially lavish bodily expenditure. This fluid idea of the body as spermatic economy or balanced menstrual evacuations was heightened by medicine's emphasis upon the body's changeableness. Of course, it was in medicine's best interest to insist upon the malleability of the body and the efficacy of any given prescription or regimen. Such a spermatic economy made effeminacy much more than an embryonic phase before the onset of real sexuality because it always accompanies and threatens to disrupt heterosexuality and masculinity. Indeed, excess heterosexuality itself could lead to effeminacy. Because he saw masculinity as being surrounded by effeminacy—boys begin as effeminate, boys can be naturally attracted to effeminate boys, and men who have too much sex can revert to being boys—Byron is rightly skeptical of masculine strength as an essence. He is also rightly skeptical about the putative naturalness of heterosexuality.

John Sinclair, for example, refutes the idea that the "bones, cartilages, muscles, and other solid parts, being once formed, are permanent, because the identity of the individual is permanent" (Appendix 2:83). Rather, he insists, "every part and particle of the firmest bones, is successively absorbed and deposited again. The solids of the body, whatever their form or texture, are incessantly renewed. The whole body is a perpetual secretion, as the saliva that flows from the mouth, or the moisture that bedews the surface" (Appendix 2:84). By emphasizing the body as a form of secretion, Sinclair highlights its essential fluidity and underscores the value of the spermatic fluid for men. That Byron's friend, the pugilist J. Jackson to whom Byron refers as his "corporeal pastor and master" (cited in Dyer 564), was the source of much of Sinclair's remarks on the role of exercise in health, meant that Byron likely would have paid especially attention to these remarks. The poet trusted Jackson enough to ask him to get another bottle of a "Lamb's-Conduit-Street remedy" so Byron could ask a physician to test it (*BLJ* 1:169). In the appendix to his first volume, Sinclair apologizes for his necessary reticence on the subject: "the semen is a discharge of infinite importance to the human frame, but for obvious reasons, cannot much be dealt with in a work of popular nature" (Appendix 1:16). He warns nonetheless that "if indulged before the body is fully formed, it stints the growth, and brings on languor, debility, and various other disorders. . . . Manhood is the proper period of life for these gratifications, which are then natural and useful, but even then they ought not to be indulged into excess" (ibid.). This advice did not help Byron, who claimed that he lost his sexual innocence at the age of eight at the hands of his female servant.

In Byron's case, this threat of effeminacy was all the more serious given his epic struggles over body weight and his ideal of a slim body.[33] If slenderness was somewhat of a feminine ideal, Byron's abstemious diets perhaps were in part attempts to make him look more boyish, youthful. The poet lost fifty-eight pounds in the spring of 1807 and upon his return to Cambridge he was unrecognizable. Even his love, John Edelston, did not know him: he "told me he saw me in Trinity walks twice, & knew me not, till pointed out by him, by his Brother or Cousin" (*BLJ* 1:122).

To lose weight, Byron took up boxing. Boxing sets up another important context for thinking about Byron and effeminacy.[34] Dyer clues us in that the sport is tied to "an underclass for whom the gallows was an ever-present threat" and that Byron's sexual practices made him no less criminal (563). In one sense, boxing could enhance one's manliness and lean muscularity. At the same time, boxing, like the ancient Greek gymnasium, could allow men to ogle male bodies. Boxing, thus, paradoxically reinforced one's manliness even when it made male bodies objects of desire; because men were permitted to view muscular male bodies whereas softer male bodies were the exclusive province of the female gaze (Harvey 128), boxing enabled softer men to strengthen themselves while ogling other men.

Potter's 1795 *Dictionary of Cant and Flash Language*, which Byron owned (Munby 1:212), clearly suggests ways in which boxing could push masculinity in either direction. "Flash" designates men of sport, "men of the ring" (*OED*). Defining a "cock alley" as the private parts of a woman, and a "commodity" in terms of the "private parts of a modest woman," this dictionary showed how heterosexual activity was essential to masculinity, so much so that a woman's genitals were unambiguously the place of a man's. Nonetheless, it listed no fewer than five code terms for sodomite: backgammon player, back door gentleman, indorser, madge, and madge cull (a buggerer). A "madge cove," moreover, was "a keeper of a house for buggerers." Byron telling compares the slave mart in canto 5 to a "backgammon board" (5:10), and he thereby aligns passivity, sodomy, and commerce. Of course, Byron's point is that the marriage mart in England is little better than slavery. By implication, heterosexuality/marriage does not exclude sodomy; marriage therefore can be a closet for perversion. Despite the fact that this *Dictionary* was dedicated to the justices of the peace, promising to help the middle class avoid being victimized by such men, the *Dictionary* could let others in on an elaborate code so that one sodomite might find another. Not only did Byron himself search for William Beckford, "the great Apostle of Paederasty" (*BLJ* 1:210), but he also contemplated writing a treatise "to be entitled "Sodomy simplified or Paederasty proved to be praiseworthy from ancient authors and modern practice" (*BLJ* 1:208). The fact that a cultural ideal of athletic masculinity was inseparable from sodomy meant that boxing could provide an effective and pleasurable closet for homoeroticism if not homosexuality.

When he claims that "No lady e'er is ogled by a lover. . . . As is a slave by his intended bidder" (5:26–27), Byron stretches the simile across two stanzas to show that despite their ostensible differences, slavery can shed light on marriage. While such overt ogling might be frowned upon in the marriage market, in sober truth, the ogling is just more restrained. In a Greek context, the slave would have been expected to take the passive sexual position, and this context further stretches the simile between marriage and slavery. While it is crucial to note that Juan later protests his feminizing garb and to being circumcised, Byron invites the reader to take the subject position of the slave as well as the position of the married woman (Donna Julia, Lady Adeline). He thereby suggests some sympathy and identification with this role. We also witness Juan being reduced to a sexual object. As Byron understands only too well, human sexuality means ideally that one is both sexual agent and object of desire. If intimacy is to stand for power relations based on equality, agent must become object and vice versa. His ability to identify with the object—to take the female or slave's role—makes Byron skeptical of the claim that sodomites could clearly be divided into passive and active roles. Identification is the solvent of identity. Juan, moreover, is often actively passive, a collapse that further undermines not only the law of gender, but also the meaning of certain sexual positions. Finally, if even Lord Byron can imagine the vantage point of a slave, these positions are hardly mutually exclusive or ironclad.

If slimming suggested a modicum of mental control over the body, that sense of control was undermined by Byron's sense that too much sex was depleting his constitution. A few months later in February 1808, Byron was advised by his physician, Pearson, to stop seeing prostitutes. Byron writes, "I am at this moment under a course of restoration by Pearson's prescription, for a debility occasioned by too frequent Connection" (*BLJ* 1:158). Two days later, Byron again confesses to Hobhouse that "I am at present as miserable in mind and Body, as Literary abuse, pecuniary embarrassment, and total enervation can make me.— I have tried every kind of pleasure, and it is 'Vanity'" (*BLJ* 1:160). Enervation captures his feminized self in terms of nervous disease even as literature and money and sex combine to make him literally effeminate. One of the key evils of masturbation or of too frequent connection was that it prevented the reabsorption of the semen into the male body, thus denying it its strength. Hence, Byron "began to apprehend a complete Bankruptcy of [his] constitution" (*BLJ*

1:160). When excess heterosexuality leads to absence/bankruptcy, the norm begins to look uncannily perverse.

William Munk's *Roll of the Royal College of Physicians of London* lists two Pearsons: George and Richard. Pearson was likely George (1751–1828), not Richard. Both were practicing in London in 1807–1808 when Byron went for consultation and treatment, but George Pearson was an enthusiastic follower of John Brown, who believed that health was predicated upon the right amount of excitability. Brown adopted "excitability" from his mentor, William Cullen, but generalized it beyond the nervous system.[35] Brown believed that we begin life with a fixed quantity of excitability and that as we are exposed to stimuli, they waste excitability, and this waste was only with great difficulty restored. In his letter to the Reverend John Becher, Byron notes, "I have this moment received a prescription from Pearson, not for any *complaint* but from *debility*, and literally *too much Love*" (*BLJ* 1:157). He later confesses to Hobhouse that he is "under a course of restoration by Pearson's prescription, for a debility occasioned by too frequent Connection. —Pearson sayeth, I have done sufficient with[in] this last ten days, to undermine my Constitution, I hope however all will soon be well" (*BLJ* 1:158). In George Pearson's *Principles of Physic* (1801), he notes that, "if the organs be excited too violently, or for too long a time, the excitability becomes so far diminished, that the ordinary excitants to healthy motions cannot produce them; such a state has been called indirect debility" (18). Pearson's and Brown's emphasis upon the role of the environment upon the body was very much in keeping with Byron's sense in *Don Juan* that man was a creature of circumstance. For Brown, life is a reaction to changing stimuli (Risse "Brownian" 46). Byron would have found helpful Brown's notion that health is the balance of internal excitability and external stimulation. Finally, it was Pearson who convinced Byron that "there is no sterner moralist than pleasure" (3:65). When Byron understands "the quickening of the heart" in terms of "how much it costs us" (2:203), he shows his Brunonian understanding of excitability.

Pearson adopts Brown's idea that excessive excitement caused "sthenic diseases," but, if stimulation were increased still further, the store of excitability would become depleted, resulting in deficient excitement, "asthenic diseases," or indirect debility (*Principles* 18).[36] Brown writes, "Anyone who has lived luxuriously . . . labors not under plethora, but under indirect debility" (1:86). He continues, "To restore vigor, a debilitating plan of cure is to be avoided" (1:86), and he based this idea on the fact that deficient excitement would benefit most greatly by "reproducing the lost quantity of blood" (2:5). Curing asthenia required the "encrease [of] deficient excitement likewise all over the system" (1:286). Semen, we recall, was thought to be essentially refined blood. Not only did Brown thereby equate the upper classes with disease, but he also paradoxically suggested that the cure to high living, at least in terms of diet, was more high living. Some capitalist fantasy! Brown offers the medicinal equivalent of having one's cake and eating it, too, and he goes so far as to index abstinence with "not less immoral and irreligious than excess" (2:347). He urged physicians that in cases of debility they must "not to give way to a weakened appetite" (2:7). Lots of alcohol and opium were crucial to his therapy (Risse "Brunonian Therapeutics" 46).[37] Perhaps this helps to explain much of the popularity and influence of Brown. He was revered by no less than Hegel and Kant, and the 1788 English edition, in runs of a thousand copies, frequently was out of print (Overmier 311). Echoing Brown, Pearson writes, "By still further repeated excitation, the parts gradually lose their power of acquiring excitability" (*Principles* 16). Although rich eating and drinking were encouraged, Brown warned his patients sternly that "in every degree of debility that high force of the passions, that produced indirect debility, must be avoided" (1:304). Pearson's and Brown's debilitated patients could stimulate themselves, as long as they sublimated their stimulation from sex to food.

Brown began to link asthenic diseases to sthenic ones because of his own battles with gout. Under the care of his mentor, William Cullen, he did not get better.[38] Like most physicians, Cullen thought that gout was caused by excess vigor and as a result recommended abstemiousness with regard to food and drink especially. Frustrated with Cullen's therapy, Brown decided to begin eating and drinking richly, and, coincidentally, Brown's attacks of gout subsided. He therefore decided that gout was caused by indirect debility rather than excess vigor, and thus his mode of treatment, contrary to received wisdom, was stimulation via a high-protein diet and other stimulants such as alcohol and opium. Brown's emphasis on stimulation as the route to health was echoed by Sinclair, who insisted that "ascetics are a proof, not of the length of life, which temperance insures, but of the premature old age which abstinence brings upon us" (Appendix 2:85). The pugilist John Jackson, whom Byron referred to as his "corporeal master," also recommended wine and malt liquor (cited in Sinclair Appendix 2:101–2). Thus, when Byron links Malthus with asceticism—"but certes it conducts to lives ascetic,/Or turning marriage into arithmetic" (15:28)—he implies that the reduction of sex to math will make human beings unhealthy.

Posing as a patient without complaint, as if "complaint" might overly feminize him and undermine his aristocratic status, Lord Byron learns to read libidinous excess as indirect somatic debility, a debility that threatens to make him quite literally effeminate. He will later describe himself in terms of "total enervation" (*BLJ* 1:160). When excess is transformed into a lack, the body's symbolic economy becomes based in paradox, acting more like a text than a body. Within his epic, Byron wryly notes that although we "sneer" at physicians when in health, "when ill, we call them to attend us, / Without the least propensity to jeer" (10:42). Our skepticism therefore depends upon our condition of health. That Byron originally wrote "they teaze" and changed this to "we teaze" (Nicholson *Facsimile* 25) emphasizes the shifting grounds of our skepticism. In any case, since Brunonianism transformed an excess into a lack, it demanded an aesthetic reading of the body and its pleasures, one that might lead to unexpected consequences. In the same way that the dots connecting anatomy to destiny were far from predictable, Byron frustrates narrative teleology, going so far as to allow the contingency of rhyme to move the narrative forward.

Pearson also helps unpack the significance of Byron's stanza listing a prescription, placing this stanza in the context of Brunonian medicine. Indeed many of the ingredients are designed to treat the indirect debility Byron himself believed he suffered from: too much coitus. In the original draft of the stanza, Byron refers to what looks like "Doctor Rogeson's prescription" (S&P 3:245), and Nicholson's manuscript facsimile supports this point.[39] In any case, not only do Pearson and Rogeson sound distinctly similar, but both also treated patients who had too much sex. Byron writes,

> But here's one prescription out of many:
> "Soda-Sulphat. 3 vi. 3.s. Mannae optim.
> Aq. fervent. F. 3.ifs. 3ij. tinct. Sennae
> Haustus." (And here the surgeon came and cupped him)
> "R. Pulv. Com. gr. iii. Ipecacuanhae"
> (With more beside, if Juan had not stopped 'em.)
> "Bolus Potassae Sulphuret. sumendus,
> Et Haustus ter in die capiendus." (10:41)

Since Brunonianism argued that indirect debility had to be cured by more stimulation, Pearson prescribes a host of stimulants. According to George Pearson's *Arranged Catalogue of the Articles of Food, Drink, Seasoning and Medicine* (1801), Ipecacuanhae was the best specific stimulant to "excite secretions in certain organs, and produce evacuations" (41), the best manna was a stimulating laxative, while "dry cupping" helped to "excite Action or Motion of the Muscular Fibres, Nerves, and Mental Faculties" (32).[40] Indeed, vomiting was particularly good for "exciting peculiar action in particular organs, especially the secretory" (*Principles* 142). "Secretory" is a polite way of referring to the seminal secretions, nocturnal emissions being their most neutral form, and menstrual evacuations. Carthartics like Mannae Optim (best Manna) also helped to stimulate the secretory system (ibid.). Aqua fervent (heated water), moreover, was a "stimuli of life" (*Principles* 132–33) and helpful to the operation of other medicines (*Catalogue* 43) while Sennae Haustus was in small and limited doses another purgative stimulant, meant to increase the circulation and "stimulate the intestines" (44). This combination of excitants is in keeping with Pearson's comment that "in different parts, different kinds and degrees of action may be excited at the same time by different kinds of excitants" (*Principles* 17). Given that Rogerson, Queen Catherine's physician, was called in to treat Lanskoi, another favorite boyish lover of Catherine, Rogerson's prescription recalls Pearson's.

Byron's regimen would also include a solid diet of meat, wines, ales, beers, and gentle exercise (hence his regimen of boxing), along with a "stimulating" drug like opium or hashish. The pill of sulphurated potash was a strengthener or tonic (*Arranged* 63, 65), and Pearson recommended it "for morbidly diminished power of motion or action to usual healthy stimuli" (*Principles* 145). Sulphuric acid topped the list of his recommended chemical "external excitants" (*Principles* 134). Taken together, the ingredients for this prescription are designed to ward off enervation or a return to effeminacy and to restore the body to its original condition of excitability. Indeed, just five stanzas earlier, Byron depicts "the gentle Juan" (10:37) as a shrinking sensitive plant. Sensitive plants in eighteenth-century British erotica were complex metaphors for the penis: because they receded even from a woman's touch, sensitive plants transformed the penis from a virile member to a "tender thing of feeling" (Harvey 137).[41] Because Byron worries if Juan's "withered form" will be "further drain[ed]" (10:38), along with the poet's description of Juan's "delicate state" and "wasted cheek" (10:43), this prescription is quite likely not far from the ones Pearson actually dispensed to the poet in 1808. Lest we forget, Juan is at this point trying to satisfy Catherine the Great's voracious sexual appetites for boyish men, what Byron refers to as "her preference of a boy to men much bigger" (9:72). Brown suggests that excessive evacuations, moreover, threaten to return the body to its prepubescent, effeminate, norm. If effeminacy could be treated through prescription, this suggests that gender was much more mobile in the Romantic period than we have acknowledged. To the extent that the Romantics felt the need to "colonize the feminine," they recognized the essential tenuousness of masculinity, its likelihood of being lost (Richardson 1988 13–25). Such a link between masculinity and loss made Byron more sympathetic to the plight of women.

In 1819, Byron confessed to Douglas Kinnaird that his enervation had returned, and thus in the midst of finishing canto 2 would have had Pearson's treatment very much on his mind. "The air of this cursed Italy enervates—and disfranchises the thoughts of man after nearly four years of respiration—to say nothing of emission" (*BLJ* 6:232). Pearson furthermore suggested that the body could be in a state of "Morbid Strength" whereby "ordinary excitants produce extraordinary motions" (*Principles* 24), and this helped to push strength into the side of pathology. Pearson thus enables Byron to see strength as a pathology and, in so doing, question strength as a necessary gendered good. Finally, since the very worst climate for asthenic diseases is a frigid one, Byron has an excuse to ship Juan to a warmer clime, to England. If the climate caused the body to produce sweat, it would become further weakened by relaxation (Brown 2:8). Hence, in the same way that Pearson suggested that a change of climate and scene were good in cases of debility (*Arranged* 32), Juan's doctors recommend immediate travel (10:43).

In light of Trumbach's suggestion that prostitution was a supplement to sodomy for middle-class men and because Byron has only just been alluding to his love for Edelston in letters to his Cambridge circle, Byron's wanton display of heterosexual excesses makes it look like he doth protest too much. When coupled with Byron's sense of himself as literally depleted by heterosexual sex, so much so that a doctor has to be called in to treat him, the homosexual innuendos within his letters perhaps suggest that Byron is playing doctor. Having diagnosed himself with the symptoms of effeminacy, he attributes its cause to too frequent connection with prostitutes when in fact that cause might be a cover for his homosexual desires. When Byron refers to his seminal "Bankruptcy," might he be alluding to his friend, William Bankes?[42] In 1820, Byron admitted to Murray that he "loved Bankes" (Crompton 358). Here I want to take issue with critics like Jerome Christensen who insist that nothing happened in England so that sodomy can be equated with the journey east. Yet, in order for nothing to have happened, sexuality must be reduced to acts, leaving questions of desire behind. Louis Crompton (1985) and Fiona MacCarthy have argued that Byron did consummate his relationships with boys while in England, even going so far as to suggest the poet had a fling with his servant Rushton

(MacCarthy 78).[43] Byron himself declares his skepticism that feeling can be so easily disciplined and categorized: Juan and Haidee gaze at each other with "looks of speechless tenderness,/Which mix'd all feelings, friend, child, lover, brother" (4:26).

If Pearson helped to show Byron how important it was to moderate his sexual desires because indirect debility was not far from death, Samuel Solomon's *Guide to Health* would reinforce these lessons. Moderation thus could liberate the body from the tyranny of desire even as it situated desire within an aesthetic framework, one that could lead to meaningful choices. Originally published in 1795, Solomon's book went through sixty editions (*BLJ* note 7:229). Oft quoted is Byron's unkind remark that Keats's "writing was a sort of mental masturbation" (*BLJ* 7: 225), but Byron gets the substance of his remarks from Solomon. Writing again to John Murray, complaining of the attention Keats is getting from the critics, Byron asks, "Why don't they review & praise 'Solomon's Guide to Health'? it is better sense and as much poetry as Johnny Keates" (*BLJ* 7:229). Solomon remarked that "the great alteration which takes place in the boy of the male at the time when the semen begins to be formed and collected, is so manifest that it appears to the common observer; for the rise and continuance of the beard and cloathing of the pubes depend thereon; and a wonderful alteration takes place in the voice and passions of the mind, for hitherto crying boy now becomes bold and intrepid, despising even real danger" (94). Although Byron takes great pains to distinguish his own poetry from that of Keats, using his aristocratic status and strength as bulwarks against Keatsian onanism, Solomon reveals that neither aristocracy nor heterosexual sex can prevent emasculation.[44] Even the heterosexual "immoderate use of coition depresses the spirits, relaxes the fibres, and renders the whole frame weak and exhausted" (95).

Although Solomon allows Byron to project his own fears of emasculation upon Keats by solidifying links between Cockneyism and effeminacy, his *Guide* in the end brings the two poets down to the common level of masculinity under threat. Of course, Byron's boxing background meant that his intimate knowledge of the Cockney underclass might make him too more Keatsian than he wants to admit. Likewise, despite his sense of himself in the stronger, more active role, Byron is not beyond effeminacy. In point of fact because of the connections between luxury and effeminacy, Byron's social class makes him more vulnerable to effeminacy than Keats, not less. Perhaps this is why he converts nobility to mobility, thus aligning the mob and nobility (Haslett 153). Perhaps this is also what enables Byron to stand outside of class privilege and to see the normalizing powers of masculine strength.

Solomon also helps explain why Byron refers to eunuchs as the third sex and why he links the third sex with foppery. Byron muses, "From all the pope makes yearly t'would perplex/To find three perfect pipes of the third sex" (4:86). The poet noted that both the sultan and the pope are the "chief encouragers of this branch of trade" (S&P 3:115); by calling them castrators, he foists perversion onto Roman Catholicism even as he connects the Church with wanton Oriental sexuality. Writing about the changes in boys during puberty, Solomon argues that these changes "are prevented by destroying the organs which serve to separate the liquor that produces it: and just observations evince, that the amputation of the testicles at the age of virility has made the beard fall and the puerile voice return! After this, can the power of its operation be questioned?" (94). "Third sex" thus reifies the effeminate boy as a normal middle ground between male and female. Such a middle position implies the inadequacy of the male/female dyad.

Byron reminds us that puberty is a highly variable process, leaving some men like Juan without the most visible sign of manhood—a beard. Byron's narrator suggests that he can "find no spot where man can rest eye on,/Without confusion of the sorts and sexes" (11:3). The world, he concludes, is at the worst a "glorious blunder" (11:3). In an age that sought to make sex correspond unambiguously with gender, Byron ruptures the mapping of gender onto the body by making masculinity ineffable. All is blunder and confusion. Noteworthy is the fact that he begins a description of Juan as a negation.

> Juan was none of these, but slight and slim,
> Blushing and beardless; and yet ne'ertheless
> There was something in his turn of limb,
> And still more in his eye, which seemed to express
> That though he looked one of the Seraphim,
> There lurked a Man beneath the Spirit's dress.
> Besides, the Empress sometimes liked a boy,
> And had just buried the fair faced Lanskoi. (9:47)

In fact, this entire stanza circles around absence because not only is Juan not like any of the "nervous six-footers" in the previous stanza, but also he resembles the dead and buried Lanskoi. By alluding to the nervous six-footers that Juan is not, Byron makes him an even paler shade of masculinity because nervous men are

already under feminization by nervous diseases. Syncope (the elision of a syllable in ne'ertheless) becomes in Byron's hands an apt figure for a playful and not
entirely negative effeminacy: absence normalizes the line into pentameter.
Analogously, does effeminacy normalize men? "Seraphim," moreover, brings
Juan close to the angel of the house that will be firmly enshrined in the Victorian period even as it embroils angelicness within serpenthood. The *OED* suggests that the seraphim may or may not be aligned with the serpent. Moreover,
with his play between "ne'ertheless," "beardless," and "still more," the poet suggest that less is more. My point here is that Byron makes it difficult to localize
masculinity and makes it very difficult to map onto a sexed body. The closest
linguistic signifier we get to masculinity here is "something," and even that is
under erasure by an angelic metaphor that may hint at the presence of a burning serpent. And if "turn of limb" offers more certainty, that too is compared to
a turn in the eye which "seemed to express/. . . there lurked a Man beneath the
Spirit's dress." Indeed, manhood is itself in drag, dressed in spiritual clothing.
Yet there is one further turn. "Turn of limb" verges on the very turn of the verse,
and it is perhaps fitting that gender is itself figured as a turn, a trope. The poet
was not beyond dressing his prostitutes or lovers like boys.

Byron makes Juan more the object of conquest rather than the agent of it in
part to show agency as a gendered fiction: we are more creatures of circumstance than persons of principle. As Byron puts it, "Men are the sport of circumstances, when/The circumstances seem the sport of men" (5:17). The vagaries
of assonance reinforced in the rhyme thus drive the narrative of the poem instead of any predetermined plot. But his emphasis upon Juan's passivity along
with his status as victim of seduction rather than active perpetrator of it, is more
importantly designed to undermine the biological and legal grounding of activeness in the male body and of passivity in the female body. Initially, he
"seem'd/Active, though not so sprightly, as a page" (1:54). The poet's emphasis
on seeming and the fact that his seeming activeness is immediately negated by
his not being as active as a lower-class boy erases the power of gender to confer
activeness. Moreover, if page is also a servant, Juan's activeness is placed in the
passive role, of being at the beck and call of the upper class. Byron's depiction
of Juan as a nursing infant in the Haidee episode renders him into a most passive object of Haidee's care, just as Haidee is described as active: "in her air/
there was a something which bespoke command" (2:116). Haidee's "something"
presages Juan's "something": not only is that thing not anatomical, but also Juan
can acquire it from Haidee. Once again, both sexes are accorded the same

"something." The poet is not just being coy here; the ineffability of that some-thing deliberately undermines the notion that gender can be reduced to an anatomical locus. Trumbach demonstrates how the legal system sought to cod-ify further manhood in terms of activeness. After age fourteen, even the passive participant in sodomy was considered as guilty as his active partner (59). De-spite the legal system's efforts to instantiate a magic age when a boy became a man, and despite its efforts firmly to align activeness and manhood, Byron cel-ebrates the manifold ambiguities of puberty because it enables him to question sexual and gendered norms. Here, this questioning extends to the narratives un-derwritten by the body, the very idea of anatomic localization of sex.

Byron furthermore has little truck with the idea of female passionlessness, arguing that women have desires equal to or surpassing those of men.[45] In mak-ing most of the sexual advances come from women, Byron thought he was being true to nature (cited in Wolfson 602). Against a trend toward a biology of in-commensurability that dictated that only men need to achieve orgasm in order to procreate and women were passionless, Byron insists that the sexes are evenly passionate.[46] Byron not only makes his women characters sexual initiators, but also shows what is lost when women are reduced to sexual purity. Adeline goes through the motions of morality, in the process stultifying into a cardboard character. By contrast, the Duchess of Fitz-Fulke looks hard at Juan after his first nightmare encounter with the Black Friar and determines then that she will masquerade as the friar in order to seduce Juan. The poet most clearly argues against complementarity when he notes that man's "sympathy" with the female "estate" "has much of selfishness and more suspicion/Their love, their virtue, beauty, education,/But form good housekeepers, to breed a nation" (14:24). Here Byron suggests that the price of complementarity for women may be too high: femininity entails their domestic enslavement and reduction to breeders. As Donna Julia makes clear, men have the world at their disposal, while women are reducing to falling in love and being undone (1:194). Byron furthermore suggests that women have coded their sexual desires in terms of worship of mil-itary figures like Nelson and Wellington (Haslett 196–97). Sexual repression thus demands that both men and women closet their real desires so that they can act on them.

In *Don Juan*, Byron makes a passing reference to "soft Abernethy" (10:42). The noted physician John Abernethy helped buttress Byron's skepticism about the complementariness of the two sexes because of Abernethy's insistence that life does not depend upon organization.[47] Although historians of sexuality have paid a great deal of attention to how sexual desire gets localized in the body and within psychiatry, they have neglected to pay enough heed to how biological sex gets localized in the body.[48] The resistance to the role and importance of structure and anatomy in the Romantic period by such key figures as Abernethy and Brown points to a larger resistance to the mapping of biological sex onto a specific body part. The gap between specific anatomical parts and biological sex undermines the notion of sexual complementarity. Recall here Byron's resistance to localizing sex to an anatomic part; his refusal to specify sex in other than "something" allows him simultaneously to draw attention to the logic of metonymy—we want a sign in the place of that something—and to defer that metonymic substitution. The poet thereby asks why we want the figural work of metonymy especially when sex is at issue. Both Brown's and Abernethy's theories of the body deliberately resist that move toward metonymy, since they seek to understand the body as a coherent whole rather than in terms of anatomical localization. To the extent that the genitals no longer embody the teleology of sex, sex allegorizes Byron's overall resistance to epic purpose. Epic once again becomes epicene.

Abernethy argued that in the same way life is superadded to structure, mind is superadded to life (4:95); therefore, humankind "possesses a sensitive, intelligent, and independent mind" (4:95).[49] Although he did not specify that this was also true for women, the fact that Abernethy thought the source of most diseases was in the common digestive system meant that his pathology had little need for sexual complementarity. Abernethy's mantra that local diseases are "precipitated by general disorders . . . of which the disordered state of the digestive organs is an evidence, and may have been the cause" (1:196) further suggest skepticism about the absolute and incommensurate difference between men and women. Because John Hunter had shown that even remote parts of the body are in sympathy with one another, Abernethy believed that the "subtile substance" of life pervaded the body, bringing it into one whole (4:91). Thus, he insisted that not even diseased structures "arose from any particular organ. . . . All the digestive organs [are] concerned for during this state" (National Library of Medicine MSB 366 "Notes from Lectures by John Abernethy, 1805"). Byron alludes to Abernethy's insistence that the digestive system is at the root of most bodily illnesses when he claims that the use of the intellect "depends so much upon the gastric juice" (5:32).[50] Like John Brown, Abernethy rejected organ localization because the proximate disease was merely a symptom of a larger more generalizable condition.

Abernethy might well be the source of Byron's cryptic comment about the "confusion of sorts and sexes" (11:3). He referred to beards as "delusive signs" (4:175) and argued, based on John Hunter's claims, that "those occurrences which denote the sexual character are to be considered as the effects of sympathies existing between remote parts of the body, which like other instances of sympathy, are liable to occasional failure and considerable variation" (4:175). Beards thus get dissolved into corporeal sympathy. Abernethy further repeated Hunter's claim that "when age has annulled the sexual powers, their appropriate external evidences are not only discontinued, but sometimes those of an opposite character are displayed" (4:176).[51] The fact that women after menopause grew facial hair meant that even beards might be misleading. He continues, "The difference of form and character between the male and female of most animals, is, in general, considerable and striking, and denoted by circumstances very diversified but not reducible to any general rules. Yet this difference does not seem a consequence of necessity: for there are some species of animals in which it scarcely can be said to exist; and in others the female is the larger and stronger, partaking more of what we usually deem the masculine character" (4:176). Although sexual difference exists, it cannot be codified. Nor are these differences necessary or essential.

Byron would also have agreed with Abernethy's assessment that Gall and Spurzheim had vastly underestimated the role of "education, habit, and association" when they urged that we equate the form of the head with innate propensities (4:364). As he put it elsewhere, "Nature may have made us, she has at least given us great powers of forming and fashioning ourselves" (4:185). Abernethy anticipated "nothing but mischief" from their "Physiognomy and Cranioscopy" (4:364), and he did so because he felt that their stress on specific organization overlooked larger sympathetic relations between body parts. It is surely no accident that Byron understands Spurzheim's "philoprogenitiveness," what Spurzheim referred to as a specific and localizable organ of parenting, to mean a love of the act of generation. Byron wrote, "For my part, / I think that 'Philogenitiveness' is—/ Now here's a word quite after my own heart, . . . methinks that 'Philo-genitiveness'/Might meet from men a little more forgiveness" (12:22). In a poem whose hero believes in serial erotic encounters instead of domestic stability, Byron's perversion of Spurzheim's organ of heteronormativity into an organ of sexual bliss largely without reproduction reinforces the values of pleasure rather than of function. Then and only then can it be a word after his own heart. Pondering the strangeness of the propagation of life, Byron mused that "a bubble of Seed which may be spilt in a whore's lap—or in the Orgasm of a voluptuous dream—might (for aught we know) have formed a Caesar or a Buonaparte" (*BLJ* 9:47). Once again the poet emphasizes waste and pleasure rather than procreation. Although Haidee does give birth to Juan's only child, she is unable to explore her philoprogenitiveness for long before both she and her baby succumb to illness.

In the same breath that Byron mentions "soft Abernethy," Byron refers to "mild Baillie" (*BLJ* 10:42). Baillie was not only called in to examine the poet's club foot, but also became the poet's physician. Lady Byron tried to get him to testify to Byron's insanity or even perhaps to his sodomitic tendencies. Along with Abernethy, Hunter, Brown, and Sinclair, Baillie, too, reinforced Byron's skepticism about sexual complementarity. Matthew Baillie argued that the enlarged clitoris is a natural defect (1793 283). "At birth, the clitoris in such a case is often larger than the penis of a child of the same age" (284). He elaborates, "It has a well formed prepuce and glans, together with a fissure at its extremity, so as to resemble almost exactly the external appearance of the male organs. Females often been baptized for males" (284). The fact that men-midwives and physicians could not always tell the difference between an elongated clitoris and a penis can be partly attributed to a one-sex model, which made the clitoris an analogous penis rather than its own organ. Tellingly, Baillie moves from anatomic evidence to belief when he claims that the "clitoris enlarges as child grows, but I believe, not in the same proportion as the penis would do" (285). When inverted, the vagina sometimes allowed the child to be mistaken for a hermaphrodite (279).

If women were baptized for men, men could also be mistaken for women. Baillie notes that "labia joined together by common skin" so that "the appearance of the labia is lost entirely" (286). This defect, however, can be "remedied by art" (286). Baillie then describes a woman with a remarkably masculine look, with plain features, but no beard (Appendix 139). "The labia were more pendulous than usual, and contained each of them a body resembling a testicle of moderate size" (Appendix 139–40). Far from being unambiguous signs of sex, the genitals were prone to "natural defects." Byron's club foot made him especially sensitive to natural defects. To underscore the fluidity of the human body further, Baillie noted that "habit has considerable influence in regulating our sensations, as well as many other functions of the body . . . it can even change the nature of sensations, rendering those which were originally agreeably indifferent, or perhaps even disagreeable; and, on the contrary, rendering those at length pleasant which were originally disagreeable to us" (*Lectures* 137). Baillie insists that the bounding line between nature and culture was fine indeed, so much so that habit could have anatomical effects. In sum, Abernethy and Baillie demonstrate that even the genitals are a kind of clothing to the body in that they have the potential to hide the body's sex. Beneath Byron's fascination with cross-dressing, then, is a body that refuses to unambiguously take on sex. This is exacerbated by the fact that ambiguous genitalia can be considered "natural defects," which only makes the ground of sex all the more tenuous. If sex made bodies intelligible, it also threatened to falsify bodies into neat categories.

The Roman poet Horace further enables Byron to step outside of complementarity and compulsory heterosexuality. From the beginning of the poem, when Byron alludes to Horace's having made "medias res" the "heroic turnpike road" (1:6), Byron alludes to Horace in *Don Juan*. In 1820, he revives his interest in Horace and publishes his *Hints from Horace*, his translation of Horace's *Ars Poetica*. Perhaps reading Horace was literally part of his treatment from the enervation from four years in the hot climate of Italy, not to mention his emissions. John Brown recommends wit as an additional stimulant for debility; in particular, the odes of Horace. Brown waxes, "How fine was that feeling in Julius Caesar Scaliger, when he declared he would rather be the author of Horace's few stanzas of Lydia and Telephus. . . . How delightful must the feelings of Horace have been, in whose works every Ode is an effort of the most beautiful, and, frequently, of the most sublime, conceptions of human genius!" (1:304–5). In light of Horace's refusal to commit to a single woman as well as his serial encounters with women and the boys Gyges and Ligurinus, Horace as cure could easily become poison. Even Adam Smith noted that the "gallantry of Horace [is] always agreeable" (29). To which we might ask: even when directed toward boys?[52]

In keeping with the eighteenth-century's understanding of Horace as a classical model of aristocracy, Byron identifies himself with Horace.[53] Horace not only defines the summer and autumn of one's life as the proper time for erotic pursuits of both men and women—summer and autumn being the analogous season to puberty—but also in advocating retirement from public life as a gentlemanly pursuit of manhood, he and his Sabine farm could undermine the gendering of the separate spheres since the private life was not necessarily antithetical to manhood. In book II, ode 5, Horace notes that Lalage is not yet "ready for the obligations of a wife," and he invokes oncoming autumnal imagery to suggest it will soon be time. "Soon vari-colored autumn / will tinge for you these blackish clusters/to purple red" (Alexander 63). In his "Epistle to Augustus," Horace, moreover, urged that "what they learned erstwhile as beardless boys/ Must now be put away with other toys" (Kraemer 369). To the extent that privacy and retirement could become legitimate male pursuits, the idea of complementarity could be shown to be incoherent. Horace makes retirement from the public sphere and ironic distance suitable for masculinity. Byron thus quotes Horace, " 'Beatus ille procul!' from negotiis" (14:77): blest is he who is free from business.

In the same way that Horace deflated the epic values of warfare, replacing martial battles (*grandia*) with erotic ones, Lord Byron turns away from battle. In book I of his odes, Horace announced to Agrippa that, whereas Varius would celebrate his courage and martial achievements, "modest is the Muse who presides over my peaceful lyre,/forbidding that I praise illustrious Caesar and you, Agrippa,/diminishing them by the defect of my wit" (Ode 6, 12).[54] Horace then turns to "virgins in combat" (ode 6) and argues that this change of focus does not in any way diminish the ode. Like Horace, Byron lists military men only to claim that they are "not at all adapted to my rhymes" (1:3). Byron then considers his virgins in combat, arguing similarly that the epic form is not diminished by a turn to erotic matters considered private. As Horace claimed in his *Ars Poetica* that "Nature shapes first our inner thoughts to take the bent of circumstance" (400), so, too, does Byron insist upon the circumstantial in *Don Juan*.

But perhaps the most crucial lesson Byron would learn from Horace concerned the role and value of the middle. Byron credits Horace with having taught him that the "medias res" is the "heroic turnpike road" (1.6). Writing on love, Byron later notes the many "ways that lead there, be they near or far,/ Above, below, by turnpike great or small" (9:80). Byron sexualizes turnpikes and hints at the body's many orifices, above and below, near and far. Spatial metaphors level any moral distinctions between them; all are equally sacred. Moreover, in canto 6, stanza 17, Byron writes, "In short, the maxim for the amorous tribe is/Horatian, 'Medio tu tutissimus ibis,'" (6:17). While the line "in the middle is the safest path" comes from Ovid's *Metamorphoses*, and not Horace, the fact that Horace is now twice credited with the middle suggests that "middle" must be a kind of code. Crompton has demonstrated that among his Cambridge circle, Horace was a code for bisexuality (146). Given that the *OED* lists intermediate and intervening as possible definitions of "middle," I suggest that it encodes both puberty and bisexuality. Even in Ancient Rome, puberty not only cuts across gender with the younger male looking more feminine (C.

Edwards 78), but also if Horace defines puberty in terms of summer and autumn, puberty is literally the middle of one's life. Buffon also insisted that puberty was a middle stage between childhood and manhood. In his "Hints from Horace," Byron translated Horace's sense of the stages of one's life thusly, "Till time at length the mannish tyro weans,/And prurient vice outstrips his tardy teens!" (McGann 1: 297, lines 221–22). Byron, of course, makes Juan a mannish novice, and his coupling of tyro and weaning further suggests masculinity to be a developmental process. By converting mannishness from a noun to an adjective, he underscores that manhood is about process. "Middle" further suggests for the "amorous tribe" a position outside conventional heterosexuality: neither part of the norm nor completely outside of it. I would add that "middle" emphasizes perspective and relationality in ways that sexual acts and identities don't. The value that Byron places upon digression teases the Horatian middle beyond its decorous restraint. Hence, where Horace divides life into clear phases—for, example, beardlessness and beyond—Byron muddies the distinctions between them with phrases like "Mannish tyro."

Middle thus is code for puberty and bisexuality. By highlighting puberty, Byron is able to undermine the logic of two incommensurate sexes and suggest the costs of a mandatory heterosexuality. Thinking about bisexuality and puberty together allows Horace and Byron to insist upon change, that any rules about sexuality are contingent on the stage or season of life that the person is in. Such contingency undermines the possibility of a secure sexual or gendered identity. Puberty further suggests that bisexuality is itself natural in that in as much as the body itself moves from one sex to another, it must, like Tiresias, understand multiple sexual objects. In fact, Byron invokes Tiresias:

> There is an awkward thing, which much perplexes,
> Unless like wise Tiresias we had proved
> By turns the difference of the several sexes:
> Neither can show quite *how* they would be loved. (14:73)

Men can be like Tiresias to the extent that they recall that in puberty bodies have literally shifted from one sex to another. In getting his audience to sympathize with both the conditions of men and women, and in showing how their conditions are not necessarily mutually exclusive, Byron has been trying to get us to identify with and be like Tiresias. Because "proved" recalls Byron's own having been "proved the soft condition," Byron announced his own Tiresias-like transformations. But, whereas Tiresias was alternately man and woman,

Byron's insistence upon "several" obscures the number of sexes at the same time that it hints that even this sage's experiences might be limited. Finally, Byron underscores that despite any differences, the knowledge of the several boils down to the very same thing: "neither can show quite *how* they would be loved." The italicized "how" hints that there might be ways of love that cannot be shown. By ending his stanza with "upon whose back 'tis better not to venture" (14:73), he begins to show us what cannot be shown. Because the "how" is so various in sexual object, sexual aim, and sexual act, Byron highlights the naturalness and polymorphisms of perversity.

Although Horace insists that one must conduct oneself in ways appropriate to one's season in life, he also makes it clear that while rules may be rules, not even he, nor his ironic speakers, are immune to their infraction (Arkins 113). Thus, despite Horace's suggestion that amorousness is itself appropriate for the middle—telling Venus that he knows he is too old and "neither girls nor boys now delight" (4:1)—Horace declares that "in my nocturnal dreams I now/hold you [Ligurius] captive" (4:1). Like Horace, Byron adopts the pose of the detached viewer only to make clear that he himself is not above his own critique. Because boys and women were somewhat interchangeable objects in Roman love poetry, and because in puberty effeminate males became strong men, Horace's sense that in summer and fall a certain sexual playfulness is appropriate does not prevent him from chasing after Ligurius in his dreams even though he is in winter. That Horace refers to his "nocturnal dreams" as the time he spends chasing the cruel Ligurius connects homosexual desire once again with puberty. Nor is Byron immune from sexual behavior he satirizes. As he put it in "The Edinburgh Ladies' Petition to Doctor Moyes, and his Reply," love is "subject to no jurisdiction,/But burns the fiercer for restriction" (McGann 1:197). In Greece, Byron would soon encounter his own cruel Ligurius, Loukas Chalandritsanos, and he laments the fact that "it be my lot/To strongly—wrongly—vainly—love thee still" (cited in Gross 147). As Byron imagines it, love chafes against all forms of social restriction, even to the point of eroticizing restriction itself. He would also there encounter his own Horatian Lycus, Nicolo Giraud (see MacCarthy 129).

But Byron's Horatian code is even more specific.[55] Byron owns Richard Hurd's 1766 edition of Horace (Munby 1:219).[56] Hurd lambasted readers of Horace's epistles for not recognizing that Horace's "seeming posture of neglect and inconnexion" (ix) was really a careful method of didacticism. The "wrong explication" of it derived from "inattention to the method of it" (iii). Moreover, critics have "never looked for, or could find a consistency of disposition in the method" (iv). Method, it turns out, is a crucial term in Byron, and he used the term "*méthode*" to indicate sodomy (Crompton 1985 129, 145; Gross 136; Dyer). Seen in this light, Hurd's "inconnexion" has a decidedly sexual resonance to it, recalling Byron's illness due to too frequent connexion. If for Hurd, method is a code for a hidden didacticism that is screened by a seemingly haphazard epistolary method, for Byron, method with an "e" is a double screen for a dissident sexuality that stands outside of the usual method. Hurd wants his readers to pay attention to the unities of Horace so that method equals a kind of formalist attention. Byron, in turn, takes a method that stands for a unity, making that unity stand for puberty and the biological transition from one sex to another and for bisexuality. Hurd's formal unity thus takes on the bent of perversion because in puberty one can choose multiple sexual objects and because the very idea of unity is necessarily fractured between mobile biological states and multiple sexual objects. The *méthode*, then, of Byron's *Don Juan*, one might say, is to show that within any seeming unity are multiplicities and heterodoxa that threaten to undermine the very idea of unity. From the vantage of puberty, sex seems more of a position, a stance, a way of looking at the world, than an identity. Although *Don Juan* coheres around the idea of puberty, puberty is an unstable center that has the potential to undermine the naturalness of masculine strength and the normality of heterosexual desire.

If puberty and bisexuality provide Byron with a place to intervene in compulsory heterosexuality and gender complementarity, they also help him to see the limits of connecting sexuality with identity. Moreover, insofar as he could stand outside any one sexual identity, he could see the extent to which locating sexuality within identity was dangerous in that it allowed desire to become more effectively policed. As the law in the eighteenth century increasingly narrowed its definition of "sodomite" to capture sexual acts between men from a label that originally encompassed all forms of sex that did not lead to intercourse, it struggled to find ways of making sodomitic desire visible. The legal proof required for sodomy was both penetration and emission (Crompton 1985 21), and emission was very difficult to prove in an era before DNA testing and blue dresses. Thus, undercover agents had to resort to the lesser charge of "assault with an attempt to commit sodomy," and this could be proven by a solicitation invited by a plainclothes man who had gone to a homosexual rendezvous precisely to entrap someone (Crompton 21). Because of the need to make semen biologi-. cally present to convict for sodomy, the law turned to an effeminate identity and the molly house, collapsing male effeminacy with sodomitic desire. Trumbach documents that, although many men and boys charged with sodomy and sodomitic assault showed no conventional signs of effeminacy, they were represented as "mollies" at trial (59–62). Acts did not provide enough prosecutions. Identities did. Because the Romantic period is the one in which effeminacy is pushed closer to sodomy (Elfenbein 1999 21), proving that one was effeminate became a crucial step in proving sodomy (Trumbach 101). My point here is that, as sexual acts get consolidated into identities, perverse sexualities become more easily policed. At the same time, this condensation of desire into identity could be useful to a coterie of sodomites who could turn to an elaborate code, as Byron and his Cambridge circle did, to escape surveillance and to begin to recognize the potential for sodomitical desire in others.

Byron's example thus suggests a new approach to the acts versus identity debate in the historiography of sexuality. Rather than understanding the absence of sexual identity as an ontological given before 1869 when the word homosexual was invented, we need to think about the obstacles and disincentives to thinking about a sexual identity. Because one could not claim a homosexual identity for fear of capital punishment, this means that homophobia is almost a baseline position. To the extent that homophobia becomes a necessary screen for homoerotic desire, the presence of homophobia does not discount the presence of homophilia. Because homophobia could mask homophilia, the denial of identity can paradoxically become a claiming of it. Moreover, since puberty suggested a necessary incommensurability between biological sex and the body, not to mention gender and the body, the very idea of a stable identity based on gender and sex becomes a problem. To read gender and sex in Byron is to be reminded that, although we consider the penis and vagina to be unarguable signs of sexual difference, which in turn implies incommensurablity between the genders, the genitals then could not encapsulate difference because of the recent shift from one sex to two as well as the emphasis upon secondary sexual differentiation as real differentiation. Medical theories of the body that emphasized vitality throughout the body rather than the localization of vitality further undercut the idea that sex could be localized in the body. These gaps then imply that sexuality cannot be coextensive with identity since identity is itself inchoate during puberty. The gap between the gendered body that is clothed as masculine or feminine and the physical body that is not yet fully masculine or feminine, moreover, is a place where gender distinctions unravel. Our acceptance of genital difference as the sign of difference, then, has come at the high price of forgetting the body as a site of dynamic change.

Byron's emphasis on the middle reminds us that in the Romantic period masculinity was caught between prostitution, on the one hand, and the effeminate sodomite, on the other. Masculinity is thus caught between two poles of perversion. Byron shows that rather than being an either/or decision, one could choose both, thereby displacing the erotic couple and replacing them with triangularity. My attention to the triangulation of masculine identity that takes place within puberty, a transition that Buffon thought lasted for twenty years and one that always threatened to return further supports Marjorie Garber's point that in imagining the erotic triangle, Girard and Sedgwick reduce the erotic choices to either/or instead of both.[57] In triangulated desire, a rival's desire rather than the love object itself sets into motion a complex power dynamic that captures societal relationships of power. As a form of triangulation ontologically prior to the traffic in women, puberty allows us to see how, for example, a feminized male could legitimately choose as erotic object between another feminized male and/or a masculinized male and/or a woman (Garber *Vice Versa* 426–29). Even worse, because an effeminate male might make as his erotic object another effeminate male, especially since the effeminate male is ontologically prior to the manly male, Girard and Sedgwick occlude the fact that bisexuality constitutes the dynamics of human sexuality because that sexuality contains ambiguities and interstices. As Garber puts it, these models "prove only that the shortest distance between two points is a triangle" (*Vice Versa* 428).[58]

Triangulation also made Byron increasingly resistant to the idea of a sexual identity in part because desire for him did not seem fixed into any one kind of sexual object. Brown's sense of excitability throughout the body not only undermined the power of anatomical localization to pinpoint sexuality in the body, but it also opened the door to gender equality because structures such as the penis and clitoris were only metonymies for excitability. Of course, for sexuality to subsume identity, metonymy must enable the equation of a specific bodily part with an erotic practice and consequently an erotic practice with identity. More to the point, triangulation implies that desire is subsumed beneath a web of relationships that undermine the neat labels of homosexual or heterosexual, male, female, sodomite, and molly. To the extent that one embraced the dynamism of bodily sex, one gained the capacity to see beyond normalizing categories of sex and gender. Hence, Lord Byron not only repeatedly figures manliness as a garment, but also unexpectedly explores the positive dimensions of effeminacy. Insofar as Byron's epic frustrates purpose/teleology, it is especially fitting that he celebrates sexual acts that resist the finality of reproduction. Moreover, puberty enables him to think in terms of sexual positions that shift depending upon one's vantage point rather than in terms of sexual identities. In this way, identification can be a solvent for identity, even when that identity is aristocratic strength.

# Notes

## Introduction

1. The second edition of the *OED* makes the connection between perversion and functionlessness clear: it defines perversion as "a disorder of sexual behavior in which satisfaction is sought through channels other than those of normal heterosexual intercourse." In the eighteenth century, normal heterosexual intercourse entails intercourse with the aim of reproduction. In *The Pleasure of the Text*, Roland Barthes equates the writer's perversity to "pleasure . . . without function" (17). I discuss the differences between perversion and perversity in chapter 2. This book originated with my argument in *The Visual and Verbal Sketch in British Romanticism* that women writers turned to the propriety of the sketch to license their perversions.

2. In his *Critique of Judgment*, Kant defines the beautiful in terms of "purposiveness without purpose" (Pluhar 65). Kant explains, "there can be purposiveness without a purpose, insofar as we do not posit the causes of this form in a will, and yet can grasp the explanation of its possibility only by deriving it from a will" (Pluhar 65). My references to Kant's *CJ* are from Pluhar's edition; I have used the pagination which corresponds to the German edition.

3. Though Wollstonecraft is regularly chided for her sexual prudery, she argues for a "true voluptuousness," one that "proceeds from the mind" and takes the form of "mutual affection, supported by mutual respect" (*VRW* 316). Wollstonecraft, in particular, considers the forms of passion available to women—sensibility and modesty—and concludes that women's sensibility became mere selfishness when it was "entirely engrossed by their husbands" through ignorance (*VRW* 312). Claudia Johnson notes that Wollstonecraft in *The Wrongs of Woman* not only accepts Maria's "'voluptuousness' without a sneer but even claims 'it inspired the idea of strength of mind, rather than of body'" (165). See "Mary Wollstonecraft: Styles of Radical Maternity" in *Inventing Maternity*. By showing how Wollstonecraft entwines reading with sexual intimacy, Julie Carlson, in *England's First Family of Writers*, has hopefully put to bed Wollstonecraft's alleged prudery. She argues that Wollstonecraft, in *Wrongs of Woman* wants "sex . . . to regain its mental and imaginative features" (34).

4. Wordsworth refers to the "savage torpor" of industrialism in his "Preface to the Lyrical Ballads." As Shelley puts it, Burkean custom "maketh blind and obdurate/The loftiest hearts" (*LC* 4:9).

5. In *Shelley's Textual Seductions*, Samuel Gladden argues that Shelley explores "the dismantling of oppressive rulers by posing erotic relations as paradigms for alternative social models" (159). — Godwin ?

6. Jonathan Loesberg argues that Kant's purposiveness without purpose allows him to deal with "nature as designed without presupposing a designer" (56). See his *Return to Aesthetics*. For the influence of design in the Romantic period, see Colin Jager.

7. See Redfield's *Phantom Formations*. On the linkage between illness and aesthetics, see Lawlor, chapter 3.

8. The *OED* definitions are from the on-line *OED* cited above. These definitions are dated from the second edition of 1989. Dino Felluga argues that Victorian critics of Byron would willfully misread the poet's subversions as perversions (117). Compare *The Perversity of Poetry*. Robert Stoller simultaneously defines perversion as the "erotic form of hatred" and makes perversion critical to the preservation of families; projecting sickness onto other members preserves the whole family as a unit (216).

9. *OED* on-line, definition dated December 2005.

10. Where Dollimore's study of perversion highlights dissidence, Teresa de Lauretis foregrounds *The Practice of Love* in her main title, while perversion is shunted to the subtitle. In *Libidinal Currents*, Joseph Allen Boone rejects "Toward a Poetics and Politics of the Perverse" as his title (13–14). Although the use of perversion is deeply offensive when it describes homosexuality, my point is that this offensiveness is an indication of the ability of perversion to challenge norms. This book helps explain why homosexuality became labeled as perverted.

11. Samuel Taylor Coleridge, *The Notebooks of STC*, ed. Kathleen Coburn, 1:1637.

12. See Carlson's key *England's First Family of Writers*. Carlson argues that Wollstonecraft endorses sex with mental and imaginative features because sex without mind is, for her, libertinism (34).

13. On Coleridge and divorce, see Anya Taylor's *Erotic Coleridge: Women, Love, and the Law Against Divorce*, chapter 8. Taylor details Coleridge's advice to women friends on page 140.

14. On the importance of affect to the history of sexuality, see Andrew Elfenbein's response to the essays in "Historicizing Romantic Sexuality," in *Romantic Praxis* (January 2006), and the work of George Haggerty, particularly *Men in Love*.

15. Vernon Rosario demonstrates how French medicine began to make perverse sexual desire itself so that erotic expressions threatening to the social order could be contained. See *The Erotic Imagination: French Histories of Perversity*. In *The Perversity of Poetry*, Dino Felluga shows how romance poetry in the eighteenth century became increasingly associated with sexual perversity—especially masturbation—and this meant that Victorian critics were able to contain Byron's radical poetry under the rubric of adolescent sexual perversity. On how the colonial world required "a complex negotiation of disease and desire," see Alan Bewell, *Romanticism and Colonial Disease*, 25–26, 261–62, 268–69, and 273–75. The intersections of colonialism and sexual perversion are the focus of my forthcoming essay, "Othering Sexual Perversity: England, Empire, Race, and Sexual Science."

16. For reasons I make clear in the first chapter, I disagree with David M. Halperin's claim that "the search for a 'scientific' aetiology of sexual orientation is itself a homophobic project." See his *One Hundred Years of Homosexuality* (49).

17. I am here indebted to Thomas Pfau's "'Beyond the Suburbs of the Mind' The Political and Aesthetic Disciplining of the Romantic Body" (644–47). Pfau reminds that Malthus can vindicate sexual passion so long as pleasure is not divorced from reproduction; by making sex without reproduction a vice, his cure of temporary celibacy thus begins to look more like a vice than a virtue (642–43).

18. Clark's edition of Shelley's prose is unreliable. It is, however, the only available accessible edition of the poet's later prose.

19. "Process of materialization" is Judith Butler's term. See the introduction to *Bodies that Matter.*

20. Stuart Curran, *Shelley's Annus Mirabilis* (106–8).

21. See Annette Wheeler Caffarelli's important critique of the limits of Shelley's sexual liberation, "The Transgressive Double Standard: Shelleyan Utopianism and Feminist Social History" (88–104).

22. As Anthony Appiah frames it, "equality as a political ideal is a matter of not taking irrelevant distinctions into account. People should be treated differently, . . . because there are grounds for treating them differently" (*The Ethics of Identity* 193). Here Shelley insists that sex is not a ground for unequal treatment.

23. Ruth Perry links the rise of the Gothic novel in England to a rise in incest. She points to how an "increasingly contractual nature of property relations supplanted older understanding based on lineal relations in both maternal and paternal lines" (271). The emotional power of consanguinity in Gothic novels was a reassertion of blood ties over law. See her "Incest as the Meaning of the Gothic Novel" (261–68). In "Rethinking Romantic Incest: Human Universals, Literary Representation, and the Biology of Mind," Alan Richardson wonders why Romantic sibling incest is at once idealized and yet ends so tragically. He posits that the Romantics anticipated Westermarck's hypothesis that growing up in proximity made siblings sexually unattractive. I would suggest that Shelley recognizes that if living in proximity undermines eroticism, then marriage cannot be a durable form of caring. Shelley's description of Laon and Cythna's growing up together does not inhibit their passion. Nor does Richardson take into account Shelley's reading in Zoroastrianism, which equated incest with the highest form of sex. Finally, the fact that their relationship ends badly has more to do with Shelley's sense of the cycle of history than it does with their incest. Indeed, within a Zoroastrian framework the death of the lovers is the first step to the resurrection of the world. In canto 12:38, for example, Shelley's reference to the "Sun, Moon, and moonlike lamps, the progeny of a diviner Heaven" recalls the Zoroastrian belief that the sun and moon were in fact generated by the incestuous union of Ur and Ruha. Occurring after the death of the lovers, this insistence upon cosmological incest frustrates Richardson's argument. On Zoroastrianism, see R. C. Zaehner, The *Teachings of the Magi: A Compendium of Zoroastrian Beliefs* (65).

24. As Geraldine Friedman puts it, "The asexual interpretation of romantic friendship functions as a closet for same-sex sexuality between women and does not so much so much deny women's sexual agency as subject it to preterition" (62). See her "School for Scandal: Sexual, Race, and National Vice and Virtue in *Miss Marianne Woods and Miss Jane Pirie Against Lady Helen Cumming Gordon*" (53–76).

25. I am here indebted to de Lauretis's point that "lesbian desire . . . is constituted against a fantasy of castration" (261).

26. See his preface to "Romanticism and Sexual Vice," a special issue of *Nineteenth-Century Contexts* (March 2005).

27. Elfenbein, *Romantic Genius: Towards a Prehistory of a Homosexual Role.*

28. This is Jonathan Loesberg's point. See *A Return to Aesthetics* (184).

29. Thus, for example, Jean Hagstrum's *Romantic Body* neglects science and medicine;

Nathaniel Brown's *Sexuality and Feminism in Shelley* treats sexuality as a timeless entity; and William Ulmer's sense of eroticism in Shelley is a deconstructive one. Compare *Shelleyan Eros*.

30. See Lee Edelman, *No Future: Queer Theory and the Death Drive* (13). For Edelman, "Queerness exposes sexuality's inevitable coloration by the drive: its insistence on repetition, its stubborn denial of teleology, its resistance to determinations of meaning" (27). Although I applaud his critique of how children are elided with futurity, I suggest that instead of giving up on the future, we embrace purposiveness, especially since the form of purposiveness does not automatically assume any liberation has been achieved. When Edelman defines homosexuality as that which "leads to no good and has no other end than an end to the good as such" (cited in Nyong'o 115), he might have relinquished reproductive futurity, but he does not relinquish purposiveness. Furthermore, whereas Edelman, following Bersani, links *jouissance* to antirelationality, to a self-shattering that undermines all forms of sociality, the Romantics idealize *jouissance* in terms of mutually purposive pleasure. For them, if that *jouissance* leads to self-shattering, such shattering demands unification. Bersani might respond that purposiveness amounts to a degaying of gayness, a risk that has the advantage of inviting thought about the consequences of any particular form of sexuality. See *Homos*. In *The Culture of Redemption*, Leo Bersani reminds us that "the corrective virtue of works of art depends on a misreading of art as philosophy" (2). I would reply that the Romantics assert the redemptive potential of art even when they are deeply skeptical of it. Their ability to regard even perverse sexuality as a form that may or may not lead to redemption reminds us of their wariness of the gaps between art and philosophy. Bersani himself credits the aesthetic with the possibility of critique when he claims that "art may reinstate a curiously disinterested mode of desire for objects, a mode of excitement that, far from investing objects with symbolic significance, would enhance their specificity and thereby fortify their resistance to the violence of symbolic intent" (*CR* 28). Tavia Nyong'o offers an important critique of Edelman's and Bersani's reliance and misunderstanding of antirelationality. For Nyong'o, the self-shattering of the ego in *jouissance* is not antirelationality at all since it depends upon Lacan's notion that sexual relationships are structured by a third term, the other. "There is, in other words, a relationship, but not just the one we believe there to be. I make this point to clarify that the virtues and faults of antirelationality lie in nothing so simple as the metaphysical question of whether society, the future, or relationality 'exists' but, rather, in what the theory enables us to grasp of a reality that can never truly be grasped" (113).

31. My phrasing here deliberately recalls Elizabeth Grosz's: "becoming-lesbian . . . is thus no longer or not simply a question of being-lesbian, of identifying with that being known as a lesbian, of residing in a position or identity . . . the question is . . . what kinds of lesbian connections, . . . we invest ourselves in" (*Space, Time Perversion*, 71).

32. Heather Love, *Feeling Backward: Loss and the Politics of Queer History*. My use of "waste products" is indebted to Love (71). While studies of perversion must engage the very backward feelings Love argues that queer theory has abjected, I note that Love, unlike myself, wants to think about a future without the "promise of redemption" (147). Love is blind to how denial can be a form of refusal, and refusal becomes much more difficult to include as a form of politics when it encompasses denial.

33. Jonathan David Gross, *Byron: The Erotic Liberal*.

34. Helen Bruder, *William Blake and the Daughters of Albion*.

35. Jerome Christensen, for example, argues that liberation is constrained in Byron

by regionalism and by the fact that the "liberation of homosexual desire is not a final break with a prior repression" (54–55). See *Lord Byron's Strength*. I suggest that, since liberation itself is a negation of power, not liberty, the concept does not necessarily imply even the possibility of a final break. Christensen's argument that nothing happened in England is undercut by Byron's famous letter of June 22, 1809, to Charles Skinner Matthews. The poet writes, "I do not think Georgia itself can emulate in capabilities or incitements to the 'Plen.and optabil.——Coit,' the port of Falmouth & parts adjacent,——We are surrounded by Hyacinths & other flowers of the most fragrant [na]ture, & I have some intention of culling a handsome Bouquet to compare with the exotics we expect to meet in Asia" (*BLJ* 1:207).

36. The phrase is Alan Richardson's. See "Romanticism and the Colonization of the Feminine."

ONE: Romantic Science and the Perversification of Sexual Pleasure

1. I have delivered versions of this argument at the National Library of Medicine's History of Medicine Seminar, the Wordsworth Conference in Grasmere, the Queer Romanticism Conference in Dublin, the Clark Library's "Vital Matters" Conference, and the MLA annual convention. For advice and encouragement, I thank especially Jim Mays, Michael O'Rourke, Alan Richardson, Mike Sappol, Helen Deutsch, Susan Staves, and George Haggerty. Jerome McGann's *The Romantic Ideology* has been influential in its thesis that Romantic poets offered transcendence in the place of meaningful social change. On Romantic eroticism as liberation in particular, see Hagstrum, Brown, and Frosch. But no one to my knowledge has tried to understand fully how the sciences of sexuality shape Romanticism's incipient sexual liberation: Hagstrum's "body" is emphatically not medical, and Brown ascribes to a timeless sexuality. For more on Romantic sexuality, see, among others, Binhammer, Porter and Hall, Porter, Crompton, Clarke, Dyer, Elfenbein, Felluga, Gilman, Hitchcock, Hobson, O'Donnell and O'Rourke, Rousseau, Sha, and Trumbach. See also my two edited collections of essays on Romanticism and sexuality, one for *Romanticism on the Net* 21 (2001) and another on historicizing Romantic sexuality for *Romantic Praxis* (2006). Last, but not least, see Michael O'Rourke and David Collings's "Queer Romanticism," a special double issue of *Romanticism on the Net* (2004–5).

2. Foucault defines biopower as a deployment of power at the level of life. Its two procedures of power are an "anatamo-politics of the human body"—the making of the body as a useful machine—and a species-level biopolitics of population (*HS* 1:139–41). In this chapter, I want to throw a wrench into the notion of biopower by highlighting the ways in which scientists were fascinated by functionlessness and by foregrounding the general skepticisms within science itself. In other words, science then could think of itself as a game of truth. Foucault's emphasis on how science structures knowledge, constituting objects as knowledge, makes him unable to see its liberating possibilities.

3. As Binhammer argues, "The opposition of conservative and radical masks the intricate and important ways in which this very opposition manufactured a consensus around female sexuality and gender" (410). For this reason, I think that apprehending science through a Kantian lens of purposiveness without purpose helps us to see the radical and conservative possibilities in sex.

4. We would do well to remember David Knight's caution that "the historian, rather

than searching for parallels which might indicate influences, should perhaps content himself [*sic*] with expositions, and might be well advised to explore the way in which certain terms . . . were employed in the thirty years or so [on] either side of 1800" (*Science in the Romantic Era* 79). Likewise, George Rousseau argues that neurology was everywhere in eighteenth-century culture; it had a kind of bedrock influence.

5. Cited in Owsei Temkin, "Basic Science, Medicine, and the Romantic Era," 106.

6. Hilde Hein elucidates strands of vitalism, one that insisted upon a separate vital principle irreducible to structure and later another strand that stressed structural and organizational differences between the living and the nonliving. See her "The Endurance of the Mechanism: Vitalism Controversy," 169.

7. In John Abernethy's hands, vitalism could be fundamentally conservative. See Sharon Ruston, *Shelley and Vitality* (41–49).

8. On this shift, see Lisa Forman Cody, *Birthing the Nation* (21). This paragraph is indebted to Cody.

9. On vitalism and chemistry, see Reill, chap. 2.

10. To the extent that plant sexuality allegorized human sexuality, "sexuality" has existed ever since Cowper used it in 1800 to refer to plant sexuality. Botany, therefore, plays a crucial, if underacknowledged, role in the history of sexuality.

11. Hein points out that the mechanists too believed in the purposiveness of living things. "The concept of purposiveness is in this application purely formal, a category without content . . . no particular purpose is consciously intended" (161). Nonetheless where mechanism made actions predictable because they conformed to the physical laws of the universe, vitalism suggested that life could be in defiance of the laws affecting matter. The Romantics found mechanism to be too deterministic.

12. See Maurice Florence's (alias Foucault) take on Foucault's history of sexuality in Faubion, ed. (463).

13. Foucault develops the concept of biopower at the close of the introduction to his *History of Sexuality* (139–41). He tellingly argues that the shift from mechanism to vitalism was superficial, "surface effects" of a deeper shift, one that moved away from displayed descriptability as knowledge and toward inner biological laws that organize relations between functions and organs. See his *Order of Things* (232, 237). In severing life from theology and in replacing it with principle or structure, vitalism made it possible for biological law to support republicanism and reciprocity of relationship instead of autocracy.

14. Peter Reill argues that vitalism is epistemologically modest. I do wonder how much of it is modesty and how much of it is a reliance upon metaphysics or a papering over of difficulties.

15. This point is made by James Larson in *Interpreting Nature* (157).

16. Quoted from the Huntington Library, uncataloged manuscript of William Hunter's "Two Introductory Lectures" (95). I thank Dan Lewis for making it available to me.

17. On the abuses of sociobiology, see Sahlins, *The Use and Abuse of Biology*, and Lancaster, *The Trouble with Nature*. Sahlins laments that sociobiology relies upon a reductive isomorphism between behavioral traits and social relations (14). The resurgence of interest in science and Romanticism suggests that humanists are beginning to put aside their unreflective hostility to science. Lancaster attacks "innatist claims about humans'

sexual orientation" because they are "not a legitimate scientific interest" (15). But what if innatist claims could explain flexibility?

18. David Halperin has recently shown how Foucault never meant to make rigid distinctions between sexual acts and sexual identities. See his *How To Do the History of Homosexuality*. Hence my attention to sexual subjectivities. I argue that alterity has become a postmodern form of objectivity, using Halperin and Percy Shelley's notions of ancient Greek sex, in my "The Use of Abuse of Alterity."

19. Other influential such readings besides Davidson's that make the Romantic period one of sex and not sexuality include Porter, "Perversion in the Past," Bristow, *Sexuality*, and Halperin, *How to Do the History of Homosexuality*.

20. Following Richardson and Temkin (1977), I take Romantic science to refer to an insistent collapse of mind and body dualism, a recognition of the mind as an active agent as opposed to being a passive object to be inscribed upon, and an attention to the physiology of sensibility as a counter to rationalism. Poggi insists that "a first characteristic common to all lines of thinking of the Romantic period is the postulation of the existence of an opposition of two fundamental forces within the organism—sensibility versus irritability; electricity versus magnetism" (42). David M. Knight calls the nineteenth century "the age of science" because "those engaged in the sciences took pains to make the world aware of their work and its implications (*Age of Science* 6). In *Science in the Romantic Era*, Knight links Romantic science to "concern with the processes of life" (54), a concern with "the imagination's role in art and science" (83), "an opposition to mechanical explanations" (88), and an attitude toward science in which it "is fitted into a complete frameworks including all other knowledge" (90). Robert Richards defines Romantic biologists (German only) as having synthesized teleological judgment and aesthetic judgment, and this meant that "the aesthetic comprehension of the entire organism or of the whole interacting natural environment would be a necessary preliminary stage in the scientific analysis of respective parts" (12–14). See also Hermione de Almeida's detailed study, *Romantic Medicine and John Keats*. Among the surprising claims she develops is how Romantic vitality leads to a physiological mechanism. See pages 102–5 especially. On perversification as a powerful French political rhetorical strategy, see Rosario, *The Erotic Imagination*. Rosario credits the late eighteenth century until World War I with the emergence of modern eroticism (the components of which are individualist subjectivity, medico-legal matters, nationalist rivalries, and consumer culture). Modern eroticism led to the emergence of the "sexually perverse" as the objects of "focused biomedical attention" (11).

21. For more on this, see my "Medicalizing the Romantic Libido: Luxury, Sexual Pleasure, and the Public Sphere."

22. My remarks here are indebted to Jonathan Dollimore's concept of the "paradoxical perverse." See his *Sexual Dissidence*, especially part 5.

23. See Coleridge's abundant medical writings in *Shorter Works and Fragments;* the collection of essays, *Samuel Taylor Coleridge and the Sciences of Life;* Coleridge's essay on life; and Martin Wallen's *City of Health, Fields of Disease*.

24. On anatomy lectures as a form of public entertainment in the early eighteenth century, see Anita Guerrini. On the popularity of Gall and Spurzheim, see Cooter.

25. On the connections between radicalism, electricity, and science, see also Fulford, "Radical Medicine and Romantic Politics." For a counter view, see David Knight, who

insists that "scientists tend to be conservative, preferring a firm government that will let them get on with their work" (*Age of Science* 12).

26. In a letter to me dated June 1999, Ray Stephanson insists upon Haller's uncertainty regarding erections and their relation to the will. Although it is true that Haller links the penis and breast nipple to sensibility—and only later, in his *Dissertations*, does he connect them to irritability as well—I want to emphasize here that Haller's connecting of the genitals to the brain/soul opens the door to a more strategic sexual liberation, a liberation different from the knee-jerk libertine rejection of religion and state authority. Stephanson argues in *The Yard of Wit* that "noteworthy in Haller's formulations is that the will has no direct access to or control over erection, although he does not say what part of the mind does" (71). He also makes the key point that for Whytt irritability depended upon sensibility: "bodily mechanism was ultimately informed by a soul which was in turn coextensive with the body and nervous system" (70). Despite the ambiguous relation of sexual desire to the will, an ambiguity that crops up again and again in the Romantic period, the fact that sex is thought to take place in the head and not in the genitals by the end of the eighteenth century makes it more proximate to rational control.

27. On the Hunter brothers, see *William Hunter and the Eighteenth-Century Medical World*, edited by Bynum and Porter. Hunter underscores the mind's role in male impotence in his *Treatise on the Venereal Disease*. Hunter shows quite clearly that sex and personality have come together in the Romantic period and that sexuality has emerged before the advent of sexology. See also chaps. 1, 7, and 8 of de Almeida. De Almeida rightly claims that "Hunter's genius loomed very large over the clinical medicine of England and France during the Romantic period" (32).

28. Angus McClaren argues that the condom had little role in the decline of fertility because it was used primarily against venereal disease. See his *History of Contraception* (157–58).

29. Thomas Laqueur argues that gender had "no part" in research on germ substances during the Romantic period (*Making Sex* 174–75). While he insists that debates about preformation as opposed to epigenesis were based on metaphysical principles and the politics of sciences rather than on gender, he does concede, relying on Roe, that animaculists wanted to "base some claim about gender on the nature of the sperm and egg" (n. 61, 286). I am arguing that Spallanzani's distinction between feminine motion and masculine life can only be explained by gender. I thank Laqueur for his careful reading of this chapter and for his warm encouragement of it. For more on Spallanzani, see Pinto-Correia, *The Ovary of Eve* and Capanna, "Lazzaro Spallanzani: At the Roots of Modern Biology."

30. I have checked the translation against the original Italian text, *Dissertazioni di Fisica Animale, e Vegetabile dell' Abate Spallanzani* (Tomo II, 2:161).

31. On artificial insemination in the eighteenth century, see also Poynter, "Hunter, Spallanzani, and the History of Artificial Insemination."

32. I quote from the National Library of Medicine MS B 967 vi, William Cruickshank and Matthew Baillie's "Lectures on Anatomy" located at the National Library of Medicine, Bethesda, Maryland. The manuscript is not numbered, but this quotation appears after "Physiology," toward the end of volume 1.

33. On nerves, see works by Rousseau, Logan, Oppenheim, Felluga, and Sha. In *Making Sex*, Laqueur argues that in the nineteenth century, with the rise of the science

of pathology, "sexual pleasure . . . lost its place in the new medical science" (188). His emphasis on how orgasm is used to define sexual difference makes him unable to account for how sexual pleasure could be seen as liberating. More recently, Laqueur argues that Haller's notion of sensibility helped to provide a "framework for moral physiology" (*Solitary Sex* 206). I return to Laqueur in chap. 3.

34. The Wellcome Library has manuscript letters of Spurzheim, Gall's former dissectionist, from the period of his London residence. Spurzheim announces that he will perform a brain dissection at Dr. Hunter's lecture room on Portland Street (MS 7636). Spurzheim was very concerned about his seeming materialism. On 2 July 1827, Spurzheim writes a long letter to Mrs. Rich Smith, who had written to him because she was concerned about his salvation (Wellcome MS 7636 #4). He apologizes for his "not being able to speak of the influence of Phrenology on religion" and insists that he "feel[s] warmly for the Sublime doctrine of pure Christianity," although he laments the fact that "religion is [now] a trade." He concludes the letter, "You may allways [*sic*] perceive my hesitation to decide in doubtful questions, and to leave the decision to every one's conscience in order not to trouble peace on earth and good will towards each other." John van Wyhe has recently argued that although scholars have generally accepted phrenology as a science of moral reform, it was, in fact, only a science of "personal authority." Wyhe insists that "his language of reform was a hollow bid for recognition. Spurzheim was never involved in social reforms, founded no schools or asylums, and took no part in political life in Britain, Germany, France or the USA" (322). Spurzheim's careful positioning on the subject of sexual perversion—eroticism need not lead to parenting, but propagation should be taught—makes it possible to think about sexuality as a category that can liberate from social repression, but Wyhe is right to caution us against assuming that his language of reform is more than rhetoric. Spurzheim's above letter also is ambivalent about reform: while religion is a trade, he ends the letter by saying essentially can't we all just get along?

35. See Wellcome MS 5323, "Notes on Phrenological Lectures by F. J. Gall, taken at Paris in 1810," taken by James Roberton, a Paris-based doctor. Gall claims he would have named an "organ of sodomy," but he considers it "merely a consequence of the excess of organization" of the organ of propagation (69, 79). The connection between strangling and erection is detailed on page 82. Gall further claims that "idiots are often addicted to self-pollution. Idiotism is not a consequence of this vice" (80).

36. The Latin reads, "et primis etaim ab incunabulis tenduntur seapius puerorum penes, amore nodum expergefacto" (1:46). My thanks to Michael North for this translation.

37. In *The Sexual Brain*, Simon LeVay uses the fact that the anus is littered with nerves to assert that it is a sexual organ. Darwin is perhaps part of the genealogy of such an argument.

38. According to Hera Cook, "The English did not even begin to develop the knowledge and means of effective direct control of their fertility until the publication of information about contraception began in the 1820s" (41). I would insist that one could only develop such knowledge when it was possible to imagine a split between sexual pleasure and reproduction. Cook notes that Place probably got his information from France through Robert Owen, who returned from France in 1818 with the sponge and knowledge of withdrawal (55).

39. For more on Botany, see Bewell, King-Hele, McNeil, Kelley, Teute, Schiebinger, and Shteir. Teute names Erasmus Darwin as the editor of *Families of Plants*. On Erasmus Darwin's radicalism, see McNeil, especially chaps. 3 and 4.

40. Pornotopia is Steven Marcus's term. See his *The Other Victorians* (268–71).

41. At his seminar on Romantic Natural History at the 2006 annual meeting of the North American Society for the Study of Romanticism, Alan Bewell argued that Erasmus Darwin's contribution to sexuality was his attempt to reimagine bodies that would be commensurate with a polymorphous sexual desire. This suggestive reading pushes Darwinian sexuality outside the orbit of heterosexuality and into the perverse.

42. Gad Horowitz pointedly asks, "Aren't the radical Foucaultians, in spite of their official policy of rejecting sexual liberationism, asserting a special version of it that proclaims that there is no such thing as sexual repression, and it can't be abolished, but we should resist it as hard as we can, without ever calling it repression?" (69).

43. Foucault himself succinctly captured his project in *The History of Sexuality*. Using the pseudonym Maurice Florence, Foucault described his goal as "a matter of analyzing 'sexuality' as a historically singular mode of experience in which the subject is objectified for himself and for others through certain specific procedures of 'government'" (*Essential Works* 2:465). Foucault's pseudonym allows the subject (himself) to become the object of discourse: the philosopher who warned us of the perils of the subject and subjectivity can thus de-anthropomorphize himself. The "dead" author thereby brilliantly transforms himself into discourse.

44. On this line, see Susan Wolfson, "The Strange Difference of Female 'Experience'" (266).

45. In the 1761 *Lex Coronatoria; Or, The Office and Duty of Coroners*, Edward Umfreville, Coroner for Middlesex, lists "sodomites and monstrous births and other matters [as] said to be inquirable of, by the coroner" (I:lxi).

46. See my "Uses and Abuses of Historicism: Halperin and Shelley on the Otherness of Ancient Greek Sexuality."

47. For more on what has been called moral hedonism, see Foot, "Locke, Hume, and Modern Moral Theory."

48. In "The Transgressive Double Standard: Shelleyan Utopianism and Feminist Social History," Annette Wheeler Cafarelli shows how women who tried to espouse the "sexual ideology of Romantic men" paid a heavy price. As I will argue in subsequent chapters, that the Romantics could see the sexed body as an allegory for power meant that they could also see the price of their gender attitudes. Male Romantic emphasis on female sexual expression should be placed in context of the fact that "women had no right to sexual autonomy" (Cook 3). In *A History of Bisexuality*, Steven Angelides comments that Foucault does not situate himself outside of the deployment of sexuality because he refuses sex and sexuality and experiences the delights of nonidentity only by "assum[ing] the masculinist position of self-possessing subject" (160).

TWO:  Historicizing Perversion

1. William Coleman documents the origin of the term "biology" around 1800. In 1802, Lamarck defined biology as "one of the three divisions of terrestrial physics; it includes all which pertains to living bodies and particularly to their organization, their de-

velopmental processes, the structural complexity resulting from prolonged action of vital movements, the tendency to create special organs and to isolate them by focusing activity in a center, and so on" (2). By 1820, the term biology had gained currency (1). Coleman reminds us that in the Romantic period biology had not yet emancipated itself from medicine (3).

2. Canguilhem makes the important point that Brown's distinction between sthenic and asthenic diseases "undermined all existing nosologies, yet paradoxically, the dearth of therapeutic possibilities led to an enlargement of the pharmacopoeia" (1988, 43).

3. The Romantic period then reinforces connections between Foucault's sense of sexuality as power (vol. 1 of the *History of Sexuality*) and his emphasis upon sex as an aesthetics of the self in volume 3, *The Care of the Self*. Foucault's critics have long debated the reasons for the seeming rift between the two ways of thinking about sexuality. To the degree that volume 1 is about the forms that power takes and volume 3 is about the aesthetics of the self, Foucault consistently frames sexuality as a form of aesthetics. One limitation of Sharon Ruston's otherwise helpful study, *Shelley and Vitality*, is that she does not adequately consider why Shelley might have misgivings about vitalism insofar as strands of it insisted upon a radical dualism between matter and life.

4. Canguilhem's notion of scientific ideology is fruitful here. He defines this term as "explanatory systems that stray beyond their own borrowed norms of scientificity" (1988 38). To the extent that localization is contingent upon knowledge of the organ or system—it is not productive to localize a disease into something one knows little about—localization is an important scientific means of fostering traffic between the known and unknown. Broussais, for example, knows much about the digestive tract and thus makes it the origin of disease itself. Insofar as diseases stray beyond the digestive system, Broussais can be seen to be fostering a scientific ideology. Canguilhem continues, "Scientific ideology is not to be confused with false science, magic or religion. Like them, it derives its impetus from an unconscious need for direct access to the totality of being, but it is a belief that squints at an already instituted science whose prestige it recognizes and whose style it seeks to imitate" (ibid.). Clarke and Jacyna clarify the concept of localization of brain function. Haller believed in the unitary theory of brain action, by which no localization of specific brain functions to individual regions was possible. Pierre Flourens claimed that the morphologically separate divisions of the brain—cerebellum, medulla oblongata—were functionally distinct, although each contributed to the brain's total energy. Third, various subdivisions of the brain had specific discrete functions (212–13).

5. By contrast, Blumenbach thought that "man alone is destitute of instincts, that is, certain congenital faculties for protecting himself from internal injury, and or seeking nutritious food, &c (*Anthropological Treatises* 82). In *The Future of the Brain*, neuroscientist Steven Rose notes that "the ethologist Pat Bateson has pointed out that the term 'instinct' covers at least nine conceptually different ideas, including those of: being present at birth (or at a particular stage of development; not learned; developed in advance of use; unchanged once developed; shared by all members of the species (or the same sex and age); served by a distinct neural module; and/or arising as an evolutionary adaptation. The problem with all of these—not necessarily mutually exclusive—senses of the word is that they lack explanatory power. Rather, they assume what they set out to explain, that is, an autonomous developmental sequence" (114).

6. There is no entry under "instinct" in Bartholomew Parr's 1809 *The London Medical*

*Dictionary; Including under Distinct Heads Every Branch of Medicine.* Instinct is not even in the index. Nor is there an entry under instinct in G. Motherby's 1801 *A New Medical Dictionary.* Although this might suggest a resistance of medicine to instinct, one must be cautious not to overread two absences. Whereas Foucauldians might respond that this proves the localization of sexuality to the instincts has not yet occurred, the fact is that discussions of instinct in the Romantic period, as does Smellie, often address sexuality in the guise of the instinct of love.

7. In Coleridge's annotations to Shakespeare's sonnets, he insists upon the chaste and pure love of Shakespeare. The crime that dare not speak its name "seems never to have entered even his Imagination. It is noticeable, that not even an Allusion to that very worst of all possible Vices (for it is wise to think of the Disposition, as a vice, not of the absurd & despicable Act, as a crime)" (*Marginalia* 1:42–43). Coleridge's sanitizing of Shakespeare must be placed in context of the fact that Shakespeare was made perverse in the 1790s; with the identification of the male addressee of the sonnets, Shakespeare became a potential sodomite. See Carlson, "Forever Young" (579). Likewise, Coleridge insists on the purity of the Greeks with regard to boys: those "suspected [of] Love of Desires against Nature" were "cursed."

8. Smith's "The wheat-ear" appeared in her *Conversations Introducing Poetry* (1804) and is reprinted in Stuart Curran's edition of her poems.

9. Whereas many read this text as a Thomsonian jeremiad for liberty, Robert Gleckner argues that *Edward the Third* is not without irony, and he reads the character William as the surrogate for Blake in the play. Gleckner's reading then supports a positive valence to instinct here.

10. See Hilde Hein's important article, "The Endurance of the Mechanism: Vitalism Controversy," which argues that both mechanism and vitalism sought to understand life in terms of purposiveness rather than purpose (161).

11. For more on Monstrosity in the Romantic period, see Paul Younquist's important study. While I agree that the singularity of monsters "disappears into the normative truth of physiological function" (21), I think that this tells only part of the story. Youngquist underestimates in my view the beholdeness of physiology to perversity or monstrosity. Moreover, he does not pay sufficient attention to how scientists sought to normalize monsters; nor does he acknowledge the plethora of proper bodies in the period. Appel makes clear the political stakes of the differences between Cuvier and Geoffroy. Cuvier "feared that speculative theories . . . would be exploited in the name of science and undermine religion and promote social unrest" (52–53).

12. On the pathology of the imagination, see George Rousseau's essay on the imagination reprinted in *Nervous Acts.*

13. I am grateful to Stuart Peterfreund for urging my attention to Bell's later treatise.

14. Clarke and Jacyna argue that Gall "remained skeptical of a universal correlation between mental processes and mental topography, and believed that an acceptable association could be found in only a small number of individuals, who possessed particularly well-developed 'organs'" (223–24).

15. Fancher attributes this term to Freud (380).

16. That Freud speaks of language in terms of a "verbal residue" implies that even language is being localized in the brain tissues (23–24). Likewise his phrase "tissue of memory" provides an anatomical basis for his concept.

THREE: One Sex or Two?

1. In the June 2003 issue of *Isis,* Michael Stolberg challenged Laqueur's claim that the idea of incommensurable sexual difference was a product of the eighteenth century. Stolberg argues that such a model began in the 1600s, and he points to illustrations of the female genitals and skeleton of the Renaissance to prove his case. Laqueur responded that Stoller's cases had "minimal impact" and that stray examples do not undermine world views. More crucially, Laqueur argues that, in the Enlightenment, "biology as opposed to metaphysics became foundational" (*Isis* 306). The Romantic period is so interesting precisely because it wavers between the foundations of biology and metaphysics. Stolberg's objections were reinforced by Wendy D. Churchill, who demonstrates that doctors treated women differently from 1600–1740, based on their sex and age, which was itself linked to physiological changes in the sexed body. See her "Medical Practice of the Sexed Body" (3–22). Karen Harvey suggests that the kind of cultural history that Laqueur writes is better equipped to deal with the synchronic as opposed to the diachronic; her study of pornography and erotica in the eighteenth century reveals his linear chronology to have underestimated synchrony (7). My point is two-fold: that since the debate between the models was not yet resolved in the Romantic period, sex could become the groundwork for liberation; furthermore, because puberty suggested that sexual dimorphism unfolded diachronically but universally, sexual difference is diachronic even within Romanticism at the same time it is erected upon the foundation of one sex.

2. G. J. Barker-Benfield notes that "the promise that the new psychoperceptual paradigm [of sensibility] held for women's equal mental development was recognized immediately" (xvii).

3. My framing of this issue is indebted to Eve Kosofsky Sedgwick, *The Epistemology of the Closet* (45–47).

4. Offen demonstrates that we have been too quick to separate feminism and the Enlightenment along with feminism and the French Revolution. She reminds us how serious the challenge to male aristocracy was in the eighteenth century, calling attention to actual petitions for women's citizenship among other things in the Revolution. See particularly her chaps. 2 and 3. It was only when domesticity became synonymous with public utility (around 1793) that the cause for women's citizenship was doomed (58–61). Susan Wolfson is far less sanguine about the French Revolution's attention to gender. See *Borderlines* (5–9).

5. On women's genitals as the inverse of men's see Laqueur, *Making Sex,* chap. 3.

6. Bruno Latour analyzes how science relies upon black boxes to do its conceptual work. See his *Science in Action* (2–7).

7. Andrew Elfenbein shows how effeminacy and sodomy are closely aligned in the Romantic period in *Romantic Genius.* I am suggesting that sodomites and effeminates were really a third sex in the Romantic period, not a third gender as Randolph Trumbach argues.

8. See Jonathan Dollimore, *Sexual Dissidence* (especially 101–30).

9. John Keats attended Astley Cooper's lecture on the nerves while he was training at Guy's Hospital. Keats's *Anatomical and Physiological Note Book* mentions that "we need not say any thing about the sympathy between the Breast and the uterus. Upon this most of the diseases of the Body depend" (57). It is hard to reconcile this statement with

Cooper's "nine-tenths of surgical diseases we meet with are in the Male Organs of Generation" (Wellcome MS 7096). The Wellcome notes were taken by Robert Pughe at almost precisely the same time that Keats is at St. Guy's Hospital: 1815–17. That Cooper restricts his comments to "surgical disease" in the second example may account for the difference.

10. When John Brown describes the causes of menstruation as being an increased excitability brought on by the awakening of sexual desire in puberty, his system offers much more ambiguous results for the cause of sexual equality. Menstruation depends upon the venereal emotion: the more women have sexual desires, the more they menstruate. Too little menstruation leads to chlorosis, a debilitating disease. The remedy is "gratification in love" (1:199). See volume 1:185–99. On the one hand, this naturalizes female sexual desire. On the other hand, too much excitability leads to disease, and menstruation becomes a visual sign of sexual desire. Christopher Lawrence has made the important point that Brown's theories were not essentially radical, that they were appropriated by radicals and conservatives alike. Again, my point is not to make any medical theory essentially radical or conservative; rather, I want to call attention to the radical potentiality of medical theories, and I do so because Foucauldian accounts have neglected these radical possibilities.

11. I develop these issues in my "Medicalizing the Romantic Libido" (41–46 in the *Nineteenth-Century Contexts* version and in paragraphs 30–36 of the *Romanticism on the Net* version).

12. In his forward to Peter Logan's *Nerves and Narratives*, Roy Porter comments that "the nervous narrative was automatically considered feminine, even when [it was] associated with males" (xiii). What interests me about nervous narratives, by contrast, is their potential to disrupt gender codes by making sex a tenuous ground for gender. Logan comments that "the new nervous medicine continued to associate the female body with a greater susceptibility to nervous disorders by ascribing to it a nervous system more impressionable than that of the male body" (23). But even this is to make sexual difference a matter of degree, not kind. Difference of degree undermines the idea of sexual complementarity. That Logan's history of nerves is in service of a cultural history of hysteria perhaps blinds him to the radical potential of nerves in the nineteenth century. Barker-Benfield credits the novel with diffusing a nerve-paradigm in the eighteenth century (15). Although I find much of what Adriana Craciun has to offer about how Robinson and Wollstonecraft revalue women in terms of strength helpful, I note that she does not link this redefinition to neurology (see her chap. 2). Wollstonecraft exploits a common nervous body to undermine sexual complementarity. I agree with Craciun's point that Robinson and Wollstonecraft saw inequality as preceding and constituting corporeal difference (68) and that both turned to mental strength as a demand that women's political agency not be confined to the domestic sphere (60). In my treatment of Wollstonecraft and nerves, I argue against Michelle Faubert, who insists that Wollstonecraft represents feminine sensibility as an affliction of female madness. Faubert does point out that Wollstonecraft in her letters presents herself as a victim of disturbed feminine sensibility (139). Although I recognize that the nerves eventually became a way to discipline femininity, I am interested in the potential of the neurology in the Romantic period to heal the Cartesian rift, and thus ameliorate the gender divide. This potential, I believe, accounts for Wollstonecraft's redefinition of female strength as mental and bodily. I also want to question Logan's argument that Wollstonecraft articulates a "separate social role

for woman that is founded on biological difference but is no longer limited by a disabling sexuality" (70).

13. See, for example, George Rousseau's "Nerves, Spirits, and Fibres," which argues that Thomas Willis gave rise to "a radically new assumption . . . about man's essentially nervous nature" (150). According to Claudia Johnson, "men's natural superiority in point of physical strength was hardly a matter of consensus in the political theory of the seventeenth and eighteenth centuries" (40). For an extended mediation on how Wollstonecraft can help us to reconfigure the relationships between Romanticism and gender, see Orrin Wang, *Fantastic Modernity* (110–25). I agree with Wang that Wollstonecraft allows "gender assignation [to] operate as localized semantic moments, dependent on the situational strategy of a fluid political polemic" (126). I would add that such mobile gender assignation is due to the mobility of sexual difference. Finally, unlike Paul Youngquist, who insists that the body is idealism's albatross, and thus paradoxically reads Wollstonecraft's emphasis on women's physical fitness as a form of "bodily independence" (152), I insist that Wollstonecraft takes advantage of nervous embodiment to redefine the parameters of the body, not to leave it behind. I find much more helpful his sense that Wollstonecraft "challenges the silent assumption of liberalism that bodily life indebts women to men" (151) and that Wollstonecraft turns to motherhood to "liberate the body from the incommensurability of its biological sex" (152). But even here I caution that complementarity is still not a somatic fact.

14. On the limitations of female strength, see Craciun (70–75).

15. Elfenbein puts it thusly in his essay on Wollstonecraft and genius: "she also uses biological and scientific phrases like 'animal spirits' and 'subtle electric fluid' to avoid locating genius obviously in one gender" (239). Also suggestive is his point that Wollstonecraft links normative sexual relations with imprisonment (242). In the context of Wollstonecraft's antidualism, Wollstonecraft's repeated use of the "soul"—as when she asks if men would deprive women of souls too—exploits a metaphysical vocabulary to the end of breaking down gender differences.

16. Claudia Johnson argues that "Wollstonecraft's refrain about the excellence of male strength is thus not a concession, but an admonition she feels compelled tirelessly to repeat, for current practices with respect to rank and sex, far from bolstering men's superiority, have threatened their bodily dignity" (41). While Johnson's insistence that Wollstonecraft must be understood in light of notions of Republican manhood—under the tyranny of Kings, men cannot live up to their manhood because they are not free— is important, it underestimates the costs of such Republicanism, costs that I suggest Wollstonecraft is well aware of. Republican manly strength runs the danger of licensing patriarchy.

17. On Wollstonecraft's ambivalence to sensibility, see chap. 7 of G. J. Barker-Benfield's *Culture of Sensibility*. "Wollstonecraft's distinction was to take 'Sense' further in her defense of woman's mind, and to be still more damning in her analysis of what an exaggerated 'Sensibility' could do to women" (362).

18. I borrow Claudia Johnson's phrasing. See her "Mary Wollstonecraft: Styles of Radical Maternity" (169).

19. For more on the role of the French Revolution in shaping Wollstonecraft, see Tom Furniss, "Mary Wollstonecraft's French Revolution." He shows how Wollstonecraft's "own attitudes towards sexuality underwent a revolution as she witnessed the

political revolution around her" (65). He quotes Wollstonecraft thinking about remaining in post-Terror France where her illegitimate daughter "would be freer" (68).

20. In *Romantic Genius*, Elfenbein argues that genius increasingly came to be associated with pushing gender boundaries. Elfenbein argues in his later essay on genius in Wollstonecraft that here is a small glimpse of her connecting genius with sexual daring (240). For the most part in the *Vindications*, Wollstonecraft avoids genius because she must address ordinary folk (Elfenbein 240). Elfenbein is at odds with Johnson, who sees Wollstonecraft's homophobia in her phrase "equivocal beings."

21. Craciun writes, "Robinson argues that, since some women are stronger than some men, relative strength and weakness are found along a continuum, not necessarily according to sexual difference" (54).

22. "Resisting nerves" in Mary Robinson's lexicon are not always positive. In her *Memoirs*, for example, she refers to the "resisting nerves" of her father's mistress, and these nerves allow this adulterous lover to "brave the story ocean," and to "consent" to remain two years with her father in "the frozen wilds of America" (17). More troubling is the fact that Robinson claims that too much thinking has destroyed her health; nerve specialists thought that too much thinking could be especially dangerous to women. "Alas! How little did I then know either the fatigue or the hazard of mental occupations!" she cries (125). Although Linda Peterson shows how Robinson displayed herself as both a good mother and a genius in her *Memoirs*, Peterson ignores Robinson's uses of nerves. Perhaps her ill health and weak nervous system along with motherhood is a way for Robinson to display her appropriate femininity, one that might garner sympathy from her readers, a sympathy she would need given her status as mistress to the prince of Wales. Her *Letter*, by contrast, does not broach women's weakness but rather insists on feminine strength. These differences indicate that Robinson is not so much a postmodern subject as some have claimed, but rather she is acutely aware of the rhetorical needs of each situation. She uses whatever female essence that will be persuasive.

23. In her edition of *A Letter to the Women of England*, Sharon Setzer notes that Fox was potentially Robinson's lover after her affair with the Prince of Wales (64).

24. Laurinda Dixon argues that, in the eighteenth century, the "French Court actively practices contraception; as a result of such views, medical writers began to argue that too much sex rather than not enough was a prime factor in women's illness" (226). Of course, the caricaturists insisted that French women of the court practiced the wrong kinds of sex: lesbianism and incest.

25. Laqueur points out that female castration "both assumed and did not assume incommensurate sexual difference" (*Making Sex* 176). On the one hand, women had female testicles. On the other hand, female testicles were not considered "sacrosanct" (177).

26. In January 1801, Coleridge suffered from a hydrocele, the painful swelling of his left testicle. Thus, his letters show his intimate familiarity with the anatomy of the testicle and spermatic chord. See his *Collected Letters* (II: 662–67).

27. How immersed Coleridge was in the political intrigues of St. Thomas's Hospital, where his own Doctor Green was trying to become elected as surgeon, can be seen in Coleridge's letter to Thomas Allsop of early June 1820. Coleridge speculates on why Cooper voted against Green. See the *Collected Letters of Coleridge* (5:54). Ruston notes that Cline treated Mary Shelley when she was ill as a child (when she was fourteen) (Ruston 88). Cline Jr. was also Keats's teacher (de Almeida 5).

28. In the *Chirurgical Works of Benjamin Gooch*, he notes that in complicated cases of

the schirrous testicle, castration can be immediately performed; but to have to do that after the eschar (scab caused by a burn) is separated, "would be a very discouraging circumstance to the patient, as well as very disagreeable to the surgeon, whose character as well as mind might suffer by it" (2:224).

29. On the biology of castrati in the Romantic period, see J. Jennifer Jones (paragraphs 8–20). She argues that castrati are an analogue for transcendence in sound, the embodiment of Longinian height.

30. In his "Philosophical View of Reform," Shelley figures priests as eunuchs who want to foist their own unmanly disqualifications upon others through slavery (D. Clark 237). The denial of liberty is thus a form of literal emasculation, though it does not look like one. For Shelley, castration is a figure for the deprivation of liberty.

31. This manuscript follows Cullen's lectures of 1777 at the University of Edinburgh and conforms to his *Practice of Medicine.* I thank the Wellcome Library for permission to quote from MS 6036.

32. This quotation appears in Wellcome MS 7601, "William Hunter's Lectures on Anatomy," circa 1780. The notes cover seventy-nine lectures given at Hunter's Great Windmill Street School. The student was likely John Power, later a surgeon in Market Bosworth, Leics. I thank the Wellcome for giving me permission to quote from this manuscript. The analogousness of the clitoris to the penis is everywhere in the medical literature of the Romantic period. See, for instance, John Burns's *Principles of Midwifery,* where he comments that "the clitoris is a small body resembling the male penis, but has no urethra. . . . When distended with blood, it becomes erected and considerably longer, and is endowed with great sensibility" (38–39). In his medical lectures, William Hunter noted the "extreamly analogous" nature of the penis to the clitoris (Glasgow MS GEN 771, vol. 3). The suppressed ground of complementarity, thus, is similitude and resemblance. For more, see Valerie Traub's key article "Psychomorphology of the Clitoris."

33. On the ambiguous sex of the man-midwife, see Ludmilla Jordanova's *Nature Displayed* (22–29 especially). In William Hunter's manuscript notes "Draft of final? Lecture on Midwifery" (Glasgow MS Hunter H37), he refreshingly admitted that of the three kinds of diseases men-midwives would encounter, only one was clearly discernable, another could not be understood "with any degree of certainty," and still another "are of so dark a nature . . . we are not able even to form a probable conjecture about them. Such were many diseases which it has been my misfortune to see and I am afraid you will meet too often. They are more common than some of the profession would wish to believe." Of course, all this uncertainty meant that professional knowledge was not necessarily better than women's knowledge. Lisa Cody argues that the debates over man-midwifery encapsulated larger crises in gender. In particular, the man-midwife's gender ambiguity was compounded by a shift in fatherhood toward feeling and away from harsh patriarchy. Cody shows also how Hunter's Scottishness meant that he could symbolize foreign penetration into the Queen's body. See chaps. 6 and 7 of *Birthing the Nation.*

34. The debate between Osborn and William Bland/Thomas Denham is quite instructive: Bland claimed that labor was far from necessarily difficult, and Osborn's insistence that the pelvis was "badly designed" was disproved by the flexibility of the pelvic bone (21). Bland called attention to Osborn's motive: Osborn wanted to justify the man-midwife's active intervention in labor, insisting that the man-midwife's job was to slow down labor so the woman would not tear her perineum (56–57). If women's bodies were not managed by men, they would tear themselves badly. Very recently, doctors have de-

termined that the regular practice of cutting the perineum to prevent tearing is ineffective and unjustified. Osborn also sought to diminish any loss felt in the loss of an unborn child: wealthy families did not really feel parental loss; rather they felt only the pangs of "disappointment" in the loss of an heir (210). And parents in general "may, I think, be literally said to suffer nothing, by the loss of an unborn child" (209).

35. According to the *New Medical Dictionary* a hermaphrodite was: "one who is supposed to be of both sexes; but the truth is, the clitoris of a woman being of an extraordinary size, is all the peculiarity in this supposed species of the human kind."

36. For background on the medical history of puberty, see Helen King, *The Disease of Virgins*, especially pages 83–90. She focuses mostly on puberty in women. For an historical treatment of adolescence in Britain, see John Springhall's *Coming of Age*, 22–25. Springhall reminds us that Rousseau referred to adolescence as a "second birth, prolonging childhood, including the condition of innocence as long as possible" (22). He also quotes a 1789 diary of John Tennent, an apprentice to a merchant, who refers to the fact that he has been "so alter'd in stature, knowledge and ideas" from the ages of fourteen to seventeen that he can hardly recognize himself (23). In *The Adolescent Idea*, Patricia Spacks provides a literary perspective, noting that in the eighteenth century adolescence was a vague idea but was associated with vulnerability and passions. Since middle- and upper-class adolescents had no customary activities, society worried about how to keep them occupied. See chap. 4 especially.

37. Buffon, by contrast, traced the common signs of puberty in both sexes, including changes in voice, enlargement of the body and engorgement of the groin. He also listed the changes as a result of puberty in the separate sexes: namely, menstruation and the development of breasts in women and the growth of beards and the seminal emissions in men (488–89). Women arrive at puberty before men: the greater size and strength of men meant that the changes in puberty in them simply took longer. Buffon further dismissed the hymen and caruncles as imaginary signs of virginity. After puberty, the natural state was marriage (502). According to the *Index-Catalogue of the Library of the Surgeon-General's Office*, French medical writers on puberty seem much more interested in the changes in women than their English counterparts: The index lists 14 titles on puberty in women during the Romantic period. During the years of Revolution, puberty in France is often referred to as a natural revolution.

38. In John Bell's *Anatomy of the Human Body* (1802), sexual difference is primarily skeletal (pelvis). In his chapter "Generation, Anus, and Perinaeum," Bell insinuates sexual difference when he talks about the male parts of generation under the muscles and entirely neglects to discuss the uterus and vagina. Such a division supports the superiority of masculine strength, and female passivity over male activeness. Bell attended Percy and Mary Shelley in Rome.

39. The appearance of female skeletons in the eighteenth century alongside male ones leads Londa Schiebinger to support Laqueur's narrative of the transition from one sex to two. See her *Nature's Body*.

40. Peter Reill argues that, around 1750, chemists argued that chemical affinity was based on difference. Before then, like particles were thought to seek like. See chapter 2 of *Vitalizing Nature*.

41. In *The Body and the French Revolution*, Dorinda Outram argues that writers on hygiene during the revolution denied that virtue and vice were directed to spiritual ends, allowing the body to become self-referential (51).

42. Wollstonecraft does claim that "it is time to effect a revolution in female manners" (132), and revolution may in fact take on a French hint of puberty as a natural process. That she alludes in the above passage to the French *physiognomie* makes this claim seem less of a stretch. On how Wollstonecraft thinks women are deformed into women, see Barbara Taylor's *Mary Wollstonecraft and the Feminist Imagination* (87–91). Finally, we should remember Angela Keane's caution that "the critique of Wollstonecraft as an advocate of the restriction of sexuality to productive maternity, then, tells only a partial story. . . . She is alert to the fragile border between plenitude and deprivation, delight and abjection: a border marked most strongly in the maternal body itself, that productive object of the power of sex" (121–22).

43. In her *Memoirs*, Mary Robinson figures her puberty in terms of a change of dress. Robinson writes, "as soon as the day of my wedding was fixed, it was deemed necessary that a total revolution should take place in my external appearance. I had till that period worn the habit of a child, and the dress of a woman so suddenly assumed sat rather awkwardly upon me" (46). Her "revolution in dress" perhaps obliquely refers to how French medical writers of the period of the Revolution figured puberty as revolution. That the revolution was in dress, and not in body, moreover, hints that her husband-to-be was really robbing the cradle. This argument is reinforced by Robinson's claim that she was only fourteen at this time. Mary was really sixteen at the time of her marriage (Runge 564, n. 3), and it is also possible that she speaks of herself as a child so that she can further undermine the marriage's legitimacy. Robinson may also be pointing out a gap between how the law defined puberty—when one is sexually ready for marriage—and how medicine understood puberty, a gap that undermines generally the institution of marriage. Runge situates the *Memoirs* within the context of the period's adultery debates, arguing that Robinson shows the ineffectiveness of gallantry as a form of male protection; for Robinson, gallantry really only facilitates seduction (581).

44. Jorgensen argues that Hunter's primary interest in these transplants was to "elucidate the properties of the vital principle" (17). While I agree, I do want to point out that sexuality so fascinated Hunter precisely because it was intimately connected to vitality. So the two purposes were more aligned than Jorgensen suggests.

45. Marilyn Butler identified Lawrence of this long article on generation in Rees's *Cyclopedia*. See her edition of Mary Shelley's *Frankenstein*. Neil Fraistat reminds us that Rees's *Cyclopedia* was published in weekly numbers, starting in 1778 (2:660); thus this article circulated well before the publication of the set. It is therefore possible that Wollstonecraft could have read it.

46. On homophobia in the Romantic period, see Robert Corber's "Representing the 'Unspeakable'" and Crompton's biography of Byron. Corber argues that Godwin sought to stigmatize aristocratic patronage as a pernicious form of male bonding (96). See also Sedgwick's *Between Men* (83–117).

47. See Anne Mellor, *Blake's Human Form Divine* (128–29).

48. See Nelson Hilton, *Literal Imagination* (79–101). I will develop some of these claims in my Blake chapter; these paragraphs are meant to be suggestive rather than definitive.

49. Elfenbein reminds us, for example that "Ololon is a 'they' with both male and female members" (*Romantic Genius* 152).

50. In *Homosexuality and Civilization*, Crompton claims that Voltaire's entry on "Amour nommé socratique" "was probably the eighteenth century's most widely read

pronouncement on the subject [of homosexuality]." Curiously, Crompton omits Voltaire's inference that sodomy is only a crime of convenience: since boys are educated around boys—the culture is homosocial—they can conceivably choose other boys as the object of their awakening sexual desire because no other objects are available.

51. See Diane Long Hoeveler's important study, *Romantic Androgyny*. Hoeveler limits androgyny to a "literary device," one that is "limited by the parameters and ideological content of mythology itself" (17). This book argues, by contrast, that androgyny was not a myth and that it was based on competing ways of understanding sex in the period.

52. My remarks here are indebted to Richard Terdiman's perceptive study *Body and Story*, especially chapter 6. Terdiman traces a productive tension between bodies and signs, whereby bodies resist semiotization and language needs bodies (27). But his acute sense of the tensions is even more provocative than he imagines: eighteenth-century medical understandings of the body made it an especially important sign/signified in this debate. On the flexible materiality of the sexed and gendered body, see Roughgarden, chapter 12. She argues that, "although the XX/XY system of sex determination is widely believed to define a biological basis for a gender binary, this system allows for a sharp binary and a great overlap between XX and XY bodies, as well as gender crossing" (212).

53. On sodomy in the Romantic period, the literature is enormous. Sodomy, of course, can refer to all sexual acts that are not heterosexual intercourse. See Crompton's two books, Trumbach, Elfenbein, Rousseau's *Perilous Enlightenment*, articles by Gilbert, Harvey, Kimmel, and Morris, among others.

54. The only critic I know who mentions Shelley's connection of puberty to homoeroticism is Eric Clark in *Virtuous Vice*. Clark mentions this only in passing. I consider Shelley's essay on the Greeks more fully in my "Uses and Abuses of Alterity: Halperin and Shelley on the Otherness of Ancient Greek Sexuality" in *Romantic Praxis* (January 2006). In his generous response to my essay, Elfenbein points out that the psychologizing of male sexual threat may sidestep Shelley's intent of staving off his audience's rejection of the whole of *The Symposium*. Elfenbein further argues that Shelley may have used class respectability to suggest that genteel Greeks would have had nothing to do with something as operose as sodomy. See his "Romantic Loves: A Response to Historicizing Romantic Sexuality." Following Foucault on friendship, I would argue that love between men is precisely what puts male friendship in the orbit of the perverse.

55. I treat the sexologists more fully in "Othering Sexual Perversity: England, Empire, Race, and the Science of Sex," forthcoming, in *The History of the Human Body in an Age of Empire*, ed. Michael Sappol.

56. Alice Dreger's important study of hermaphrodites ignores the literature before the 1860's. Yet her insight that medical men "struggled to come up with a system of sex difference that would hold" is an important one (16). On William Cowper's hermaphroditism, see Elfenbein, *Romantic Genius* (83–88).

57. Rodin credits Baillie's *Morbid Anatomy* with being the first to relate cirrhosis of the liver to alcoholism, and the first to "grossly delineate" emphysema (29). Coleridge comments on "Bayley's" [*sic*] Morbid Pathology in His *Letters* (4:614).

58. On racialization in the Romantic period and its connections to beauty, see Paul Youngquist, *Monstrosities: Bodies and British Romanticism*, chap. 3.

59. Roughgarden made this comment in a lecture "Gender and Evolution" given at the National Institutes of Health on 18 April 2007.

FOUR: The Perverse Aesthetics of Romanticism

1. Marc Redfield explains why the *Bildungsroman* and aesthetics share the same fate: they are but "tropes for the aspirations of aesthetic humanism" (39).

2. Terry Eagleton's sweeping generalization that "aesthetics is born as a discourse of the body" (13) blinds him to how the sexual body functions in aesthetic discourse. See his *Ideology of the Aesthetic.*

3. See Walter Kendrick's splendid *The Secret Museum* for more on obscenity and neo-classicism.

4. Zizek bases this claim on the fact that the human brain "wastes a lot of energy, time, and effort" on art and on the fact that even prehistoric stone handaxes were produced by males as sexual displays because their symmetry had no direct use value (247–48).

5. In *Erotism: Death and Sensuality,* Georges Bataille provides a model for thinking about how eroticism enables readers to experience an excess that defies philosophical theoretical tools. See chap. 1 especially.

6. On Wordsworth's "perverse rewriting of the normative oedipal tale" in *The Prelude,* see David Collings, *Wordsworthian Errancies* (chap. 5).

7. While looking through the holdings of the Kinsey Library, I was surprised find three volumes by Charlotte Smith. See the microfilm collection *Sex Research: Early Literature* (reel 99, number 791).

8. Altieri appropriates Kant's concept of purposiveness without purpose to think about the value of emotional investments without necessarily being trapped within them. He tellingly, however, must apologize repeatedly for seeming "vulgar" interpretations of an aesthetics that tries to understand emotional rapture: "It may seem vulgar to speak of this kind of cultivation as "aesthetic" (24). Altieri's magnificent book would have been strengthened by a greater engagement with the work of Alphonse Lingis: Altieri cites one of Lingis's essays, but does not do much with it (109–10). He also, in my view, underestimates the resistance between Kant and affect.

9. I borrow this suggestive term from David M. Halperin; see his response to my essay, "The Use and Abuse of Alterity" in *Romantic Praxis* (January 2006).

10. This is Danny O'Quinn's perspicuous insight. See his forward to *Romanticism and Sexual Vice,* a special issue of *Nineteenth-Century Contexts.* Herbert Marcuse defined the perversions as the revolt against the reality principle (44–45); he reads aesthetics in terms of a more muted liberation: a "liberation of sensuousness from the repressive domination of reason" (164). Kant's aesthetics mediates between nature and reason. This chapter, by contrast, looks at how both sexual perversion and aesthetics have a mutual distrust of function, and what happens when sexuality can be understood as a purposiveness without purpose.

11. For help with Kant's concept of purposiveness without purpose, I thank David Krell, Marc Redfield, William Flesch, and Jonathan Loesberg. All references to Kant's *Critique of Judgment* are from the Pluhar edition, and I cite the pagination that corresponds to the German text.

12. Susan Meld Shell is especially helpful on this concept. "'Purposiveness without purpose' defines our experience of 'kinship' with nature, yet in a manner that resists, through the explicit fictiveness of its device, the twin pitfalls of vitalism (or the confu-

sion of matter and reason) and mysticism (the confusion of truth and illusion)" (208–9). She adds, "the regulative or reflective concept of objective purposiveness in nature is thus a way of attributing to nature something more than 'blind mechanism' without going so far as to credit it with causes that act intentionally" (236).

13. On *Sinnlichkeit*, see Marcuse (166).

14. See Richards (232–39).

15. On this, see Andrew Elfenbein's response to "Historicizing Romantic Sexuality" in *Romantic Praxis* (January 2006), as well as the work of George Haggerty, especially, *Men in Love*.

16. On the sexual contract and its invisibility to social contract theory, see Carole Pateman.

17. For more on Coleridge and science, see, among others, Wallen, and Pamela Edwards (chaps. 6 and 7), and Vickers. For Coleridge, localizing function into organs ran the danger of missing "the efficient cause of disease" (cited in P. Edwards 153).

18. Jonathan Loesberg argues that Coleridge in his earlier aesthetic writings "takes purposiveness and attributes it to an integral aspect of nature—organicism." He then uses Schiller's opposition between mechanism and organicism as an opposition between organization from without and organization from within—rather than Schiller's actual contrast between perceiving nature as random and perceiving it as organized according to a purpose. Finally, he connects symbolic immanence with organization from within and takes the whole complex as a natural reality upon which art could be modeled. He thus creates a "vaguely defined and internally contradictory empirical entity out of a difficult conceptual maneuver in Kant" (26). I am suggesting that Coleridge got closer to Kant by the time of Green's lectures.

19. According to Russell, "the author of On Sublimity is unknown. The manuscript attributes it in one place to 'Dionysius Longinus,' in another to 'Dionysius or Longinus'" (x). The accepted dating for the text is the first century A.D.

20. Because Snyder's translation is attentive to lesbianism, I cite it rather than Russell's. While the 1751 London translation uses Philips' translation of Sappho into couplets, a translation that ignores completely the sex of the addressee, the 1762 Dublin translation by Reverend Charles Carthy and the 1800 London William Smith translation also turn to Philips but add notes that make it clear that Sappho is addressing Dorica. Carthy writes, "Sappho address'd this ode to Dorica, and that she was likewise beloved by Charaxis, Sappho's brother," while Smith quotes Plutarch's comment that "Sappho says, that at the sight of her beloved fair, her voice was suppressed." Payne Knight read Longinus in the Greek; see below.

21. Snyder's translation. *Epei kai peneta* has not been translated because it is "largely unintelligible" according to Snyder. It means something like "even the poor."

22. My thanks to Michael North for breaking down this line for me. He cautioned that the comma is of course an editorial intervention, but that there were six stresses in each syntactical unit. North agreed that the phrase following the comma does not quite make sense. Although Sappho's poem is a fragment, Longinus does not emphasize its fragmentary status. In a private e-mail to me, Alice Browne notes that "the line divides sharply after *pan tolmaton*, so that bears out the emphasis on control, as does the mastery of the poem itself." She cautions that the *pan* is neuter singular in the Greek, a fact that I think emphasizes a kind of unity in totality.

23. I cite Snyder's translation. In Russell's translation, the enjambment is severely curtailed, but the lady's sweet voice still spills into her lovely laughter. The Ambrose Philips translation, popular in the eighteenth century, transforms Sappho into mostly end-stopped couplets.

24. Foucault notes that Greek physicians generally distrusted *phantasia*, largely because it could stimulate sexual desires not strictly necessary to the bodily economy (136–37). Longinus's embrace of *phantasia* thus can be seen as another means of reconciling the sexual with the aesthetic.

25. Potts argues that Wincklemann's *History of Ancient Art* borrows from Plato's negation of the image in *The Statesman*, only to revalue the vividly sensuous. (109). Whereas Potts finds Winckelmann in the *History* being mastered by desire (127), I foreground Winckelmann's need to master desire in his *Reflections*.

26. Winckelmann may also be thinking about Plato when he writes about Alcibiades, though the specific detail is not in Plato. Winckelmann praises Alcibiades for having "in his youth, refused to blow the flute (*die Flöte*) for fear of distorting his face" (9). Frances Grose's *Dictionary of the Vulgar Tongue* provides a possible sexual gloss (fluting was an idiomatic expression for fellatio). I have no idea if this was the case in Germany, too. If it was, the point I would emphasize here is that it is not so much the sexual act that is denigrated as it is the ugliness of the face while doing it.

27. Since Blake read Winckelmann, could Winckelmann help explain why Blake's infant is "struggling against my swaddling bands" in "Infant Sorrow" (28)? Blake's image here of the infant does have a trace of classical musculature. Winckelmann's disgust at wrinkles on the skin in Enlightenment art may also have influenced Blake's represented bodies that seem transparent.

28. Where Theresa Kelley stresses the sufficiency of Greek art in Wincklemann (*Reinventing Allegory* 171), Jonah Siegel highlights an erotics of absence in Winckelmann (chap. 2). I want to think about how the aesthetics of Winckelmann's theories help to bridge the divide between this debate. Siegel underestimates the role of the sexual in Winckelmann. Potts mistakenly argues that the Burkean sublime has no erotic appeal and uses this to distinguish Winckelmann from Burke (127). I will counter this below. And, whereas Potts is perhaps right that in the *History* there is no aesthetic education into self-mastery, I demonstrate that such mastery is indeed the goal of the *Reflections*.

29. All references to Burke are to part and section number.

30. Ronald Paulson, for example, situates the Burkean sublime in an Oedipal narrative; see his *Representations on Revolution* (69–73). Frances Ferguson takes as a given the slippage between sensation and idea, sensation and language and thus does not attend to the role of sex in arresting this slippage. See her *Solitude and the Sublime*. Jules David Law examines how figures of reflection in Burke enable discoveries about the functioning of language in *The Rhetoric of Empiricism* (134–64).

31. Hume made the love of beauty the medium between lust and kindness because "one who is inflamed with lust, feels at least a momentary kindness towards the object of it" (*Treatise* 443). Eagleton notes that, in Burke, "if the aesthetic judgment is unstable, then so must be the social sympathies founded on it, and with them the whole fabric of political life" (52).

32. I am alluding to Claudia Johnson's marvelous *Equivocal Beings*.

33. Burke, by contrast, addresses the power and influence of pleasure in *A Vindication*

*of Natural Society*. Artificial society like aristocracy has created "Pleasures incompatible with Nature," pleasures that render "millions utterly abject and miserable" (86).

34. In *Phallic Worship*, Robert Allen Campbell comments that "in its origin and early use, [phallic worship] was as pure in its intent and as reverent in its ceremonies, as far removed from anything then looked upon as trivial or unclean in its symbolism, as is the worship and symbolism of today" (16). For more on Knight's lack of interest in relations with women, see Rousseau, "Sorrows of Priapus." Rousseau claims Byron defended Knight's anticlericalism (133). Jonah Siegel writes on Knight's *Discourse*: "rather than succumbing to the crush of information . . . these writers sought in the accumulation of objects a pattern indicative of an acceptable unitary moment of origin" (76). That source was the representation of human sexuality.

35. Although Burke worried that aesthetic sensation might cut itself off from empirical sensation, Knight turns to the principle of association to separate the physical senses from the mind. For Knight, "the faculty of improved or artificial sensation . . . continues to improve throughout the subsequent stages of our lives as long as our minds retain their vigour; and becomes so far independent of the organ of sense, from which it is derived, that it often exists in its highest state of perfection, when those organs are enfeebled by age, and verging to decay" (*Taste* 99). Knight nonetheless emphasizes the sexual within the aesthetic.

36. Knight chided Hugh Blair for censuring Longinus and for having "confounded the effect of poetical description or expression of a passion, with the effect of the passion itself" (338). In so doing, of course, Blair is merely being transported by the erotic sublime.

37. On manifold connections between antiquities, the Grand Tour, Italy, and sodomy, see Rousseau, *Perilous Enlightenment* (172–99).

38. I have checked Shearer's transcriptions against the pencil manuscript notes in the Huntington Library Copy, Rare Book 11577.

39. For an overview of these debates, see Bradford Mudge, *The Whore's Story*, as well as his essay on historicizing pornography in *Romantic Praxis*.

40. My colleague Jonathan Loesberg argues that pornography is inherently aesthetic given its status as representation. See his note 47, 259–60, in *A Return to Aesthetics*.

41. In the British Library's Private Case, its holdings of pornography, there is an anonymous volume, *Veneres Uti Observantur in Gemmis Antiquis*, circa 1790. The cataloger speculates that it might be by Pierre d'Hancarvilles. Where Knight is silent on Ganymede, this author comments on a depiction of *Jupiter in love with Ganimede, refuses the ardent solicitations of young Hebe* that "several of our readers would have done otherwise, but this God was more fantastick than he was powerful" (entry to number 6). The claim that only "several" readers would have done otherwise hints that such a work was written for a sodomitic subculture, and reminds us of the sodomitic links to neoclassicism. Peter Funnell suggests that Knight may be arguing for toleration for eighteenth-century Hindu religious groups in the *Discourse;* they too worshipped obscene objects (59–60).

FIVE:  Fiery Joys Perverted to Ten Commands

1. Christopher Hobson's concept of perversion in Blake does not in my view account for its radical instability, nor does it deal with how Blake actually uses the term. Finally, while I am sympathetic to Hobson's claim that we are all sexually perverse—Freud made

the departure from normal sexual aims (sexual intercourse between a man and a woman) and objects both forms of perversion—I worry that if we are all perverts then perversion cannot do the work of liberation because it is everywhere (see 32–36). This chapter is better for Mark Lussier's generous yet critical reading of it. Blake and Catherine did not have children. Greer speculates this was deliberate (81–83).

2. In *Milton* (plate 27, lines 8–10), Blake explicitly links the wheels of the wine press with the printing press.

3. On history in Blake as trauma, see Rajan.

4. On the role of sexuality in Blake, see Hagstrum, *The Romantic Body*. Hagstrum shows the sexual resonances of Blake's words, but his body is divorced from science and medicine. He also equates sexual pleasure with liberation, when in fact Blake was far more cautious about liberation. Roy Porter considers Blake in *Flesh in the Age of Reason*, but he suggests that Blake wants to transcend sexual energy into a "higher aesthetic" (442). This ignores the role of sexual desire within Blake's aesthetic. Porter's suggestion that orthodoxy is "systematic moral perversion" (439) in Blake captures only partly how Blake understands perversion.

5. I should note that textualism is predicated upon a misprision of Derrida. Although Derrida recognized that one could never escape logocentrism, textualism operates under the assumption that by acknowledging the inevitable textuality of all signs, one can liberate language from materiality.

6. Some uses of perversion are straightforward, as, for example, when Blake claims that Pity "in perverse and cruel delight" fled from Los's arms in *Urizen* (E 79). Pity perversely takes delight in sexual deferral.

7. Saree Makdisi argues that antinomianism gave Blake the ability to think outside of the radical hegemonic position that socioeconomic egalitarianism was liberty. See chap. 2 of *William Blake and the Impossible History of the 1790s*.

8. See Robert Essick, *William Blake and the Language of Adam*. Essick argues that Blake's literalization of the figurative attempts to unite conception with execution and to return to the Logos. I would, by contrast, insist on the limits of the Logos, its capacity for tyranny. Essick also suggests that, although a deconstructive method is appropriate for Blake's *Urizen*, it fails to account for Blake's reclaiming of the Logos in *Jerusalem*. Behind the debate on whether logocentrism is a good or bad thing is a larger debate about whether a deconstructive awareness of language liberates us from false representation, or whether logocentrism liberates us from our fallen condition. For the purposes of my argument here, that both deconstruction and logocentrism declare liberation means that neither can be intrinsically liberating.

9. Blake uses "unperverted" again when referring to "the Word of God, the only light of antiquity that remains unperverted by War" ("On Virgil" E 270). Note that he is not claiming that the word of God is unperverted: it is unperverted by war (unlike the works of Greece and Rome).

10. My sense that materiality of printing is a form of critical deferral is confirmed by the Princeton edition of Blake's *Early Illuminated Books*, which begin their discussion of the individual books with the plate and printing history of the books to follow only then to offer plate by plate readings. The will to truth that informs how Blake produced the texts only defers the huge blindnesses in Blake criticism. To the substantial credit of the editors of this edition, they generally make us aware of those blindnesses. Nonetheless, particularity in Blake criticism is a necessary symptom of unknowing.

11. On Blake and Paine, see Mee (139–42) and Goldsmith (178–82).

12. Porter argues rightly that "this remark was intended to say more about Watson than about Paine" (2004 438).

13. Goldsmith notes that although Paine's *Age of Reason* is highly derivative, Paine does inaugurate a genuinely new idea, that of subversive reading (179). Because Blake gets to Paine via Watson, and because Blake uses the concept of perversion and not subversion, I examine these points in some detail.

14. This line is often cited as if this were Blake's point. But Blake begins this passage by listing "Paine's Arguments . . . One for instance, which is that. . . . That the Bible is all a State Trick" (E 616). This bracketing is crucial to my argument that irony allows Blake to distinguish between Watson's perversion of Paine and Paine, and Paine's perversion of the Bible and the Bible. It also enables Blake's identification with Paine and his critique of him.

15. See, for example, Eugene Goodheart, whose criticisms of sexual liberation were anticipated by the Romantics. Goodheart might have considered how skepticism about sexual liberation enhances the commitment to sexual liberation. In Blake, the expression of sexual desire can be a form of tyranny, as Beulah, Rahab, and Tirzah make clear. As Orc's rape of the nameless shadowy female in America highlights, Blake knows that desire can convert women into objects and sex into tyranny. Beulah further shows the dissatisfaction in the concept of illimitable desire. Hence, Blake insists upon the difference between liberation and liberty.

16. On the "Song of Liberty" as being originally a separate leaflet, see Viscomi's *HLQ* essay. The word "liberty" in the marriage appears once before the "Song," and that is in Blake's description of Milton as being "at liberty" when he wrote of devils and hell but did not know it.

17. See, by contrast, Harold Bloom, who uses sexual perversion as if it were a self-explanatory thing to be avoided in Blake: "War and sacrificial religion are founded upon the perversion of the sexual energies" (279). But if generation is itself potentially a perversion of the sexual energies in Blake, perversion is a much more complex category.

18. For more on Blake and the state of falleness, see Frosch (chap. 2). While Albion's creative failure is the human body itself, the body for Blake does not necessarily take on failure.

19. In *Flesh and the Age of Reason*, Porter describes David Hartley's concept of annihilation in such a way that suggests Blake's notion of self-annihilation may owe something to Hartley. Although Hartley refers to annihilation as the spiritualization of matter after death, something that Blake would have abhorred because for him, matter is already spiritualized, Porter suggests that annihilation for Hartley was tied to "the psychological development in life from a self purely selfish to one which became progressively more benevolent, even altruistic or spiritual" (359).

20. Morton Paley argues that regeneration in Blake is essentially imaginative, and he argues that Boehme shapes Blake's concept (see chap. 6). He does not, however, connect the importance of generation to regeneration (1970).

21. Here and elsewhere, I adopt Blake's own rather unconventional punctuation.

22. On Milton's use of perversion, see Dollimore, *Sexual Dissidence* (126–28). In Milton, "the perverse not only departs from, but actively contradicts the dominant in the act of deviating from it, and does so from within, and in terms of inversion, distortion, transformation, reversal, subversion" (125).

23. Lincoln's speculation that the speaker's words can represent the triumph of Tirzah is at odds with Blake's concept of self-annihilation. Self-annihilation actively repudiates the mere physical, mortal body and the triumph of the five senses over the imagination. Yet the speaker's need to divorce itself from the mortal body is wrong in that such a divorce perpetuates a binary opposition between body and spirit rather than breaks it down. See Lincoln (201). On typology and Blake, see Tannenbaum (86–123).

24. Hobson makes the case for the first part of this statement most eloquently; see *Blake and Homosexuality* (chap. 5). Hobson does not agree that Blake's Satan here stands for Blake's view of homosexuality because Satan offers a negative view of homosexuality. Rather, he insists that this is Leutha's interpretation and that Leutha represents moral condemnation (93). But if self-annihilation demands the embrace of one's sins, Leutha cannot rescue Blake in the way Hobson argues. Hobson is incorrect in his statement that "judges, juries, satires, polemics, and mobs showed no . . . interest in distinguishing between [dominant and submissive sodomitical] roles." See *The Phoenix of Sodom; Or, the Vere Street Coterie*, which highlighted the fact that these sodomites first staged a marriage, and "make their wives, who they call tommies, topics of ridicule" (11). I note here how the travesty/mimicry of marriage roles is supposed to heighten the reader's homophobia. Even worse, although the author notes "it is a very natural opinion, that the prevalency of this passion has for its object effeminate delicate beings only, . . . Fanny Murry, Lucy Cooper, and Kitty Fisher are now personified by an athletic bargeman, an Herculean Coalheaver, and a deaf tyre smith: the latter of these monsters has two sons, both very handsome young men, whom he boasts are fully depraved as himself" (13). While athletic men may not correlate to the gender role, there is nonetheless an obsession with connecting gender role with sexual role.

25. Elfenbein argues that effeminacy and sodomy were not equivalent since effeminacy could mean simply civic decay (20–21). Yet his example showing effeminacy being distinguished from sodomy strongly suggests that the very need to make the distinction suggests that effeminacy implies a predisposition to sodomy, should it be allowed to develop further.

26. On Blake's phallocentrism, see William Keach, *Arbitrary Power* (133–43). In neglecting to think about how the various characters speaking might inflect this phallocentrism, Keach underestimates Blake's aesthetic embodiment of sexuality.

27. Hobson argues that Blake eventually manages to see masturbation as prolific in *Ahania* (see 36–45). Arguments that put Blake squarely within the camp of approving perverse sexuality are undercut by the poet's clear misgivings about certain acts and certain identities, not to mention the fact that self-annihilation queers the notion of identity itself. If identity is a logical or ontological necessity, it is pretty pointless either to subscribe to it or give it up. It is there, regardless. One could choose to attend to it or not, though.

28. Such textualism is perhaps a logical outcome of a Romantic-period democratic rhetoric that, "in its fundamental drive to negate power" must "enhance language" so that "to be able to speak is to be free" (Goldsmith 168). If democratic ideas helped make language the site of freedom, textualism then turns to linguistic deferral to undermine authority.

29. See, for example, Robert Essick's "How Blake's Body Means," which assumes that Blake's texts are his only possible bodies.

30. I have not done justice to Connolly's fine book, which suggests a number of important medical contexts for Blake's works.

31. For a description and black-and-white facsimile of this manuscript, see Essick, *The Works of William Blake in the Huntington Collections* (88–115).

32. Essick helps me further differentiate Blakean incarnation from naive logocentrism by showing how Blake's "multiple compound images" of incarnation are "nearly impossible to visualize . . . as a stable entity" (*Adam* 203). He credits Blake's "dynamic syntax."

33. On Blake and medicine, see F. B. Curtis and Tristanne Connolly. My research for this section of the essay was funded by an NEH summer stipend.

34. See Spallanzani's (1769), *An Essay on Animal Reproductions.* Spallanzani endeavors to discover "whether the regenerative power existed in the whole length of the worm" (7). In a later essay published in his *Tracts on the Nature of Animals and Vegetables,* Spallanzani would describe wheel-animals after having been killed as being "regenerated" and "resurrected" (260–61). On regeneration in seventeenth-century science, see Simon Schaffer, "Regeneration." Scientists in Blake's time were fascinated by nervous regenerations.

35. Blake speaks of hermaphrodites disparagingly for the reasons detailed by Frosch (81–86) and Hobson (167–72). Yet Blake still accords them two-fold form, a step above single vision and Newton's sleep. I do not agree with Hobson's claim that the Satan-Palamabron plot has nothing to do with hermaphroditism. Blake does not use the word "hermaphrodite" to describe this episode, but Hobson wants to isolate Blake's treatment of homosexuality from his negative treatment of hermaphrodites. And he thus insists that the Satan-Palamabron episode does not reveal anything about Blake's attitude toward homosexuality, since this represents Leutha's take on it, not Blake's.

36. Henry writes, "The work in which M. Haller published these discoveries, formed the aera of a revolution in anatomy. It taught us that there exists in the living body a particular power, which may be regarded as the immediate principle of motion, as a quality diffused through the organs, which enables them all to perform their respective functions" (75–76). The memoir concludes with Henry attesting to Haller's declared faith in the Book of Revelation on his deathbed, something that would have made Blake sympathetic to Haller.

37. He once uses the term, "generated organs" (Laocoön), but there it refers to the senses as generated organs.

38. For this insight, I am indebted to my student, Amy Moran-Thomas, and her dazzling senior honors thesis on "Hookworm and History."

39. For a less optimistic reading of midwifery in the Romantic period, see Andrea Henderson, *Romantic Identities* (chap. 1). Henderson argues that behind a mysterious nature and a willful fetus in William Hunter's obstetrical work "loomed a system of economic relations that perpetually threatened to make a child merely a commodity in the world of commodities" (37). Blake's distinction between regeneration and generation meant that even in the world of commodities, regeneration was possible.

40. For information about this work, signed by Blake, see John Windle's Catalogue 32 devoted to William Blake (San Francisco 2001). Essick and Bentley confirm that the copy for sale was Blake's.

41. For more on aqua fortis and Blake, see Viscomi (1993 79–81). Quincy writes that "vitriol and nitre should be mixed together, placed on a fire for three hours, in that time there will come some red fumes into the receiver; which will again disappear" (288). Perhaps this would serve as a metaphor for Blake's Orc, turning a wreath into wrath, or the generation of Urizen.

42. On this, see King-Hele, McNeil, and Bewell's articles on botany.

43. Mitchell's article "Chaosthetics" comes closest to my understanding of Blake's perverse aesthetics. Mitchell's use of a "headless allegory" to describe Blake is enormously helpful; I would quibble with him to say that we are given heads, but they are regularly beheaded. Jerome McGann's argument that Blake mounts an "aesthetics of deliberate engagement" is also suggestive. See "Blake and the Aesthetics of Deliberate Engagement," in *Social Values and Poetic Acts*.

44. As Jonathan Loesberg aptly puts it, "Any interpretation or analysis of an artwork that works under a theory of embodiment must hold some skeptical or constrained version of that embodiment—either knowingly or not—since the fact of interpretation automatically undoes a full claim to embodiment" (116).

45. I find helpful here Essick's point that the divine in Blake "reveals itself in the 'expression' of the literal, in the acts of writing, hearing, reading, and not as Boehme would have it, in the structure or sounds of the written letter" (*Adam* 203).

46. For *The Book of Thel*, I am using the Princeton Facsimile, edited by Eaves, Essick, and Viscomi. Plate numbers correspond to their plate numbers, given atop their typescript of the text in the square brackets. Nancy Bogen's reading of Thel as heroine has been helpful. However, she neglects the significance of the ending motto. Moreover, she makes some strange interpretive moves in order to arrive at her positive assessment of Thel. She assumes, for example, that the context of pastoral elegy makes Thel into a heroine (21–22). But Blake had little truck with nature, and thus pastoral could seem to him mere error. To make Thel positive, she parallels her acts to Oothoon's, but this is simply to defer the question of heroism, not answer it (20).

47. Robert Glecker situates *Thel* alongside the Book of Job, arguing that Job is the primary context for Thel and Ecclesiastes is secondary. Gleckner unfortunately treats the relationship between Blake and the Bible as essentially passive.

48. I realize this is a contentious claim. For counter-positions, see Mitchell and Linkin. Mitchell argues that since the moral structure of *Thel* is based on self-annihilation, then we cannot judge Thel because only someone who has undergone this process can judge her (95). I argue, by contrast, that we must see the stages of her sexual self-awareness, and if her sexual awakening is not spiritual, then she has not achieved sexual liberty. Mitchell's incisive comments on the staging of *Thel* ignore the role of the motto. Linkin argues that the form of the dialogue suggests that Thel has absorbed more than she is usually given credit for.

49. Mitchell sees Thel as embodying a rational skeptical attitude, one that leads her to revelation. Her fault for him is not in her questioning, but in her inability to become a stronger thinker. I argue that she strengthens her questioning abilities as she gains sexual knowledge. His argument that Blake structures the book in terms of self-annihilation can only hold up if Thel has begun to understand how sexuality can lead to self-annihilation. Certainly, her own recognition of herself as food for worms is part of self-annihilation, but the fact remains that this is still a relentlessly vegetative approach to human sexuality. See chapter 3 of *Blake's Composite Art*.

50. Connolly argues that mole refers to a growth in the womb that is not a fetus and that Thel questions the "facts" of who is responsible for what in human generation (see 134–35).

51. Hagstrum's claim that Blake's design derives from ancient Priapian design further insinuates that the liberation of sexuality must occur on two levels (*Poet and Painter* 89):

at the natural level of recognizing the importance of the body's pleasures and at the spiritual level. Blake would define that spiritual level in terms of bringing pleasure to the point of self-annihilation, although priapic sex purchases orgasm at the expense of erection. Blake nonetheless may have found priapus helpful for making generation once again within regeneration in that "spirit" is a pun on semen.

52. While my recognition of the pun between resurrection and erection may seem to suggest that Blake only thinks males can be regenerated, I note that Albrecht von Haller defines erection in terms of both the breast nipple and penis (*Dissertation* 30). Physicians also regularly mentioned clitoral erections. Any criticism of the negative portrayal of women in Blake must take into account that Leutha undergoes self-annihilation first in *Milton*, and her example leads Milton to do the same. Moreover, Blake depicts the soul unambiguously as female as it hovers over the male body in "The Soul Hovering over the Body reluctantly parting with life," one of his illustrations to *The Grave*.

53. On metrical irregularity as a potential Sapphic code, see Susan Lanser, "Put to the Blush."

54. Another symptom of the limits of Blake's metrical contract is the need for scholars to argue that one should think of the verse in the prophetic books as verse and not prose (Ostriker, chapter 8). Ostriker points out that Blake in *Jerusalem* uses enjambment yet "allows the final foot to be accented," a "metrical disjunction" that "supports the theme of apocalyptic uprooting" (135).

55. If Blake's slap at Hayley, that "his Mother on his Father him begot" (E 506), connects with Blake's charge of Hayley's homosexuality, then sex acts were far from necessarily neutral in value to Blake. To the extent that this is the case here, female sexual assertiveness, being on top, explains Hayley's perversity, the fact that he likes to domineer, but in a feminizing way. If we connect this to Blake's comment that "Unappropriate execution is the Most nauseous of all affectation & foppery" (E 576), keeping in mind Elfenbein's sense that effeminacy draws close to sodomy in the Romantic period, we have to ask ourselves why Blake sexualizes bad execution.

56. On prophecy, see Mee (chap. 1); on democracy, see Goldsmith (chap. 3); and on the sublime, see De Luca (chap. 2 especially).

57. For a subtle revision of the relationship of Enlightenment to Romanticism, see Marshall Brown's "Romanticism and Enlightenment."

58. I use the Princeton facsimile, volume 4 of *The Illuminated Books of William Blake*, edited by D. W. Dorrbecker, because it reproduces *America* recto/verso.

## SIX: Byron, Epic Puberty, and Polymorphous Perversity

1. See Christopher Ricks, *Keats and Embarrassment*. More recently, see *Keats's Boyish Imagination* by Richard Marggraf Turley. I reviewed this in *WWC* (2007). Unless otherwise noted, all citations from *Don Juan* are from the standard edition of *Lord Byron: The Complete Poetical Works*. Volume 5: *Don Juan*, edited by Jerome J. McGann. On occasion, because I am interested in an earlier version of the poem, I cite the T. G. Steffan and W. W. Pratt *Byron's Don Juan: A Variorum Edition* (abbreviated S&P). Guy Hocquenghem reminds us that through his use of " 'polymorphously perverse,' Freud expresses the fact that . . . desire is fundamentally undifferentiated and ignorant of the distinction between homosexuality and heterosexuality" (74).

2. Linking homosexuality with puberty is fraught with dangers. Psychoanalysis has a

long and damaging legacy of understanding homosexuality in terms of immature sex or narcissism; no one thus has to take homosexuality very seriously because it is just a phase, one that will be outgrown. Despite this risk, I believe that in Romanticism, thinking about puberty can lead to provocative questioning of what gets to count as maturity and who gets to decide this. As a vehicle for destabilizing bodily sex, moreover, Romantic puberty resists the pathology of perverse sex. I will show how Byron elongates puberty below.

3. Terry Castle notes that adolescence was one moment when lesbian desire could flourish because erotic triangulation has not yet begun. See *The Apparitional Lesbian* (84). Moyra Haslett reminds us that Byron situates the poem before the turn of the century to a time when sexual libertinism could be equated with political libertinism (see 158–66, especially). In canto 6, Byron tries to turn the clock back on Caesar and Cleopatra: "I wish their years had been fifteen and twenty" (6:5). It is as if puberty will make "worlds but a sport" (6:2).

4. John Brown links the onset of puberty with menstruation in women (2:189). Yet he also connects the frequency of menstruation after puberty and before menopause with women's orgasm: "the energy of stimulus which produces menstruation" (2:188). Moreover, "menstruation depends upon venereal emotion" (2:190). "The less addicted to love women are, the less they menstruate" (2:188). Brown is working within a one-sex model that insists because men have orgasm, women must have them too. And just as men acquire "indirect debility" with too much loss of semen, women suffer the same if they menstruate or experience orgasm too often (2:192). Yet depriving women of orgasm was detrimental to their health. On Brown, see also Martin Wallen, *City of Health, Fields of Disease* (chaps. 4 and 5), and Vickers.

5. The standard nosology grouped women's irregular evacuations under chlorosis or greensickness, giving menstruation a sexually specific pathology. See Helen King, *The Disease of Virgins*. For Brown, menstruation is grouped under a rubric common to both sexes, indirect debility, and the specific locale of the disease is much less important than the generalizable condition.

6. Byron incidentally was a schoolmate of Sir John's son, George, and the poet thrashed other boys on his behalf. Byron's Library is documented in A. N. L. Munby's *Sale Catalogues of Libraries of Eminent Persons* (1:203–49). Sinclair cites John "Brown's Works" on page 38 of volume 1. While researching Byron's interest in medicine at the National Library of Medicine in Bethesda, Maryland, I happened upon a collection of medical pamphlets owned by H. Drury, Harrow. Drury was likely Byron's tutor at Harrow (1751–1834), and Byron became quite close to him after leaving Harrow. Drury was assistant master of Harrow from 1801 (*DNB*). The volumes are dated 1823 and 1824 but encompass a range of medical literature from 1748–1813. Some especially relevant titles include *Letters on Indigestion* (1813), Gordon's *Complete English Physician* (1779), An *Essay on Public Medicines*, and *Tweedie's Hints on Temperance and Exercise* (1799). I found a total of three volumes of medical pamphlets inscribed "H. Drury. Harrow": W6 P3 v.432, W6 P3 v. 431, and W6 P3 v. 434. Since Drury's ownership is not indexed in the National Library of Medicine catalogs, the only way to find them was to do a hand search of the shelves.

7. I will discuss Byron and gender in relation to Wolfson, Franklin, Crompton, and Haslett below. William Galperin argues that writing in *Don Juan* is "aligned with the memory of contingency (and vice versa) and with the theoretically ungendered, undifferentiated state it recalls" (281).

8. Christensen's point that liberation promises liberation for both the agent and object of desire is harder to refute. Christensen also shows that Byron's "liberation" of young boys was driven by aristocratic patronage, making those boys beholden to him. Gary Dyer argues that Christensen is too quick to deemphasize persecution, and that Byron's literary sense of identity is also a "gay sense of identity shaped by wariness" (570).

9. Jonathan Gross argues that Byron's libertinism in 1813 involved a turning away from the public sphere and a retrenchment into class privilege (50). The poet's attraction to softness implies ambivalence to class privilege.

10. I am here indebted to Valerie Traub's work on the clitoris because it makes clear how central metonymy is to sexuality. She traces the means by which body part = embodied desire = erotic identity (see 100–103 especially).

11. I cite Niall Rudd's translation of *Juvenal: The Satires* (9, lines 15, 18–19). In canto 1:43 of *Don Juan*, Byron writes, "I can't help thinking Juvenal was wrong . . . in being downright rude." Given Byron's praise of softness, Byron may be indicating that Juvenal was wrong to condemn effeminate sodomites.

12. For more on Byron's interest in cross-dressing, see Garber, *Vested Interests* (316–21), and Wolfson.

13. On "mobility" as ventriloquism, see McGann's "Byron, Mobility, and the Poetics of Historical Ventriloquism" in *Byron and Romanticism* (36–51). Wolfson reminds us that Byron makes Lady Adeline "the poem's definitive figure of mobility" (590), thus making even it an unreliable index of gender.

14. I survey much of the literature on impotence in "Medicalizing the Romantic Libido: Sexual Pleasure, Luxury, and the Public Sphere."

15. Harvey traces how eighteenth-century erotica mapped women's bodies in terms of unknowability (106).

16. On what Byron may or may not have known concerning Castlereagh's suicide, see Crompton, *Byron and Greek Love* (302–6).

17. To make matters worse, as part of becoming an adult, young males are educated in Greek and Latin and classical eroticism and then warned that the price of sodomitic desire is the pillory (Gross 138). If such an education is to be a normal part of growing up, how can boys later be punished for doing what these classical writers have been advocating?

18. Mimi Yiu argues that epicene in the seventeenth century became "more vague, more promiscuous, and thus truer to its epicene nature by ambivalently indexing the androgynous, hermaphroditic, or effeminate" (72). Her point still holds in the Romantic period. See her "Sounding the Space between Men."

19. Later, Krafft-Ebbing will turn to "third sex" to encompass the homosexual.

20. On how modern critics use the term "third sex" and its limitations, see Garber, *Vested Interests* (10–11). Garber makes the case that "third" moves binaries beyond complementarity and toward contextualization (12).

21. On homosexual coding, in addition to Dyer and Crompton, see T. A. J. Burnett, *The Rise and Fall of a Regency Dandy* (36–39).

22. For an interesting reading of why the "femme" lesbian must be erased in eighteenth-century literature, see Sally O'Driscoll, "The Lesbian and the Passionless Woman: Femininity and Sexuality in Eighteenth-Century England" (103–31). She argues that antimasturbation literature focused its panic on the mannish lesbian, leaving

the femme to occupy a position between the passionless woman and the mannish lesbian, one that points out the contradictions in the idea of the passionless woman (104–5). Byron's ambivalence to softness meant that he did not dismiss the "femme" subject position.

23. C. Edwards reminds us that Roman *mollitia* is not necessarily sexual. Roman effeminacy refers to excess of all kinds. That one could be a mollitia and an adulterer, for example, shows that heterosexuality and effeminacy were both possible at once. See her chap. 2.

24. H. Montgomery Hyde, in *The Strange Death of Lord Castlereagh*, argues that Castlereagh followed a companion to a nearby brothel. As his companion undressed, he was horrified to discover that the person who brought him there was not a woman, but a boy dressed in woman's clothes and disguised to pass as a woman. At this moment, witnesses rushed in and threatened to make public an accusation (see 184–88). It is noteworthy that Castlereagh did not think he could cling to a stable notion of heterosexual identity as a defense. Nor did he think he could expose his blackmailers. Byron compares Castlereagh to Eutropius (Ded. 15). According to Gibbon, "The subjects of Arcadius were exasperated by the recollection that this deformed and decrepit eunuch, who so perversely mimicked the actions of a man, was born in the most abject conditions of servitude; that before he entered the Imperial palace he had been successively sold and purchased by an hundred masters" (2:196). Gibbon links effeminacy to the downfall of the Romans.

25. On the historical meanings surrounding effeminacy, see chap. 2 of Thomas King's *The Gendering of Men* (64–88).

26. Although the *OED* does acknowledge that "ass" can be a variant form or pronunciation of "arse," it does not date this kind of use until 1860.

27. I am indebted here to Leo Bersani, *Homos* (18).

28. Elfenbein's claim that genius in the Romantic period becomes associated with pushing gender boundaries and erotic transgression is worth remembering here. Yet in making Byron the moment when the prehistory of homosexuality becomes history, Elfenbein has his cake and eats it, too (1998 203).

29. Sinclair reprints Benjamin Waterhouse's "Public Lecture," which rehearses key ideas of Brunonian Medicine without crediting Brown. Waterhouse comments that "perfect health requires the temperate action of the vital influence through every part of the system" (4:536). He warns that "an imprudence in youth lays a foundation for hypochondriasis" (4:541), and that a "rakish life" will lead to illness (4:548–49). Waterhouse further points to the central role of the gastric juice and makes "the energy of the whole system" a remote cause of changes in the quality and quantity of this liquid (4:543).

30. Harvey shows how older men in erotica of the period were depicted as turning to flagellation in order to stimulate them (138). As men age, then, the ass becomes a legitimate site of sexuality so long as heterosexuality is the ultimate goal.

31. Elfenbein argues in *Romantic Genius* that effeminacy is pushed closer to sodomy in the Romantic period (21).

32. Crompton reminds us that Bentham refutes the idea that homosexuality undermines military strength, and shows how Byron himself celebrates the military band of Thebes (*Byron and Greek Love* 49–50). Wolfson calls attention to how "he-man muscle was keyed to national security" (*Borderlines* 149), thus making Byron's depiction of Sardanapalus even riskier.

33. Byron is likely consulting *Stark's Medical Works* (1788) for advice on dieting. Munby shows that Byron owned this work (1:228). The full title is *The Works of the Late William Stark, MD.* Stark outlined various diets and stipulated how much weight loss could be expected per week.

34. On Byron's sexuality and its coding in terms of flash, see Gary Dyer. Dyer shows how blackmail and robbery can be codes for sodomy. Dyer was not able to find the flash dictionary that Byron owned.

35. W. R. Trotter suggests that Brown's approach may prove useful especially in the fields of senescence and psychiatry, where the localization of diseases or the specificity of diseases have not been very helpful concepts. Trotter further suggests that Brown's excitability might better be understood as "responsiveness" (260).

36. Although Pearson's *Principles of Physic* shows him to be solidly in the Brunonian camp, Pearson does disagree with Brown that life is itself a forced state (8). Pearson also gives more credit to localization of diseases, insisting that "the number, figure, size, weight, texture, connection, colour, &c of the different parts . . . should be investigated in healthy, and diseased states, by anatomy" (20). I must thank Virginia Murray for looking in the Murray Archives for any documents relating to Pearson; unfortunately, there were none.

37. Risse argues in "Brunonian Therapeutics" that Brown's "recourse to alcohol as both a stimulant and restorative broke no new ground" (49). He adds that "like many Scottish physicians, Brown used [pubs] to see patients and make the contacts necessary to upward social mobility, especially membership in learned societies and perhaps a position at the local university" (49).

38. My discussion of Brown has benefited enormously from the works of Risse, Lawrence, Overmier, and an anonymous article, "John Brown—Founder of the Brunonian System of Medicine," which appeared in the *Journal of the American Medical Association* in 1965.

39. Nicholson identifies "Rogeson" as Dr. John Rogerson, a Scottish doctor from Edinburgh who was Catherine's chief physician from 1769 until 1796 (Facsimile 180). The DNB lists his dates as 1741–1823 and notes that Rogerson was called in too late to treat Catherine's favorite, Lanskoy, who died. Catherine seemed to regard Rogerson as her most capable physician. He had a "predeliction for phlebotomies and laxatives" but was a doctor "who recognized the particular needs of his patients, and a good diagnostician" (47:595). Rogerson helped Catherine get over Catherine's depression at Lanskoi's demise (Alexander 195).

40. On the off chance that Byron's doctor was Richard Pearson, I checked this prescription against Richard's *New Collection of Medical Prescriptions* (1794). Richard likewise lists Sennae and Mannae as evacuants, but Richard relies upon Cullen and Boerhaave, warning against those who are "ignorant of the structure and oeconomy of the human body, who are ignorant of the seats and causes of diseases" from using this manual to prescribe medications willy nilly (xiii). Since Byron's Pearson seems so concerned with the poet's debility, and with tending to his enervation, I think the likelier candidate is George. The fact that Richard does not seem to be a Brunonian further supports my claim. For more on Brown's courses of treatment, see Guenter Risse, "Brunonian Therapeutics: New Wine in Old Bottles" (48).

41. See, for example, Edmund Curll's *Arbor Vitae, or the Tree of Life.* "The stem seems to be of the sensitive tribe, tho' herein differing from the more common Sensitives; that whereas they are know to shrink and retire from even the gentlest touch of a lady's hand,

this rises on the contrary, and extends itself, when it is so handled" (2). Byron's attention to Juan's withered sensitive plant implies that Juan's is more like the plant.

42. On Bankes, see Crompton, *Byron and Greek Love* (100, 108, 347, 357–58). Bankes was later twice arrested for sexual misconduct, once with a guardsman.

43. MacCarthy writes, "At Newstead Rushton slept in a little cubbyhole adjoining Byron's bedroom. The probability that his services included sex emerges in a coded exchange of correspondence between Byron and Hobhouse over the well-known portrait by George Sanders showing Byron and Rushton standing in a rocky landscape . . . Hobhouse teases Byron for his sexual recklessness" (78). MacCarthy also details Hobhouse's sense that Byron had nothing to learn about sexual relationships "when he came from Harrow" (40).

44. For a fascinating account of Byron's adolescence at Harrow School, and the implications of this for Lord Byron's strength, see Paul Elledge's *Lord Byron at Harrow School*. In my review of Elledge (*KSJ* 2002), I pointed out that he had done for Byron what Christopher Ricks did for Keats. Elledge does not treat the biology of puberty.

45. On this, see Caroline Franklin. While Franklin also demonstrates that Byron resisted complementarity, she focuses upon Byron's readings about the history and social condition of women, not the biological notion of complementarity.

46. Here we should remind ourselves of Karen Harvey's warning that "a language of mutuality did not mean men's and women's sexual pleasures and behaviour was in any way symmetrical" (111).

47. Byron's epithet "soft" is sarcastic. Abernethy had a reputation for roughness, especially among his well-heeled clients. On Abernethy's famous roughness when dealing with patients, see Stephen Jacyna, "'Mr. Scott's Case'" (258–61).

48. An important exception here is Valerie Traub's wonderful essay, "The Psychomorphology of the Clitoris." Traub traces how metonymy asserts "the commensurability of body part(s) and erotic identity" (101).

49. Abernethy delivered these lectures in 1815 and in 1817 before the Royal College of Surgeons in London.

50. Bernard Beatty glosses this line with "such an epigram, though dismissing intellects, promotes the intellect-based poise of the speaker" (18).

51. Hunter, we recall, treated Byron for his clubfoot.

52. According to the *OED* (1989), gallantry was more than men's devotion to women. Gallantry could mean simply "amorous intercourse," with no sex specified.

53. On the importance of Horace as a stylistic model for *Don Juan*, see McGann, *Don Juan in Context* (69–73). On the ambivalences of Byron's Horatian allegiance, see Jane Stabler, *Byron, Poetics and History* (chap. 3). Stabler shows how Byron's digressions unsettle Horatian decorum.

54. Brian Arkins argues that Horace's turn is in fact modeled after Callimachus and the Greek lyric poet Alcaeus (107).

55. Horace's use of Sapphic meter in his Odes, along with making Sappho and Alcaeus two of his main predecessors, may serve as another context for Byron's interest in Horace. See Tony Woodman, "Biformes Vates" (54–55).

56. I have not been able to locate a 1766 two-volume edition of Hurd's Horace. ECCO lists a fourth edition three-volume version published in 1766. The closest I have been able to come is a 1768 two-volume Dublin edition of the *Epistolae ad Pisones, et Augustum with an English commentary and Notes: to which are added critical dissertations by the*

*Reverend Mr. Hurd* (Dublin, 1768). Yet the three-volume edition also contains Hurd's essay on the method of the "Art of Poetry." The auction records of Byron's library lists "Hurd's Horace, 2 vol. 1766" together with "Ovid's Metamorphoses, Garth" (Munby 1: 219). This may help explain why Byron credits Horace with "medio tu tutissimus ibis" when he means Ovid.

57. In *Vice Versa*, Garber provides a helpful survey of Girard's, Sedgwick's, and Castle's takes on triangulated desire (see 424–28).

58. Steven Angelides criticizes Garber on the grounds that she automatically accords bisexuality with the power to disrupt sexuality. Angelides shows in example by example, by contrast, how the speciation of bisexuality is resisted because it "disrupts the very classificatory alliance of sex/gender and sexuality" (47). See his *A History of Bisexuality*.

# Works Cited

Abernethy, John. *Introductory Lectures Exhibiting Some of Mr. Hunter's Opinions Respecting Life and Diseases.* London, Longman, 1815.
———. "Notes from Lectures by John Abernethy, 1805." National Library of Medicine MS B 366.
———. *Physiological Lectures.* London, 1817.
———. *The Surgical and Physiological Works of John Abernethy.* 4 vols. London: Longman, Rees, Orme, Brown, 1830.
Adair, J. M. *An Essay on Diet and Regimen.* London: James Ridgway, 1812.
Adams, George. *An Essay on Electricity, Explaining the Principles of the Useful; Science with a Letter to the Author from Mr. John Birch, Surgeon.* London: R. Hindmarsh, 1792.
Alexander, J. T. "Medicine at the Court of Catherine the Great of Russia." In *Medicine at the Courts of Europe, 1500–1837.* Ed. Vivian Nutton. London: Routledge, 1990.
Altieri, Charles. *The Particulars of Rapture: An Aesthetics of the Affects.* Ithaca: Cornell UP, 2003.
Angelides, Steven. *A History of Bisexuality.* Chicago: U Chicago P, 2001.
[anonymous] "John Brown: Founder of the Brunonian System of Medicine." *JAMA* 192, 6 (May 10, 1965): 225–26.
Appel, Toby A. *The Cuvier–Geoffroy Debate.* New York: Oxford UP, 1987.
Appiah, Anthony. *The Ethics of Identity.* Princeton: Princeton UP, 2005.
Arendt, Hannah. *On Revolution.* New York: Viking, 1963.
*Aristotle's Masterpiece.* Glasgow, 1776.
Arkins, Brian. "The Cruel Joke of Venus: Horace as Love Poet." In *Horace 2000: A Celebration.* Ed. Niall Rudd. Ann Arbor: U Michigan P, 1993.
Armstrong, Isobel. "Textual Harassment: The Ideology of Close Reading; or, How Close Is Close?" *Textual Practice* 9, 3 (1995): 401–20.
Arnauld, George. *A Dissertation on Hermaphrodites.* London: A Millar, 1750.
Baillie, Matthew. *Lectures and Observations on Medicine.* London: Richard Taylor, 1825.
———. *The Morbid Anatomy of Some of the Most Important Parts of the Human Body.* London: J. Johnson, 1793.
———. *The Works of Matthew Baillie, M.D.* 2 vols. London: Longman, Hurst, Rees, Orme, Brown, and Green, 1825.
Baillie, Matthew, with William Cruickshank. "Lectures on Anatomy." National Library of Medicine MS B 967 v.1. circa 1790.
Barker-Benfield, G. J. *The Culture of Sensibility.* Chicago: U Chicago P, 1992.
Barthes, Roland. *The Pleasure of the Text.* Trans. Richard Miller. New York: Hill and Wang, 1975.

Bataille, Georges. *Eroticism: Death and Sensuality*. Trans. Mary Dalwood. San Francisco: City Lights Books, 1986.

Beatty, Bernard. *Byron's Don Juan*. London: Croom Helm, 1985.

Beer, John. "The Impact of the Book of Enoch." In *Historicizing Blake*. Ed. Steve Clark and David Worrall. New York: St. Martin's, 1994.

Bell, Andrew. *Anatomia Britannica*. Edinburgh: Andrew Bell, 1798.

Bell, Charles. *Bridgewater Treatise on the Power Wisdom and Goodness of God as Manifested in the Creation: The Hand: Its Mechanism and Vital Endowments*. London: William Pickering, 1833.

———. *Idea of a New Anatomy of the Brain*. London: 1811.

———. *The Nervous System of the Human Body*. 3rd ed. London: Henry Renshaw, 1844. [1833]

Bell, John. *The Anatomy of the Human Body*. London: A. Strahan, 1802.

Bell, T. *Kalogynomia; or, the Laws of Female Beauty*. London: J.J. Stockdale, 1821.

Benjamin, Walter. "Theses on the Philosophy of History." In *Illuminations*. Ed. Hannah Arendt. Trans. Harry Zohn. New York: Schocken, 1977.

Bentham, Jeremy. "Jeremy Bentham's Essay on Paederasty Part 2." Ed. Louis Crompton. *Journal of Homosexuality*. 4, 1 (fall 1978): 91–107.

———. *A Table of the Springs of Action*. London: R. Hunter, 1817.

Bentley, Gerald E. *Blake Records*. 2nd ed. New Haven: Yale UP, 2004.

Bersani, Leo. *The Culture of Redemption*. Cambridge: Harvard UP, 1990.

———. *The Freudian Body Psychoanalysis and Art*. New York: Columbia UP, 1986.

———. *Homos*. Cambridge: Harvard UP, 1995.

———. "Is the Rectum a Grave?" In *AIDS: Cultural Analysis Cultural Activism*. Ed. Douglas Crimp. Cambridge: MIT P, 1988.

Bewell, Alan. "'Jacobin Plants': Botany as Social Theory in the 1790s." *Wordsworth Circle* 20 (1989): 132–39.

———. "'On the Banks of the South Sea': Botany and Sexual Controversy in the Eighteenth Century." In *Visions of Empire: Voyages, Botany and Representations of Nature*. Ed. David Miller and Peter Reill. Cambridge: Cambridge UP, 1996.

———. *Romanticism and Colonial Disease*. Baltimore: Johns Hopkins UP, 1999.

———. "Romantic Natural History Workshop." North American Society for the Study of Romanticism conference. West Lafayette, IN. September 2006.

Bianchi, Giovanni. *Dissertation on the Case of Catharine Vizzani, Containing the Adventures of a young gentlewoman, a native of Rome, who for many years past [sic] in the habit of a man, was killed for an amour with a young lady; and found, on dissection, a true virgin, narrowly escaped being treated as a saint by the populace. With some curious anatomical remarks on the nature and existence of the hymen*. London: W. Meyer, n.d. [BL Shelfmark 1174c21].

Bindman, David, gen. ed. *Blake's Illuminated Books*. 6 vols. Princeton: William Blake Trust, 1991–95.

Binhammer, Katherine. "The Sex Panic of the 1790s." *Journal of the History of Sexuality* 6, 3 (1996): 409–34.

Birch, John. *Essay on the Medical Application of Electricity*. London: J. Johnson, 1802.

Blake, William. *America*. London: Trianon, 1963.

———. *Blake's Illuminated Works*. Gen. ed. David Bindman. 6 vols. Princeton: Princeton UP, 1991–95.

———. *The Complete Poetry and Prose of William Blake.* Ed. David Erdman. Garden City: Anchor Books, 1982. [E]

———. "Illustrated Manuscript of Genesis." Huntington Library and Art Gallery. Accession nos. 000.32, 000.33, 000.34, 000.35, 000.36, 000.37, and 000.38.

Bland, Robert. *Observations on Human and Comparative Parturition.* London: J. Johnson, 1794.

Bloom, Harold. *Blake's Apocalypse: A Study in Poetic Argument.* Ithaca: Cornell UP, 1963.

Blumenbach, Johann. *The Anthropological Treatises of Johann Friedrich Blumenbach.* Trans. Thomas Bendyshe. London: Longman, 1865.

Bogen, Nancy, ed. *The Book of Thel.* Providence: Brown UP, 1971.

*The Bon Ton Magazine.* Vol. 11. London: D. Brewman, 1792. British Library Private Case. Cup 820m22.

Boone, Joseph Allen. *Libidinal Currents: Sexuality and the Shaping of Modernism.* Chicago: U Chicago P, 1998.

Bostock, John. *An Elementary System of Physiology.* 3 vols. London: Baldwin, Cradock, and Joy, 1824.

Bristow, Joseph. *Sexuality.* London: Routledge, 1997.

British Museum. Department of Greek and Roman Art. Collection of Richard Payne Knight.

Brown, John. *Elements of Medicine.* 2 vols. London: J. Johnson, 1788 and 1795.

Brown, Marshall. "Romanticism and Enlightenment." In *The Cambridge Companion to Romanticism.* Ed. Stuart Curran. Cambridge: Cambridge UP, 1993.

Brown, Nathaniel. *Sexuality and Feminism in Shelley.* Cambridge: Harvard UP, 1979.

Browne, Janet. "Botany in the Boudoir and Garden: the Banksian Context." In *Visions of Empire: Voyages, Botany and Representations of Nature.* Ed. David Miller and Peter Reill. Cambridge: Cambridge UP, 1996.

Bruder, Helen. *William Blake and the Daughters of Albion.* New York: St. Martin's, 1997.

Buffon, Compte de. "Histoire Naturelle de L'Homme. De la Puberté." In *Histoire Naturelle, Générale et Particulière.* Vol. 2. Paris: Imprimerie Royale, 1749.

———. *Natural History, General and Particular.* Vol. 2. Trans. William Smellie. London: A. Strahan and T. Cadell, 1791.

Burke, Edmund. *A Philosophical Enquiry into the Origins of Our Ideas of the Sublime and Beautiful.* In *The Harvard Classics: Edmund Burke.* Ed. Charles Eliot. New York: P. F. Collier & Son, 1937.

———. *A Vindication of Natural Society.* Ed. Frank Pagano. Indianapolis: Liberty Classics, 1982.

Burnett, T. A. J. *The Rise and Fall of a Regency Dandy: The Life and Times of Scrope Berdmore Davies.* Boston: Little, Brown, 1981.

Burns, John. *The Principles of Midwifery; including the Diseases of Women and Children.* Philadelphia, 1820 (5th American ed. from the 3rd London ed.).

Butler, Judith. *Bodies that Matter: On the Discursive Limits of Sex.* New York: Routledge, 1993.

Butler, Marilyn, ed. *Mary Shelley Frankenstein.* Oxford: Oxford UP, 1993.

Bynum, W. F. *Science and the Practice of Medicine in the Nineteenth Century.* Cambridge: Cambridge UP, 1994.

Byron, George. *Byron's Don Juan: A Variorum Edition.* Eds. Truman Guy Steffan and Willis W. Pratt. 4 vols. Austin: U Texas P, 1971. [S & P]

————. *Byron's Letters and Journals.* 12 vols. Ed. Leslie Marchand. Cambridge: Harvard UP, 1973–82.

Cafarelli, Annette Wheeler. "The Transgressive Double Standard: Shelleyan Utopianism and Feminist Social History." In *Shelley's Poetry and Prose.* Ed. Donald Reiman and Neil Fraistat. New York: Norton, 2002.

Campbell, Robert Allen. *Phallic Worship.* London: Kegan Paul, 2002.

Canguilhem, Georges. *Ideology and Rationality in the History of the Life Sciences.* Trans. Arthur Goldhammer. Cambridge: MIT P, 1988.

————. *The Normal and the Pathological.* Trans. Carolyn Fawcett. New York: Zone Books, 1989.

Capanna, Ernesto. "Lazzaro Spallanzani: At the Roots of Modern Biology." *Journal of Experimental Zoology* 285 (1999):178–196.

Carlisle, Richard. *Every Woman's Book; or, What Is Love?* London: Richard Carlisle, 1828.

Carlson, Julie. *England's First Family of Writers: Mary Wollstonecraft, William Godwin, Mary Shelley.* Baltimore: Johns Hopkins UP, 2007.

————. "Forever Young: Master Betty and the Queer Stage of Youth in English Romanticism." *South Atlantic Quarterly* 95, no. 3 (summer 1996): 575–602.

Cash, Arthur. *John Wilkes: The Scandalous Father of Civil Liberty.* New Haven: Yale UP, 2006.

Castle, Terry. *The Apparitional Lesbian: Female Homosexuality and Modern Culture.* New York: Columbia UP, 1993.

Caton, T. M. Surgeon. *Popular Remarks, Medical and Literary, on Nervous, Hypochondriac, and Hysterical Diseases.* London: W. Neelly, 1815.

Cheyne, George. *The English Malady; or, a Treatise of Nervous Diseases of All Kinds.* 4th ed. London: G. Strahan, 1784.

Christensen, Jerome. *Lord Byron's Strength.* Baltimore: Johns Hopkins UP, 1993.

Churchill, Charles. "The Times." Proof Sheets Annotated by Churchill and John Wilkes. [British Library Shelfmark c61.c3. 1764]

Churchill, Wendy D. "The Medical Practice of the Sexed Body: Women, Men, and Disease in Britain, circa 1600–1740." *Social History of Medicine* 18, 1 (2005): 3–22.

Clark, Anna. *Scandal: The Sexual Politics of the British Constitution.* Princeton: Princeton UP, 2004.

Clark, David Lee, ed. *Shelley's Prose.* London: Fourth Estate, 1988.

Clarke, Edwin, and Jacyna, L.S. *Nineteenth-Century Origins of Neuroscientific Concepts.* Berkeley: U California P, 1987.

Clarke, Eric O. *Virtuous Vice: Homoeroticism and the Public Sphere.* Durham: Duke UP, 2000.

Cline, Henry. "Cline's Surgery." National Library of Medicine MS B 400. Circa 1790.

Cody, Lisa Forman. *Birthing the Nation: Sex, Science, and the Conception of Eighteenth-Century Britons.* Oxford: Oxford UP, 2005.

Coffman, Ralph. *Coleridge's Library: A Bibliography of Books Owned or Read by Samuel Taylor Coleridge.* Boston: G. K. Hall, 1987.

Cohen, William. *Sex Scandal: The Private Parts of Victorian Fiction.* Durham: Duke UP, 1996.

Coleman, William. *Biology in the Nineteenth Century: Problems of Form, Function, and Transformation.* New York: Wiley, 1971.

Coleridge, Samuel Taylor. *Collected Letters of Samuel Taylor Coleridge.* Ed. Earl Leslie Griggs. Vol. 5. Oxford: Clarendon, 1971.

———. "Contributions to a Course of Lectures Given by J. H. Green." In *Shorter Works and Fragments.* Vol. 2. Ed. H. J. Jackson and J. R. de J. Jackson. Princeton: Princeton UP.

———. "Contributions to J. H. Green's Lectures on Aesthetics." In *Shorter Works and Fragments.* Vol. 2. Ed. H. J. Jackson and J. R. de J. Jackson. Princeton: Princeton UP, 1995.

———. *Hints towards the Formation of a More Comprehensive Theory of Life.* London: John Churchill, 1848.

———. *Marginalia.* I. Ed. George Whalley. *The Collected Works of Samuel Taylor Coleridge.* Princeton: Bollingen Series, 1980.

———. *The Notebooks of Samuel Taylor Coleridge.* Vols. 1–3. Ed. Kathleen Coburn. Princeton: Princeton UP, 1957–73.

———. *Shorter Works and Fragments.* Ed. H. J. Jackson and J. R. de J. Jackson. 2 vols. Princeton: Princeton UP, 1995.

Collings, David. *Wordsworthian Errancies.* Baltimore: Johns Hopkins UP, 1994.

Compston, Alastair. "The Convergence of neurological anatomy and pathology in the British Isles: 1800–1830." In *A Short History of Neurology: The British Contribution 1660–1910.* Ed. Clifford Rose. Oxford: Butterworth Heinemann, 1999.

Connolly, Tristanne. *William Blake and the Body.* Houndmills: Palgrave, 2002.

Cook, Hera. *The Long Sexual Revolution.* Oxford: Oxford UP, 2004.

Cookson, A. "Case of Premature Puberty." *Medical and Physical Journal* 25 London (January–June 1811): 117–18.

Cooper, Astley. "History of a Case of Premature Puberty." *Medico-Chirugical Transactions* 4 London, 1813.

———. *Lectures on the Principles and Practice of Surgery.* 3 vols. London, 1824.

———. *Observations on the Structure and Diseases of the Testis.* London: Longman, Rees, 1830.

———. "Notes on Astley Paston Cooper's Lectures." Taken by Robert Pughe, student at St. Thomas's and St. Guy's Hospitals. 1815–17. Wellcome Library MS 7096. [My pagination refers to Pughe's, not the archival pagination.]

Cooter, Roger. *The Cultural Meanings of Popular Science.* Cambridge: Cambridge UP, 1984.

Corber, Robert. "Representing the 'Unspeakable': William Godwin and the Politics of Homophobia." *Journal of the History of Sexuality* 1, 1 (1990): 86–101.

Couper, R. *Speculations on the Mode and Appearances of Impregnation in the Human Female.* Edinburgh, 1789.

Craciun, Adriana. *Fatal Women of Romanticism.* Cambridge: Cambridge UP, 2003.

Cranefield, Paul F. *The Way in and the Way Out: Francois Magendie, Charles Bell and the Roots of the Spinal Nerves with a Facsimile of Charles Bell's Annotated Copy of his* Idea of a New Anatomy of the Brain. Mount Kisco: Futura Publishing, 1974.

Crompton, Louis. *Byron and Greek Love.* London: Faber and Faber, 1985.

———. *Homosexuality and Civilization.* Cambridge: Harvard UP, 2003

Cruickshank, William. "Lectures on Anatomy." MS B 967 VI. National Library of Medicine, Bethesda.

Cullen, William. "Cullen's Manuscript Text of the Practice of Medicine." Wellcome Library MS 6036. Circa 1777.

———. *First Lines of the Practice of Physic.* 4 vols. London: T. Cadell, 1786.

———. *A Treatise of the Materia Medica.* 2 vols. Edinburgh, 1789.

Cunningham, Andrew. "The Pen and the Sword: Recovering the Disciplinary Identity of Physiology and Anatomy before 1800. I. Old Physiology: The Pen." *Studies in History and Philosophy of Biological and Biomedical Sciences* 33 (2002): 631–65.

———. "The Pen and the Sword: Recovering the Disciplinary Identity of Physiology and Anatomy before 1800. II. Old Anatomy: The Sword." *Studies in History and Philosophy of Biological and Biomedical Sciences* 34 (2003): 51–76.

Curll, Edmund. *Arbor Vitae, or the Tree of Life.* 1741. [BL PC25.b.17]

———. "Horace's Integer Vitae." In *The Potent Ally.* Bath: Edmund Curll, n.d. [British Library Private Case PC 20b7].

Curran, Stuart. *Shelley's Annus Mirabilis.* San Marino: Huntington Library, 1975.

Curtis, F. B. "William Blake and Eighteenth-Century Medicine." *Blake Studies* 8, 2 (1979): 187–99.

Cuvier, Georges. *Introduction to the Study of Animal Economy.* Trans. John Allen. Edinburgh, 1801.

———. *Leçons D'Anatomie Comparée* Paris: Baudoin, Annee 8. 2 vols.

———. *Lectures on Comparative Anatomy.* Trans. William Ross. 2 vols. London: Longman and Rees, 1802. [CA]

Dante Alighieri. *The Divine Comedy of Dante Alighieri. Inferno.* Trans. John D. Sinclair. New York: Oxford UP, 1967.

Darnton, Robert, with Daniel Roche, eds. *Revolution in Print: The Press in France 1775–1800.* Berkeley: U California P, 1989.

Darwin, Erasmus. *The Botanic Garden.* London: Joseph Johnson, 1791.

———. *Zoonomia; or, the Laws of Organic Life.* 3 parts. London: Joseph Johnson, 1801.

Davidson, Arnold. *The Emergence of Sexuality.* Cambridge: Harvard UP, 2001.

Davy, Humphrey. *A Discourse, Introductory to a Course of Lectures on Chemistry.* London: J. Johnson, 1802.

De Almeida, Hermione. *Romantic Medicine and John Keats.* New York: Oxford UP, 1991.

De Bolla, Peter. *The Discourse of the Sublime.* Oxford: Basil Blackwell, 1989.

De Lauretis, Teresa. *The Practice of Love: Lesbian Sexuality and Perverse Desire.* Bloomington: Indiana UP, 1994.

De Luca, Vincent. *Words of Eternity: Blake and the Poetics of the Sublime.* Princeton: Princeton UP, 1991.

De Man, Paul. *Aesthetic Ideology.* Ed. Andrzej Warminski. Minneapolis: U Minnesota P, 1996.

———. *The Resistance to Theory.* Minneapolis: U Minnesota P, 1986.

———. "The Rhetoric of Temporality." In *Blindness and Insight.* Minneapolis: U Minnesota P, 1983.

Dean, Carolyn. "The Productive Hypothesis: Foucault, Gender, and the History of Sexuality." *History and Theory* 33, 3 (1994): 271–96.

Denham, Thomas. *Introduction to the Practice of Midwifery.* 2 vols. London: Joseph Johnson, 1794.

*Dictionary of National Biography.* 60 vols. Oxford: Oxford UP, 2004.

Dixon, Laurinda. *Perilous Chastity: Women and Medicine in Pre-Enlightenment Art and Medicine.* Ithaca: Cornell UP, 1995.

Dollimore, Jonathan. *Sex, Literature, and Censorship.* Cambridge: Polity, 2001.

———. *Sexual Dissidence: Augustine to Wilde, Freud to Foucault.* Oxford: Clarendon P, 1991.

Dreger, Alice Domurat. *Hermaphrodites and the Medical Invention of Sex.* Cambridge: Harvard UP, 1998.

Duncan, Philip Bury. *On Instinct.* London, 1820.

Dyer, Gary. "Thieves, Boxers, Sodomites, Poets: Being Flash to Byron's *Don Juan*" *PMLA* 116, 3 (2001): 562–78.

Eagleton, Terry. *The Ideology of the Aesthetic.* Oxford: Basil Blackwell, 1990.

Eaves, Morris. *The Counter-Arts Conspiracy: Art and Industry in the Age of Blake.* Ithaca: Cornell UP, 1992.

Eaves, Morris, Robert Essick, and Joseph Viscomi, eds. *William Blake: The Early Illuminated Books.* Princeton: Princeton UP, 1993.

Edelman, Lee. *No Future: Queer Theory and the Death Drive.* Durham: Duke UP, 2004.

Edwards, Catharine. *The Politics of Immorality in Ancient Rome.* Cambridge: Cambridge UP, 1993.

Edwards, Pamela. *The Statesman's Science: History, Nature, Law in the Political Thought of Samuel Taylor Coleridge.* New York: Columbia UP, 2004.

*Elements of Botany.* London, 1775.

Elfenbein, Andrew. "Mary Wollstonecraft and the Sexuality of Genius." *The Cambridge Companion to Mary Wollstonecraft.* Ed. Claudia Johnson. Cambridge: Cambridge UP, 2002.

———. *Romantic Genius: Towards a Prehistory of a Homosexual Role.* New York: Columbia UP, 1999.

———. "Romantic Loves: A Response to Historicizing Romantic Sexuality." In *Historicizing Romantic Sexuality.* Special issue of *Romantic Praxis* (January 2006) [www.rc.umd.edu/praxis/sexuality/elfenbein/elfenbein.html].

Elledge, Paul. *Lord Byron at Harrow School.* Baltimore: Johns Hopkins UP, 2000.

*Encyclopedia Britannica.* 3 vols. Edinburgh: Bell and Macfarquhar, 1771.

Essick, Robert. "How Blake's Body Means." In *Unnam'd Forms: Blake and Textuality.* Ed. Nelson Hilton and Thomas A. Vogler. Berkeley: U California P, 1986.

———. *William Blake, Printmaker.* Princeton: Princeton UP, 1980.

———. *William Blake and the Language of Adam.* Oxford: Clarendon P, 1989.

———. *The Works of William Blake in the Huntington Collections.* San Marino: Huntington Library, 1985.

Fancher, Raymond. E. *Pioneers of Psychology.* 2nd ed. New York: Norton, 1990.

Farr, Samuel. *Elements of Medical Jurisprudence.* London: T. Becket, 1788.

Faubert, Michelle. "A Gendered Affliction: Women, Writing, Madness." In *Cultural Constructions of Madness in Eighteenth-Century Writing.* Allan Ingram with Michelle Faubert. Houndmills: Palgrave Macmillan, 2005.

Faubion, James, ed. *Michel Foucault: Aesthetics, Method, and Epistemology.* Trans. Robert Hurley and others. New York: New P, 1994.

Fausto-Sterling, Anne. *Sexing the Body: Gender Politics and the Construction of Sexuality.* New York: Basic Books, 2000.

Felluga, Dino. *The Perversity of Poetry.* Albany: SUNY P, 2005.

Ferguson, Frances. *Solitude and the Sublime.* New York: Routledge, 1992.

Ferrier, P. M. "De la puberté considerer comme crise des maladies de l'enfance." Essay Presented to the School of Medicine at Montpelier. Montpelier, 1799.

Figlio, Karl. "Theories of Perception and the Physiology of Mind in the Late Eighteenth Century." *History of Science* 13 (1975): 177–212.

Fletcher, Anthony. *Gender, Sex and Subordination in England 1500–1800.* New Haven: Yale UP, 1995.

Foot, Phillipa. "Locke, Hume, and Modern Moral Theory: A Legacy of Seventeenth- and Eighteenth-Century Philosophies of Mind." In *The Languages of Psyche.* Ed. George Rousseau. Berkeley: U California P, 1990.

Foucault, Michel. *Abnormal.* Trans. Graham Burchell. New York: Picador, 2003.

———. *Essential Works of Foucault, 1954–1984.* Vol. 2. Ed. James Faubion. Trans. Robert Hurley and others. New York: New P, 1998.

———. *The History of Sexuality: An Introduction.* Trans. Robert Hurley. New York: Vintage Books, 1978.

———. *The History of Sexuality: The Care of the Self.* Vol. 3. Trans. Robert Hurley. New York: Vintage Books, 1988.

———. *The Order of Things.* New York: Pantheon Books, 1970.

Fraistat, Neil and Don Reiman, eds. *The Complete Poetry of Percy Bysshe Shelley.* Vol. 2. Baltimore: Johns Hopkins UP, 2004.

Franklin, Caroline. *Byron's Heroines.* Oxford: Clarendon P, 1992.

Freedberg, David. *The Power of Images.* Chicago: U Chicago P, 1989.

Freud, Sigmund. *The Ego and the Id.* Trans. Joan Riviere. London: Hogarth, 1927.

Friedman, Geraldine. "School for Scandal: Sexual, Race, and National Vice and Virtue in *Miss Marianne Woods and Miss Jane Pirie against Lady Helen Cumming Gordon.*" In "Romanticism and Sexual Vice." Ed. Daniel O'Quinn. Special issue of *Nineteenth-Century Contexts* 27, 1 (March 2005): 53–76.

Frosch, Thomas. *The Awakening of Albion.* Ithaca: Cornell UP, 1984.

Fulford, Tim. "Radical Medicine and Romantic Politics." *Wordsworth Circle* 35, 1 (winter 2004): 16–20.

Funnell, Peter. "The Symbolical Language of Antiquity." In *The Arrogant Connoisseur: Richard Payne Knight, 1751–1824.* Manchester: Manchester UP, 1982.

Furniss, Tom. "Mary Wollstonecraft's French Revolution." In *The Cambridge Companion to Mary Wollstonecraft.* Ed. Claudia Johnson. Cambridge: Cambridge UP, 2002.

Gall, Franz. *Manual of Phrenology: Being an Analytical Summary of the System of Doctor Gall on the Faculties of Man and Functions of the Brain.* Philadelphia: Carey, Lea & Blanchard, 1835. [Manual]

———. "Notes on Phrenological Lectures, taken at Paris in 1810." Welcome MS 5323.

———. *On the Functions of the Brain and Each of its Parts: With Observations on the Possibility of Determining the Instincts, Propensities, and Talents, or the Moral and Intellectual Dispositions of Men and Animals by the Configuration of the Brain and Head.* Trans. Winslow Lewis, 6 vols. Boston: Marsh, Capen, and Lyon, 1835.

———. *On the Functions of the Cerebellum.* Trans. George Comb. Edinburgh: Maclachlan and Stewart, 1838. [Cerebellum]

———. *On the Origin of the Moral Qualities and Intellectual Faculties of Man and the Conditions of their Manifestation.* 6 vols. Trans. Winslow Lewis. Boston: Marsh, Capen, and Lyon, 1835.

Galperin, William. *The Return of the Visible in British Romanticism.* Baltimore: Johns Hopkins UP, 1993.

Garber, Marjorie. *Vested Interests: Cross-dressing and Cultural Anxiety.* London: Routledge, 1992.

———. *Vice Versa: Bisexuality and the Eroticism of Everyday Life.* New York: Simon and Schuster, 1995.

Gasking, Elizabeth. *Investigations into Generation, 1651–1828.* London: Hutchinson, 1967.

Geoffroy Saint-Hilaire, Étienne. *Philosophie Anatomique: Des Monstruosités Humaines.* Paris, 1822. [PA]

Gibbon, Edward. *The Decline and Fall of the Roman Empire.* 3 vols. New York: Modern Library, n.d.

Giddens, Anthony. *The Transformation of Intimacy.* Stanford: Stanford UP, 1992.

Gilbert, Arthur. "Conceptions of Homosexuality and Sodomy in Western History." *Journal of Homosexuality* 6, 1/2 (fall/winter 1980–81): 57–68.

———. "Sexual Deviance and Disaster during the Napoleonic Wars." *Albion* 9 (1977): 98–113.

Gilman, Sander. *Sex: An Illustrated History.* New York: Wiley, 1989.

Gladden, Samuel. *Shelley's Textual Seductions.* New York: Routledge, 2002.

Gleckner, Robert. *Blake's Prelude: Poetical Sketches.* Baltimore: Johns Hopkins UP, 1982.

———. "Blake's *Thel* and the Bible." *Bulletin of the New York Public Library* 64 (1960): 573–80.

Goldsmith, Steven. *Unbuilding Jerusalem: Apocalyse and Romantic Representation.* Ithaca: Cornell UP, 1993.

Golinski, Jan. *Science as Public Culture: Chemistry and Enlightenment in Britain, 1760–1820.* Cambridge: Cambridge UP, 1992.

Gooch, Benjamin. *The Chirurgical Works of Benjamin Gooch, Surgeon.* 3 vols. London: J. Johnson, 1792.

Goodheart, Eugene. *Desire and Its Discontents.* New York: Columbia UP, 1991.

Goodwin, C. James. *A History of Modern Psychology.* New York: Wiley, 1999.

Gould, Stephen Jay. *The Structure of Evolutionary Theory.* Cambridge: Harvard UP, 2002.

Greer, Germaine. "'No Earthly Parents I Confess': the Clod, the Pebble and Catherine Blake." In *Women Reading William Blake.* Ed. Helen Bruder. Houndmills: Palgrave Macmillan, 2007.

Gregory, John. *Comparative View of the State and Faculties of Man with Those of the Animal World.* London, 1766.

Grose, Frances. *A Classical Dictionary of the Vulgar Tongue.* Menston: Scolar P, 1968 [1785].

Gross, Jonathan David. *Byron The Erotic Liberal.* Lanham: Rowman & Littlefield, 2001

Guerrini, Anita. "Anatomists and Entrepreneurs in Early Eighteenth Century London." *Journal of the History of Medicine and Allied Sciences* 59, 2 (April 2004): 219–39.

Haggerty, George. *Men in Love: Masculinity and Sexuality in the Eighteenth Century.* New York: Columbia UP, 1999.

Hagstrum, Jean. *The Romantic Body: Love and Sexuality in Keats, Wordsworth, and Blake.* Knoxville: U Tennessee P, 1986.

———. *William Blake Poet and Painter.* Chicago: U Chicago P, 1964.

Hall, Lesley, and Roy Porter. *The Facts of Life: The Creation of Sexual Knowledge in Britain, 1650–1950.* New Haven: Yale UP, 1995.

Haller, Albrecht von. *Dissertation on the Sensible and Irritable Parts of Animals.* Baltimore: Johns Hopkins UP, 1936 [London, 1755].

———. *First Lines of Physiology.* Trans. William Cullen, MD. London, 1786.

Halperin, David M. *How to Do the History of Homosexuality.* Chicago: U Chicago P, 2002

———. *One Hundred Years of Homosexuality.* New York: Routledge, 1990.

———. "That Obscure Object of Historical Desire." In *Historicizing Romantic Sexuality.* Special issue of *Romantic Praxis* (January 2006) [www.rc.umd.edu/praxis/sexuality/halperin/halperin.html].

Hamilton, James. *Observations on the Seats and Causes of Diseases.* Edinburgh: 1795.

Hancock, Thomas. *Essay on Instinct, and Its Physical and Moral Relations.* London: William Phillips, 1824.

Harris, John. "Coleridge's Reading in Medicine." *Wordsworth Circle* 3 (1972): 85–95.

Harvey, Karen. *Reading Sex and Gender in the Eighteenth Century.* Cambridge: Cambridge UP, 2004.

Haslam, John. *Observations on Madness and Melancholy.* London: J. Callow, 1809.

Haslett, Moyra. *Byron's Don Juan and the Don Juan Legend.* Oxford: Clarendon P, 1997.

Hazlitt, William. *Liber Amoris: or, the New Pygmalion.* Ed. Gerald Lahey. New York: NYU P, 1980.

Hegel, Georg Wilhelm Friedrich. *Introductory Lectures on Aesthetics.* Trans. Bernard Bosanquet. Harmondsworth: Penguin Books, 1993.

Hein, Hilde. "The Endurance of the Mechanism: Vitalism Controversy." *Journal of the History of Biology* 5, 1 (spring 1972): 159–88.

Henderson, Andrea. *Romantic Identities.* Cambridge: Cambridge UP, 1996.

Henry, Thomas. *Memoirs of Albert de Haller.* Warrington: J. Johnson, 1783.

Hertz, Neil. *The End of the Line: Essays on Psychoanalysis and the Sublime.* New York: Columbia UP, 1985.

[Hill, John]. Uvedale, Christian [pseudonym]. *The Construction of the Nerves, and the Causes of Nervous Disorders.* London, 1758.

Hilton, Nelson. *Literal Imagination: Blake's Vision of Words.* Berkeley: U California P, 1983.

Hitchcock, Tim. *English Sexualities, 1700–1800.* New York: St. Martin's, 1990.

Hobson, Christopher Z. *Blake and Homosexuality.* New York: Palgrave, 2000.

Hocquenghem, Guy. *Homosexual Desire.* Ed. Michael Moon. Durham: Duke UP, 1993.

Hoeveler, Diane Long. *Romantic Androgyny: The Women Within.* University Park: Pennsylvania State UP, 1990.

Hollander, John. *Vision and Resonance: Two Sense of Poetic Form.* New Haven: Yale UP, 1985.

*Holy Bible.* Authorized King James Version. New York: Oxford UP.

Home, Everard. "An Account of the Dissection of an Hermaphrodite Dog." *Philosophical Transactions.* Vol. 69, part 1. London: Royal Society of London, 1799.

Horace Flaccus, Quintus. *The Complete Odes and Satires of Horace.* Trans. Sidney Alexander. Princeton: Princeton UP, 1999.

———. *The Complete Works of Horace.* Ed. Casper Kraemer, Jr. New York: Modern Library, 1936.

———. *Q. Horace Flacci Epistolae ad Pisones, et Augustum with an English Commentary and Notes: to which are added critical dissertations by the Reverend Mr. Hurd.* 2 vols. Dublin: Sarah Stringer, 1768.

Horowitz, Gad. "The Foucaultian Impasse: No Sex, No Self, No Revolution." *Political Theory* 15 (1) (February 1987) 61–80.

Hume, David. *A Treatise of Human Nature*. Ed. Ernest Mossner. Harmondsworth: Penguin Classics, 1984.

Hunt, Lynn, ed. *The Invention of Pornography*. New York: Zone Books, 1993.

Hunter, John. "An Account of an Extraordinary Pheasant." In *The Works of John Hunter*. 4 vols. Ed. James Palmer. Philadelphia: Haswell, Barrington, and Haswell, 1841.

———. "An Account of the Free-Martin." *Royal Society of London Philosophical Transactions*. London, 1779.

———. *The Case Books of John Hunter FRS*. Ed. Elizabeth Allen, J. L. Turk, and Sir Reginald Murley. London: Royal Society of Medicine Services, 1993.

———. *Essays and Observations on Natural History, Anatomy, Physiology, Psychology, and Geology*. 2 vols. London: John Van Voorst, 1861. [EO]

———. "Medical Lectures of 1784–5." 3 vols. National Library of Medicine, Bethesda, Call Number MS B 22.

———. *Observations on Certain Parts of the Animal Oeconomy*. London, 1786.

———. *A Treatise on the Venereal Disease*. 1st ed. London: Joseph Johnson, 1786.

Hunter, William. "Doctor Hunter's Anatomical and Chirurgical Lectures, October, November, and December 1768." 4 vols. Glasgow University Library. MS Gen 769–772.

———. "Draft of Final? Lecture on Midwifery, Mainly on Diseases Peculiar to the Sex." Glasgow University Library MS Hunter H37.

———. "Fair Copy of Lecture Notes on Midwifery. 1783." Glasgow University Library MS Gen 775.

———. Uncataloged manuscript of "Two Introductory Lectures on Anatomy." Huntington Library.

———. "William Hunter's Lectures on Anatomy." Circa 1780. Wellcome Library MS 7601.

Hyde, H. Montgomery. *The Strange Death of Lord Castlereagh*. London: William Heinemann, 1959.

Jacyna, Stephen. "'Mr. Scott's Case': A View of London Medicine in 1825." In *The Popularization of Medicine 1650–1850*. Ed. Roy Porter. London: Routledge, 1992.

Jager, Colin. *The Book of God*. Philadelphia: U Pennsylvania P, 2007.

Jameson, Fredric. "Pleasure, a Political Issue." In *The Ideologies of Theory*. Vol. 2. Minneapolis: U Minnesota P, 1989.

Jenkinson, James. *A Generic and Specific Description of British Plants*. Kendal, 1775.

Johnson, Claudia. *Equivocal Beings: Politics, Gender, and Sentimentality in the 1790s*. Chicago: U Chicago P, 1995.

———. "Mary Wollstonecraft: Styles of Radical Maternity." In *Inventing Maternity*. Ed. Susan Greenfield and Carol Barash. Lexington: U Kentucky P, 1999.

Jones, Frederick, ed. *The Letters of Percy Bysshe Shelley*. 2 vols. Oxford: Clarendon P, 1964.

Jones, J. Jennifer. "Sounds Romantic: The Castrato and English Poetics around 1800." In *Opera and Romanticism*. Ed. Gillen D'Arcy Wood. Special issue of *Romantic Praxis* (May 2005) [www.rc.umd.edu/praxis/opera/jones/jones.html].

Jordanova, Ludmilla. *Nature Displayed: Gender, Science and Medicine, 1760–1820*. London: Longman, 1999.

Jorgensen, C. Barker. *John Hunter, A. A. Berthold, and the Origins of Endocrinology*. Odense: Odense UP, 1971.

Juvenal. *The Satires*. Trans. Niall Rudd. Oxford: Clarendon P, 1991.

Kant, Immanuel. *Critique of Judgment*. Trans. Werner S. Pluhar. Indianapolis: Hackett Publishing, 1987. [CJ]

Keane, Angela. *Women Writers and the English Nation in the 1790s*. Cambridge: Cambridge UP, 2000.

Keach, William. *Arbitrary Power Romanticism, Language, Politics*. Princeton: Princeton UP, 2004.

Keats, John. *John Keats's Anatomical and Physiological Notebook*. Ed. Maurice Buxton Forman. New York: Haskell House, 1970.

Kelley, Theresa M. *Reinventing Allegory*. Cambridge: Cambridge UP, 1997.

———. "Romantic Exemplarity: Botany and 'Material' Culture." In *Romantic Science: The Literary Forms of Natural History*. Ed. Noah Heringman. Albany: SUNY P, 2003.

Kendrick, Walter. *The Secret Museum: Pornography in Modern Culture*. New York: Viking, 1987.

King, Helen. *The Disease of Virgins: Green Sickness, Chlorosis, and the Problems of Puberty*. London: Routledge, 2004.

King, Thomas. *The Gendering of Men, 1600–1750*. Vol. 1. Madison: U Wisconsin P, 2004.

King-Hele, Desmond. *Erasmus Darwin Doctor of Revolution*. London: Faber and Faber, 1972.

Kipnis, Laura. *Bound and Gagged: Pornography and the Politics of Fantasy in America*. Durham: Duke UP, 1999.

Klonsky, Milton. *Blake's Dante: The Complete Illustrations to the Divine Comedy*. New York: Harmony Books, 1980.

Knight, David M. *The Age of Science*. Oxford: Basil Blackwell, 1986.

———. *Science in the Romantic Era*. Aldershot: Ashgate, 1998.

Knight, Richard Payne. *An Account of the Remains of the Worship of Priapus*. London: T. Spilsbury, 1786.

———. *An Analytical Inquiry into the Principles of Taste*. London: T. Payne, 1808.

Kramnick, Isaac. *The Rage of Edmund Burke*. New York: Basic Books, 1997.

Krell, David Farrell. *Contagion: Sexuality, Disease, and Death in German Idealism and Romanticism*. Bloomington: Indiana UP, 1998.

Laclau, Ernesto, and Chantal Mouffe. *Hegemony and Socialist Strategy: Towards a Radical Democratic Politics*. London: Verso, 1985.

Lancaster, Roger. *The Trouble with Nature: Sex in Science and Popular Culture*. Berkeley: U California P, 2003.

Lanser, Susan S. "'Put to the Blush': Romantic Irregularities and Sapphic Tropes." In *Historicizing Romantic Sexuality*. Special issue of *Romantic Praxis* (January 2006) [www.rc.umd.edu/praxis/sexuality/lanser/lanser.html].

Laqueur, Thomas. *Making Sex: Body and Gender from the Greeks to Freud*. Cambridge: Harvard U P, 1990.

———. "Sex in the Flesh," *Isis* 94, 2 (June 2003): 300–306.

———. *Solitary Sex: A Cultural History of Masturbation*. New York: Zone Books, 2003.

Larson, James L. *Interpreting Nature: The Science of Living Form from Linnaeus to Kant*. Baltimore: Johns Hopkins UP, 1994.

Latour, Bruno. *Science in Action*. Cambridge: Harvard UP, 1987.

Lavater, John Caspar. *Essays on Physiognomy*. 3 vols. London: John Murray, 1789–98.

Law, Jules David. *The Rhetoric of Empiricism*. Ithaca: Cornell UP, 1993.

Lawlor, Clark. *Consumption and Literature: The Making of the Romantic Disease.* Houndmills: Palgrave Macmillan, 2006.

Lawrence, Christopher. "Cullen, Brown and the Poverty of Essentialism." In *Brunonianism in Britain and Europe.* Ed. W. F. Bynum and Roy Porter. London: Wellcome Institute, 1988.

[Lawrence, William]. "Generation." *Rees's Cyclopedia of Arts and Sciences.* London, 1819.

———. *Lectures on Physiology, Zoology, and the Natural History of Man.* London: Benbow, 1822.

Le Cat, Mr. "An Account of the Extraction of three inches and ten Lines of the Bone of the upper Arm, which was followed by a Regeneration of the bony Matter." *Philosophical Transactions.* 56: 270–77. London: Royal Society, 1766.

Levinson, Jerrold. *The Pleasures of Aesthetics.* Ithaca: Cornell UP, 1996.

Levinson, Marjorie. "'The Book of Thel' by William Blake: A Critical Reading." *ELH* 47, 2 (summer 1980): 287–303.

Lincoln, Andrew, ed. *Songs of Innocence and of Experience.* Princeton: Princeton UP, 1991.

Lingis, Alphonse. *Libido: The French Existential Theories.* Indiana: Indiana UP, 1985.

Linkin, Harriet Kramer. "The Function of Dialogue in the *Book of Thel.*" *Colby Library Quarterly* 23 (1987): 66–76.

Linne, Carl von. *Families of Plants.* London: J. Johnson, 1787.

Loesberg, Jonathan. *A Return to Aesthetics: Autonomy, Indifference, and Postmodernism.* Stanford: Stanford UP, 2005.

Logan, Peter Melville. *Nerves and Narratives: A Cultural History of Hysteria in 19th-Century British Prose.* Berkeley: U California P, 1997.

Longinus. *Longinus on Sublimity.* Trans. D. A. Russell. Oxford: Clarendon P, 1965.

———. *Dionysius Longinus on the Sublime.* London, 1751.

———. *Dionysius Longinus on the Sublime.* London, 1800.

———. *A Treatise of Dionysius Longinus upon the Sublime.* Trans. Rev. Charles Carthy. Dublin, 1762.

Love, Heather. *Feeling Backward: Loss and the Politics of Queer History.* Cambridge: Harvard UP, 2007.

MacCarthy, Fiona. *Byron Life and Legend.* New York: Farrar, Straus and Giroux, 2002.

McClaren, Angus. *A History of Contraception.* London: Basil Blackwell, 1990.

———. *Reproductive Rituals.* London: Methuen, 1984.

McGann, Jerome. *Byron and Romanticism.* Ed. James Soderholm. Cambridge: Cambridge UP, 2002.

———. *Don Juan in Context.* Chicago: U Chicago P, 1976.

———, ed. *Lord Byron: The Complete Poetical Works.* Vol. 5: *Don Juan.* Oxford: Clarendon P, 2003.

———. *The Romantic Ideology.* Chicago: U Chicago P, 1976.

———. *Social Values and Poetic Acts.* Cambridge: Harvard UP, 1988.

McNeil, Maureen. *Under the Banner of Science: Erasmus Darwin and His Age.* Manchester: Manchester UP, 1987.

Makdisi, Saree. *William Blake and the Impossible History of the 1790s.* Chicago: U Chicago P, 2003.

Marchand, Leslie. *Byron: A Biography.* 3 vols. New York: Knopf, 1957.

Marcus, Steven. *The Other Victorians: A Study of Sexuality and Pornography in Mid-Nineteenth-Century England.* New York: New American Library, 1974.

Marcuse, Herbert. *Eros and Civilization*. New York: Vintage, 1962.

Mayr, Ernst. *The Growth of Biological Thought: Diversity, Evolution, and Inheritance*. Cambridge: Harvard UP, 1982.

Mee, Jon. *Dangerous Enthusiasm: William Blake and the Culture of Radicalism in the 1790s*. Oxford: Clarendon P, 1992.

Mellor, Anne Kostelanetz. *Blake's Human Form Divine*. Berkeley: U California P, 1974.

Milton, John. *Complete Poems and Major Prose*. Ed. Merrit Hughes. Indianapolis: Bobbs-Merrill, 1957.

Mitchell, W. J. T. *Blake's Composite Art*. Princeton: Princeton UP, 1978.

———. "Chaosthetics." *Huntington Library Quarterly* 58, 3/4 (1997): 119–27.

Modiano, Raimonda. "The Legacy of the Picturesque: Landscape, Property and the Ruin." In *The Politics of the Picturesque*. Ed. Stephen Copley and Peter Garside. Cambridge: Cambridge UP, 1994.

Moore, Wendy. *The Knife Man*. London: Bantam, 2005.

Moran-Thomas, Amy. "Hookworm and History." Senior honors thesis. American University. May 2005.

Morgagni, Giambattista. *The Seats and Causes of Diseases Investigated by Anatomy*. Trans. Benjamin Alexander. 3 vols. London: A Millar, 1769.

Motherby, G. *A New Medical Dictionary; or, General Repository of Physic*. London: J. Johnson, 1801.

Mudge, Bradford. *The Whore's Story*. Oxford: Oxford UP, 2000.

Munby, A. N. L. *Sale Catalogues of Libraries of Eminent Persons*. Vol. 1. London: Scholar, 1971.

Munk, William. *The Roll of the Royal College of Physicians of London*. Vol. 2. London: College of Royal Physicians, 1818.

*A New Medical Dictionary*. London: Joseph Johnson, 1801.

Nicholson, Andrew, ed. *Lord Byron Volume IX Don Juan, Cantos X, XI, XII, and XVII Manuscript Facsimile*. New York: Garland, 1993.

———. *Lord Byron: The Complete Miscellaneous Prose*. Oxford: Clarendon P, 1991.

O'Donnell, Katherine and Michael O'Rourke, eds. *Love, Sex, Intimacy, and Friendship between Men, 1550–1800*. London: Palgrave, 2003.

O'Driscoll, Sally. "The Lesbian and Passionless Woman: Femininity and Sexuality in Eighteenth-Century England." *Eighteenth Century: Theory and Interpretation* 42, 2–3 (2003): 103–31.

Offen, Karen. *European Feminisms, 1700–1950: A Political History*. Stanford: Stanford UP, 2000.

Oppenheim, Janet. *Shattered Nerves*. New York: Oxford UP, 1991.

O'Quinn, Danny. Preface to "Romanticism and Sexual Vice." Special issue of *Nineteenth-Century Contexts* 2, 1 (March 2005).

O'Rourke, Michael and David Collings, eds. "Queer Romanticism." *Romanticism on the Net* 36–37 (November 2004–February 2005) [www.erudit.org/revue/ron/2004v/n36-37/].

Orsini, Gian. *Coleridge and German Idealism*. Carbondale: Southern Illinois UP, 1969.

Osborn, William. *Essays on the Practice of Midwifery, in Natural and Difficult Labours*. London: Cadell and Johnson in St. Paul's Church-yard, 1792.

Ostriker, Alicia. *Vision and Verse in William Blake*. Madison: U Wisconsin P, 1965.

Outram, Dorinda. *The Body and the French Revolution*. New Haven: Yale UP, 1989.

Overmeier, Judith. "John Brown's *Elementa Medicinae:* A Introductory Bibliographical Essay." *Bulletin of the Medical Library Association* 70, 3 (1982): 310–7.

Paine, Thomas. *The Age of Reason.* New York: Citadel, 1991.

Paley, Morton. *Energy and Imagination: A Study of the Development of Blake's Thought.* Oxford: Clarendon P, 1970.

———, ed. *William Blake: Jerusalem.* Princeton: Princeton UP, 1991.

Parr, Bartholomew. *The London Medical Dictionary; including under Distinct Heads Every Branch of Medicine.* 2 vols. London: J. Johnson, 1809.

Pateman, Carol. *The Sexual Contract.* Stanford: Stanford UP, 1988.

Paulson, Ronald. *Representations of Revolution, 1789–1820.* New Haven: Yale UP, 1983.

Pearson, George. *Arranged Catalogues of the Articles of Food, Drink, Seasoning, and Medicine.* London: Wilson and Co., 1801.

———. *Principles of Physic.* London: Wilson & Co, 1801.

Pearson, Richard. *A New Collection of Medical Prescriptions.* London: R. Baldwin, 1794.

Perry, Ruth. "Incest as the Meaning of the Gothic Novel." *Eighteenth Century: Theory and Interpretation* 39, 3 (1998): 261–78.

Persaud, T. V. N. *Basic Concepts in Teratology.* New York: Alan R. Liss, 1985.

Peterson, Linda. "Becoming an Author: Mary Robinsons's Memoirs and the Origins of the Woman Artist's Autobiography." In *Re-Visioning Romanticism.* Ed. Carol Shiner Wilson and Joel Haefner. Philadelphia: U Pennsylvania P, 1994.

Pfaff, Donald. Drive: *Neurobiological and Molecular Mechanisms of Sexual Motivation.* Cambridge: MIT P, 1999.

Pfau, Thomas. "'Beyond the Suburbs of the Mind': The Political and Aesthetic Disciplining of the Romantic Body." *SAQ* 95, 3 (summer 1996): 644–47.

*Philosophical Transactions of the Royal Society of London.* Vols. 62–69. London, 1772–79.

*The Phoenix of Sodom; or, the Vere Street Coterie* London: J. Cook, 1813. [BL Private Case 364 p13.]

Pinker, Steven. *How the Mind Works.* New York: Norton, 1997.

Pinto-Correia, Clara. *The Ovary of Eve.* Chicago: U Chicago P, 1997.

Place, Francis. *Illustrations and Proofs of the Principle of Population.* Ed. Norman Himes. New York: Augustus Kelley, 1967. [1822]

Poggi, Stefano. "Mind and Brain in Medical Thought During the Romantic Period." *History and Philosophy of the Life Sciences.* 1998 (suppl. vol. 10): 41–53.

Polidori, J.W. *An Essay Upon the Source of Positive Pleasure.* London: Longman, 1818.

Porter, Roy. "The Eighteenth Century." In *The Western Medical Tradition.* Ed. Lawrence Conrad and others. Cambridge: Cambridge UP, 1995.

———. *Flesh in the Age of Reason.* New York: Norton, 2004.

———. *The Greatest Benefit to Mankind: A Medical history of Humanity from Antiquity to the Present.* London: HarperCollins, 1997.

———. "Medicine in Georgian England." In *The Popularization of Medicine 1650–1850.* Ed. Roy Porter. London: Routledge, 1992.

———. "Perversion in the Past." *Communicationes de Historia Artis Medicinae* 44 (1999): 1–4.

Porter, Roy, and Lesley Hall. *The Facts of Life: The Creation of Sexual Knowledge in Britain, 1650–1950.* New Haven: Yale UP, 1995.

Porter, Roy, and Dorothy Porter. *Patient's Progress: Doctors and Doctoring in Eighteenth-Century England.* Stanford: Stanford UP, 1989.

Potter, Humphrey Tristram. *A New Dictionary of Cant and Flash Languages.* 2nd ed. London, 1795.

Potts, Alex. *Flesh and the Ideal: Winckelmann and the Origins of Art History.* New Haven: Yale UP, 1994.

Povinelli, Elizabeth. *The Empire of Love.* Durham: Duke UP, 2006.

Poynter, F. N. L. "Hunter, Spallanzani, and the History of Artificial Insemination." In *Medicine, Science and Culture.* Ed. Lloyd Stevenson and Robert Multhauf. Baltimore: Johns Hopkins UP, 1968.

Praz, Mario. *The Romantic Agony.* London: Oxford UP, 1970.

Quincy, John. *Pharmacopoeia Officinalis & Extemporanea; or, a Complete English Dispensatory.* 10th ed. London: Thomas Longman, 1736.

Quist, George. *John Hunter, 1728–1793.* London: William Heinemann Medical Books, 1981.

Rajan, Tilottama. "(Dis)figuring the System: Vision, History, and Trauma in Blake's Lambeth Books." *Huntington Library Quarterly* 58 (3 & 4): 383–412.

Redfield, Marc. *Phantom Formations: Aesthetic Ideology and the Bildungsroman.* Ithaca: Cornell UP, 1996.

Reill, Peter Hanns. *Vitalizing Nature in the Enlightenment.* Berkeley: U California P, 2005.

Reiman, Donald, and Neil Fraistat, eds. *The Complete Poetry of Percy Bysshe Shelley.* 6 vols. Baltimore: Johns Hopkins UP, 2000.

———. *Shelley's Poetry and Prose: A Norton Critical Edition.* New York: Norton, 2002.

Richards, Graham. *Mental Machinery: The Origins and Consequences of Psychological Ideas.* Baltimore: Johns Hopkins UP, 1992.

Richards, Robert. *The Romantic Conception of Life.* Chicago: U Chicago P, 2002.

Richardson, Alan. *British Romanticism and the Sciences of Mind.* Cambridge: Cambridge UP, 2001.

———. "Rethinking Romantic Incest: Human Universals, Literary Representation, and the Biology of Mind." *New Literary History* 31, 3 (2000): 553–72.

———. "Romanticism and the Colonization of the Feminine." In *Romanticism and Feminism.* Ed. Anne Mellor. Bloomington: Indiana UP, 1988.

Ricks, Christopher. *Keats and Embarrassment.* Oxford: Clarendon P, 1984.

Ridley, Matt. *Genome.* New York: Perennial, 1999.

Risse, Gunter B. "The Brownian System of Medicine: Its Theoretical and Practical Implications." *Clio Medica* 5 (1970): 45–51.

———. "Brunonian Therapeutics: New Wine in Old Bottles." In *Brunonianism in Britain and Europe.* Ed. W. F. Bynum and Roy Porter. London: Wellcome Institute, 1988.

Roberton, John. *Observations on the Mortality and Physical Management of Children.* London: Longman, Rees, Orme, Brown, and Green, 1827.

———. *On the Generative System; Being an Anatomical and Physiological Sketch of the Parts of Generation.* 4th ed. London: J. J. Stockdale, 1817.

Robinson, Daniel N. *An Intellectual History of Psychology.* New York: Macmillan Publishing, 1976.

[Robinson, Henry Crabb.] *Some Account of Dr. Gall's New Theory of Physiognomy, Founded Upon the Anatomy and Physiology of the Brain, and the Form of the Skull.* London, Longman, 1807.

Robinson, Mary. *A Letter to the Women of England.* London: Longman and Rees, 1799 [www.rc.umd.edu/editions/robinson/mrletterjs.htm].

————. *Memoirs of Mary Robinson.* London: Gibbings and Company, 1895.

————. Sappho and Phaon in *Mary Robinson: Selected Poems.* Ed. Judith Pascoe. Ontario: Broadview Literary Texts, 2000.

Rocca, Julius. "Robert Whytt (1714–1766): The Skeptical Neuroscientist." In *A Short History of Neurology.* Ed. F. Clifford Rose. Oxford: Butterworth Heinemann, 1999.

Rodin, Alvin. *The Influence of Matthew Baillie's Morbid Anatomy.* Springfield: Charles C. Thomas, 1973.

Roe, Nicholas, ed. *Samuel Taylor Coleridge and the Sciences of Life.* Oxford: Oxford UP, 2001.

Rollins, Hyder, ed. *The Letters of John Keats.* 2 vols. Cambridge: Harvard UP, 1958.

Rosario, Vernon. *The Erotic Imagination: French Histories of Perversity.* New York: Oxford UP, 1997.

Rose, Steven. *The Future of the Brain: The Promise and Perils of Tomorrow's Neuroscience.* Oxford: Oxford UP, 2005.

Roughgarden, Joan. "Evolution and Gender." Spring Lecture Series on Evolution and Medicine. National Institute of General Medical Sciences and the Office of Science Education. National Institutes of Health, Bethesda, MD. April 18, 2007.

————. *Evolution's Rainbow: Diversity, Gender, and Sexuality in Nature and People.* Berkeley: U California P, 2004.

Rousseau, George. "Nerves, Spirits, and Fibres: Towards Defining the Origins of Sensibility." *Studies in the Eighteenth Century* 3 (1973):137–57.

————. *Nervous Acts: Essays on Literature, Culture, and Sensibility.* New York: Palgrave Macmillan, 2004.

————. *Perilous Enlightenment.* Manchester: Manchester UP, 1991.

————. "The Sorrows of Priapus: Anticlericalism, Homosocial Desire, and Richard Payne Knight." In *Sexual Underworlds of the Enlightenment.* Ed. G. S. Rousseau and Roy Porter. Chapel Hill: U North Carolina P, 1988.

Rubin, Gayle. "Thinking Sex." In *The Lesbian and Gay Studies Reader.* Ed. Henry Abelove, Michele Barale, and David Halperin. New York: Routledge, 1999

Runge, Laura. "Mary Robinson's *Memoirs* and the Anti-Adultery Campaign of the Late Eighteenth Century." *Modern Philology* (2004): 563–86.

Russell, Edward Stuart. *Form and Function: A Contribution to the History of Animal Morphology.* London: John Murray, 1916.

Ruston, Sharon. *Shelley and Vitality.* Houndmills: Palgrave, 2005.

Ryan, Michael. *Lectures on Population, Marriage, and Divorce as Questions of the State of Medicine.* London: Renshaw and Rush, 1831.

Sade, Marquis de. *Justine, Philosophy in the Bedroom, and Other Writings.* Trans. Richard Seaver and Austryn Wainhouse. New York: Grove, 1965.

Sahlins, Marshall. *The Use and Abuse of Biology.* Ann Arbor: U Michigan P, 1976.

St. Clair, William. *The Godwins and the Shelleys.* New York: Norton, 1989.

Schaffer, Simon. "Regeneration: The Body of Natural Philosophers in Restoration England." In *Science Incarnate Historical Embodiments of Natural Knowledge.* Ed. Christopher Lawrence and Steven Shapin. Chicago: U Chicago P, 1998.

Schaper, Eva. "Taste, Sublimity, and Genius: The Aesthetics of Nature and Art." In *The Cambridge Companion to Kant.* Ed. Paul Guyer. Cambridge: Cambridge UP, 1992.

Schiebinger, Londa. *Nature's Body: Gender in the Making of Modern Science.* Boston: Beacon, 1993.

Sedgwick, Eve Kosofsky. *Between Men: English Literature and Male Homosocial Desire.* New York: Columbia UP, 1985.

———. *Epistemology of the Closet.* Berkeley: U California P, 1990.

Setzer, Sharon, ed. A Letter to the Women of England *and* The Natural Daughter. Lancashire: Broadview Literary Texts, 2003.

Seward, Anna. *The Poetical Works of Anna Seward.* Ed. Walter Scott. 3 vols. Edinburgh, 1810.

*Sex Research [Microform]: Early Literature from Statistics to Erotica.* 120 reels. Woodbridge, CT: Primary Source Microfilm, 2002.

Sha, Richard C. "Medicalizing the Romantic Libido: Sexual Pleasure, Luxury, and the Public Sphere." *Nineteenth-Century Contexts* 27, 1 (March 2005): 31–52 [longer version in *Romanticism on the Net* 31 (August 2003)].

———. "Othering Sexual Perversity: England, Empire, Race, and Sexual Science." In *The New Cultural History of the Body.* Ed. Michael Sappol. Oxford: Berg, 2009.

———. Review of Paul Elledge's *Lord Byron at Harrow School. Keats-Shelley Journal* 51 (2004): 219–21.

———. Review of Richard Turley's *Keats's Boyish Imagination. Wordsworth Circle* 37, 4 (2006): 227–8.

———. "Scientific Forms of Sexual Knowledge in Romanticism." *Romanticism on the Net* 23 (August 2001) [www.erudit.org/revue/ron/2001/v/n23/005993ar.html].

———. "The Uses and Abuses of Alterity: Halperin and Shelley on the Otherness of Ancient Greek Sexuality." In *Historicizing Romantic Sexuality.* Special issue of *Romantic Praxis* (January 2006) [www.rc.umd.edu/praxis/sexuality/sha/sha.html].

———. *The Visual and Verbal Sketch in British Romanticism.* Philadelphia: U Pennsylvania P, 1998.

Sharpe, Samuel. *A Treatise on the Operations of Surgery.* London, 1769.

Shearer, Edna Aston. "Wordsworth and Coleridge Marginalia in a Copy of Richard Payne Knight's *Analytical Inquiry into the Principles of Taste.*" *Huntington Library Quarterly* 1, 1 (October 1937): 63–94.

Shell, Susan Meld. *The Embodiment of Reason: Kant on Spirit, Generation, and Community.* Chicago: U Chicago P, 1996.

Shelley, Mary. *Frankenstein; or, the Modern Prometheus.* Ed. James Rieger. Chicago: U Chicago P, 1982.

———. *The Journals of Mary Shelley.* Ed. Paula Feldman and Diana Scott-Kilvert. Baltimore: Johns Hopkins UP, 1987.

Shelley, Percy. Huntington Library Manuscript Notebook HM 2176.

———. "Hymn to Intellectual Beauty." In *Shelley's Poetry and Prose.* Ed. Donald Reiman and Neil Fraistat. New York: Norton, 2002.

———. *Laon and Cythna.* In *The Complete Poetical Works of Percy Bysshe Shelley.* Vol. 2. Ed. Neville Rogers. Oxford: Clarendon P, 1975. [LC]

———. "Life and the World." Ms. MA 408 Pierpont Morgan Library, New York.

Shteir, Ann B. *Cultivating Women, Cultivating Science: Flora's Daughters and Botany in England, 1760–1860.* Baltimore: Johns Hopkins UP, 1996.

Siegel, Jonah. *Desire and Excess.* Princeton: Princeton UP, 2000.

Sinclair, John. *The Code of Health and Longevity.* 4 vols. Edinburgh: Archibald Constable, 1807.

Smellie, William. "William Smellie on Instinct." In *Transactions of the Royal Society of Edinburgh.* Vol. 1. Edinburgh: J. Dickson, 1788.

Smith, Adam. *The Theory of Moral Sentiments.* New York: Dover, 2006.

Smith, Charlotte. *Pathetic Tales Founded upon Facts.* London, 1818.

———. *The Poems of Charlotte Smith.* Ed. Stuart Curran. New York: Oxford UP, 1993.

Smith, John Gordon. "Some Account of a Boy in whom the Generative Organs have been prematurely developed." *London Medical Repository* 17, 101 (May 1822): 353–58.

Snyder, Jane McIntosh. *Lesbian Desire in the Lyrics of Sappho.* New York: Columbia UP, 1997.

Solomon, Samuel. *A Guide to Health; or, Advice to Both Sexes.* 9th ed. London, 1797.

South, John Flint. "History of a Case of Premature Puberty." *Medico-Chirurgical Transactions.* Vol. 12. London: Longman, Hurst, Rees, Orme, Brown and Green, 1823.

Spacks, Patricia Meyer. *The Adolescent Idea.* New York: Basic Books, 1981.

Spallanzani, Abbe. *Dissertations Relative to the Natural History of Animals and Vegetables.* 2 vols. London: John Murray, 1784.

———. *Dissertazioni di Fisica Animale, e Vegetabile dell' Abate Spallanzani, Tomo II.* Modena: Presso La Societa Tipografica, 1780.

———. *An Essay on Animal Reproductions.* London, 1769.

———. *Tracts on the Nature of Animals and Vegetables.* Edinburgh: T. Cadell and W. Davies, 1799.

Spanier, Bonnie. *Im/partial Science: Gender Ideology in Molecular Biology.* Bloomington: Indiana UP, 1995.

Springhall, John. *Coming of Age: Adolescence in Britain, 1860–1960.* Dublin: Gill and Macmillan, 1986.

Spurzheim, J. G. *The Anatomy of the Brain.* London: S. Highly, 1826.

———. "Letters." Wellcome Library MS 7636, 1–4.

———. *Observations on the Deranged Manifestations of Mind; or, Insanity.* London: Baldwin, Cradock, and Joy, 1817.

———. *Phrenology; or, the Doctrine of the Mind.* London: Charles Knight, 1825.

———. *The Physiognomical System of Drs. Gall and Spurzheim.* 2nd ed. London, 1815.

Stabler, Jane. *Byron, Poetics and History.* Cambridge: Cambridge UP, 2002.

Stark, William. *The Works of the Late William Stark, MD.* London: Joseph Johnson, 1788.

Stephanson, Ray. *The Yard of Wit: Male Creativity and Sexuality, 1650–1750.* Philadelphia: U Pennsylvania P, 2004.

Stolberg, Michael. "A Woman Down to Her Bones: The Anatomy of Sexual Difference in the Sixteenth and Early Seventeenth Centuries." *Isis* 94, 2 (June 2003): 274–99.

Stoller, Robert. *Perversion: The Erotic Form of Hatred.* New York: Delta, 1975.

Tannenbaum, Leslie. *Biblical Tradition in Blake's Early Prophecies.* Princeton: Princeton UP, 1982.

Taylor, Anya. *Erotic Coleridge: Women, Love, and the Law against Divorce.* New York: Palgrave Macmillan, 2005.

Taylor, Barbara. *Mary Wollstonecraft and the Feminist Imagination.* Cambridge: Cambridge UP, 2003.

Temkin, Owsei. *The Double Face of Janus.* Baltimore: Johns Hopkins UP, 1977.

———. "The Fielding Garrison Lecture: Basic Science, Medicine, and the Romantic Era." *Bulletin of the History of Medicine* 37 (1963): 97–129.

———. "Gall and the Phrenological Movement." *Bulletin of the History of Medicine* 21 (1947): 275–321.

Terdiman, Richard. *Body and Story: The Ethics and Practice of Theoretical Conflict.* Baltimore: Johns Hopkins UP, 2005.

Teute, Fredrika. "The Loves of the Plants; or, the Cross-Fertilization of Science and Desire at the End of the Eighteenth Century." *Huntington Library Quarterly* 63, 3 (2000): 319–45.

Tissot, Samuel. *Three Essays.* Dublin, 1772.

Todd, Janet. *Mary Wollstonecraft: A Revolutionary Life.* London: Weidenfeld & Nicholson, 2000.

Tomalin, Claire. *The Life and Death of Mary Wollstonecraft.* Harmondsworth: Penguin, 1977.

Traub, Valerie. "The Psychomorphology of the Clitoris." *GLQ* 2 (1995): 81–113.

Trotter, Thomas. *A View of the Nervous Temperament.* London: Longman, 1807.

Trotter, W. R. "John Brown, and the Nonspecific Component of Human Sickness." *Perspectives in Biology and Medicine* 21, 2 (winter 1978): 258–64.

Trumbach, Randolph. *Sex and the Gender Revolution.* Chicago: U Chicago P, 1998.

Tupper, James Perchard. *An Essay on the Probability of Sensation in Vegetables; with additional observations on instinct, sensation, irritability & c.* London: 1811.

———. *An Inquiry into Doctor Gall's System.* London: Longman, 1819.

Turley, Richard Marggraf. *Keats's Boyish Imagination.* London: Routledge, 2004.

Ulmer, William. *Shelleyan Eros.* Princeton: Princeton UP, 1990.

Umfreville, Edward. *Lex Coronatoria; Or, The Office and Duty of Coroners.* 2 vols. London, 1761.

Vacherie, M. *An Account of the Famous Hermaphrodite or Parisian Boy-Girl, Aged Sixteen, Named Michael-Anne Drourt, at the Time (November 1750) upon Show in Carnaby Street, London.* London: Sam Johnson, 1750.

Van Wyhe, John. "Was Phrenology a Reform Science? Towards a New Generalization for Phrenology." *History of Science* 42 part 3, 137 (September 2004): 313–32.

*Veneres Uti Observantur in Gemmis Antiquis.* London. 1790. [BL pc 31f6].

Vere, James. *A Physical and Moral Enquiry into the Causes of the Internal Restlessness and Disorder in Man, which has been the Complaint of All Ages.* Cornhill, 1778.

[Vermeil, Francois Michel.] *Reflexions Sur Les Hermaphrodites Relativement A Anne Grand-Jean.* Lyon, 1765.

Vickers, Brian. *Coleridge and the Doctors: 1795–1806.* Oxford: Clarendon P, 2004.

Viscomi, Joseph. "The Evolution of *The Marriage of Heaven and Hell.*" *Huntington Library Quarterly* 58, 3–4 (1997): 281–344.

———. *William Blake and the Idea of the Book.* Princeton: Princeton UP, 1993.

Voltaire, Francois Marie Arouet de. *Dictionnaire Philosophique* in *Oeuvres completes de Voltaire.* 42 vols. Paris: Garnier Freres, 1878.

Walker, Sayer. *A Treatise on Nervous Diseases.* London: J. Phillips, 1796.

Wallen, Martin. *City of Health, Fields of Disease.* Aldershot: Ashgate, 2004.

Wang, Orrin N. C. *Fantastic Modernity: Dialectical Readings in Romanticism and Theory.* Baltimore: Johns Hopkins UP, 1996.

Watson, Bishop. *Apology for the Bible.* London, 1797.

Waxman, Stephen. *Form and Function in the Brain and Spinal Cord.* Cambridge: MIT P, 2001.

Webster, Brenda. "Blake, Women, and Sexuality." In *Critical Paths: Blake and the Argument of Method.* Ed. Dan Miller, Mark Bracher, and Donald Ault. Durham: Duke UP, 1987.

Weeks, Jeffrey. *Sexuality and Its Discontents.* London: Routledge and Kegan Paul, 1985.

Wesley, John. *Primitive Physic; or, an Easy and Natural Method of Curing Most Diseases.* Bemersley: J. Bourne, 1820.

White, Charles. *On the Regeneration of Animal Substances.* Warrington, 1785.

White, Deborah Elise. *Romantic Returns.* Stanford: Stanford UP, 2000.

Whytt, Robert. *An Essay on the Vital and Involuntary Motions of Animals.* Edinburgh: Hamilton, Balfour, and Neill, 1751.

———. *Observations on the Nature, Causes, and Cure of those Disorders Commonly Called Nervous, Hypochondriac, or Hysteric.* Edinburgh, 1765.

Williams, Nicholas. *Ideology and Utopia in the Poetry of William Blake.* Cambridge: Cambridge UP, 1998.

Wilson, Lyn Hatherly. *Sappho's Sweetbitter Songs. Configurations of Female and Male in Ancient Greek Lyric.* London: Routledge, 1996.

Winckelmann, Johann Joachim. *History of Ancient Art.* 4 vols. in 2. Trans. Alexander Gode. New York: Frederick Ungar, 1968.

———. *Reflections on the Imitation of Greek Works in Painting and Sculpture.* Trans. Elfriede Heyer and Roger C. Norton. La Salle, IL: Open Court, 1987.

Windle John. *William Blake. Catalogue 32.* San Francisco: John Windle, 2001.

Wolfson, Susan. "Blake's Language in Poetic Form." In *The Cambridge Companion to William Blake.* Ed. Morris Eaves. Cambridge: Cambridge UP, 2003.

———. *Borderlines: The Shiftings of Gender in British Romanticism.* Stanford: Stanford UP, 2006.

———. "The Strange Difference of Female 'Experience.'" In *Women Reading William Blake.* Ed. Helen P. Bruder. Houndmills: Palgrave Macmillan, 2007.

———. "'Their She Condition': Cross-Dressing and the Politics of Gender in *Don Juan.*" *ELH* 54, 3 (autumn 1987): 585–617.

Wollstonecraft, Mary. *Vindication of the Rights of Woman.* Harmondsworth: Penguin Books, 1985.

Woodman, Tony. "Biformes Vates: The Odes, Catullus and Greek Lyric." In *Traditions and Contexts in the Poetry of Horace.* Ed. Tony Woodman and Denis Fenney. Cambridge: Cambridge UP, 2002.

Wordsworth, William, and Samuel Taylor Coleridge. *Lyrical Ballads.* R. L. Brett and A. R. Jones, Eds. London: Routledge, 1991.

Yiu, Mimi. "Sounding the Space between Men: Choric and Choral Cities in Ben Jonson's *Epicoene; or, The Silent Woman.*" *PMLA.* 122.1 (January 2007): 72–88.

Young, Robert M. *Mind, Brain, and Adaptation in the Nineteenth Century.* New York: Oxford UP, 1990.

Youngquist, Paul. *Monstrosities: Bodies and British Romanticism.* Minneapolis: U Minnesota P, 2003.

Zaehner, R. C. *The Teachings of the Magi: A Compendium of Zoroastrian Beliefs.* London: Sheldon, 1956.

Zizek, Slavoj. *The Parallax View.* Cambridge: MIT P, 2006.

# Index